The Research Process in Nursing

THIRD EDITION

EDITED BY

DESMOND F.S. CORMACK
RMN, RGN, Dip Nurs, MPhil, Dip Ed, PhD
Honorary Reader in Health and Nursing
Department of Health and Nursing
Queen Margaret College, Clerwood Terrace, Edinburgh EH12 8TS
Scotland

b

Blackwell
Science

© 1984, 1991, 1996 by
Blackwell Science Ltd
Editorial Offices:
Osney Mead, Oxford OX2 0EL
25 John Street, London WC1N 2BL
23 Ainslie Place, Edinburgh EH3 6AJ
350 Main Street, Malden
  MA 02148 5018, USA
54 University Street, Carlton
  Victoria 3053, Australia

Other Editorial Offices:

Blackwell Wissenschafts-Verlag GmbH
Kurfürstendamm 57
10707 Berlin, Germany

Blackwell Science KK
MG Kodenmacho Building
7-10 Kodenmacho Nihombashi
Chuo-ku, Tokyo 104, Japan

First edition published 1984
Reprinted 1985, 1987, 1989
Second edition published 1991
Reprinted 1992 (twice), 1993, 1994,
1995 (twice)
Third edition published 1996
Reprinted 1996, 1997 (twice)

Set in 10/13 pt Ehrhardt
by DP Photosetting, Aylesbury, Bucks
Printed and bound in Great Britain by
Hartnolls Ltd, Bodmin, Cornwall

The Blackwell Science logo is a trade mark of
Blackwell Science Ltd, registered at the
United Kingdom Trade Marks Registry

DISTRIBUTORS

Marston Book Services Ltd
PO Box 269
Abingdon
Oxon OX14 4YN
(Orders: Tel: 01235 465500
         Fax: 01235 465555)

USA
Blackwell Science, Inc.
Commerce Place
350 Main Street
Malden, MA 02148 5018
(Orders: Tel: 800 759-6102
              617 388-8250
         Fax: 617 388-8255)

Canada
Copp Clark Professional
200 Adelaide Street, West, 3rd Floor
Toronto, Ontario M5H 1W7
(Orders: Tel: 416 597-1616
              800 815-9417
         Fax: 416 597-1617)

Australia
Blackwell Science Pty Ltd
54 University Street
Carlton, Victoria 3053
(Orders: Tel: 03 9347-0300
         Fax: 03 9347-5001)

A catalogue record for this title
is available from the British Library
ISBN 0–632–04019–X

Library of Congress
Cataloging-in-Publication Data
The research process in nursing/edited by
  Desmond F.S. Cormack.—3rd ed.
    p. cm.
  Includes bibliographical references
and index.
  ISBN 0–632–04019–X
  1. Nursing—Research.   I. Cormack,
Desmond.
RT81.5.R465   1996
  610.73'072–dc20   95-42726
                                     CIP

Contents

List of Contributors   xii
Preface   xiv

Part I: Introduction to the Research Process   1

1   The Nature and Purpose of Research   3
     Lisbeth Hockey
     The nature of research   3
     The purpose of nursing research   5
     The urgency of nursing research   7
     Research involvement   9
     Summary and speculation for the future   11
     References   13

2   Common Terms and Concepts in Nursing Research   14
     Allan S. Presly
     Research   14
     Population   15
     Sampling   15
     Correlational research   16
     Experimental research and testing hypotheses   16
     Pilot study   17
     Measurement   17
     Procedure   19
     Results   20
     Generalization   20
     References   21

3   Agencies Supportive to Nursing Research   22
     Senga Bond
     Education for research   22
     Supervision   24
     Specific advice   24
     Kindred spirits   25

Financial support   26
Information resources   27
Conclusion   28
Useful addresses   28
References   29

4 **Ethical Issues in Nursing Research**   30
   Hazel E. McHaffie
   Responsibilities of all nurses   31
   Responsibilities of the researcher   32
   Responsibilities of the educator   36
   Responsibilities of the manager   37
   Conclusion   38
   References   39

5 **An Overview of the Research Process**   40
   Desmond F.S. Cormack
   Asking the research question   41
   Searching the literature   43
   Reviewing the literature   43
   Preparing a research proposal   43
   Gaining access to the research site   44
   Research design   44
   Data collection   45
   Data handling   45
   Reporting and disseminating research   47
   Ethical issures in nursing research   47

Part II: The Research Process   49

A: Preparatory Work   51

6 **Asking the Research Question**   53
   Desmond F.S. Cormack and *David C. Benton*
   What is a research question?   53
   Do I need a research question?   54
   How do I find a research question?   55
   How can I decide which question to study?   57
   How can the research question best be described?   60
   Does the research question influence the research process?   61
   Relating the research question to the research process   61
   Can the original research question be changed?   62
   Conclusions   63
   References   63

7   Searching the Literature   **64**
David C. Benton and *Desmond F.S. Cormack*
The research literature   64
Choosing a library   67
How to search the literature   69
Manual or computerized searching   72
Conducting a search   74
References   75
Appendix 7.1: List of national libraries   76

8   Reviewing and Evaluating the Literature   **78**
David C. Benton and *Desmond F.S. Cormack*
A place to read   78
Identifying the structure of a research publication   79
Recording of critical evaluation   79
Writing a literature review   82
Structure of a literature review   83
Presentational issues   85
Identifying the anatomy of a published review   86
References   87

9   Preparing a Research Proposal   **89**
Senga Bond
The content of a research proposal   89
Final review   98
Some general comments   99
References   101

10   Gaining Access to the Research Site   **102**
David C. Benton and *Desmond F.S. Cormack*
The research site   102
Research where negotiated access is not required   103
Accessing the gatekeepers   103
Access and power relationships   105
Ethics committee approval   106
Conclusion   108
References   109

B: Research Design   **111**

11   Qualitative Research   **113**
Sam Porter
Contrasting qualitative and quantitative methods   113
The theoretical foundations of qualitative research   114
The functions of qualitative research in nursing   121

Conclusion: the increasing importance of qualitative research   121
References   122

12   Grounded Theory   **123**
David C. Benton
Grounded theory method   124
Data sources and methods of collection   124
Theoretical sampling   124
Reliability and validity of data   125
Data recording   125
Explaining terminology   126
Constant comparative method   129
Memos and memo writing   130
Sorting   131
Using literature   132
Theory writing   132
Conclusions   133
References   133

13   Quantitative Research   **135**
Diana E. Carter
Introduction   135
Reality and its measurement   136
Reductionism   136
Objectivity   137
Quantitative measurement   137
Types of quantitative research   138
Control   140
Conclusion   143
References   143

14   Experimental Research   **145**
Allan S. Presly
Comparison of independent groups   145
Repeated measures   150
Single subject   152
References   154

15   Action Research   **155**
Christine Webb
What is action research?   155
Action research in facilitating change   156
Why action research?   156
Performing action research   159
Action research in practice   161

Action research: the answer to all our problems? 163
Conclusions 164
References 165

16 **Historical Research** **166**
Anne Marie Rafferty
Shifting sands 166
Why study history? 167
Supplying sources 171
Voyage of discovery or journey without maps? 172
Social and socializing history 174
Pilgrims of progress 174
Repertoire of resources 175
Conclusion 175
References 176
Appendix 16.1: Useful addresses 177

17 **Descriptive Research** **179**
Diana E. Carter
Introduction 179
The nature of descriptive research 179
Methods of data collection 181
Descriptive designs 183
Conclusion 188
References 188

18 **Evaluation Research** **190**
Senga Bond
The purpose of evaluation 190
Comparing evaluation and research 192
Determining the evaluation approach 195
Evaluation: a small scale example 197
Conclusion 199
References 200

19 **Survey Design and Sampling** **202**
F. Ian Atkinson
Sample selection 203
Sources of error 210
Conclusion 212
References 212
Other recommended reading 212

C: Data Collection   213

20   Attitude Measurement   215
      Robert J. Edelmann
      What are attitudes?   215
      Attitude scales   216
      Assessing attitudes and normative beliefs   221
      Other methods   222
      Which measure to use?   223
      References   224

21   Interview   226
      Philip J. Barker
      General principles   226
      Training interviewers   230
      Unstructured and structured interviews   232
      Special considerations   233
      Advantages of the interview   233
      Conclusion   234
      References   234

22   Questionnaire   236
      Philip J. Barker
      The function of the questionnaire   236
      General principles   237
      Design of the questionnaire   238
      Scaling methods   244
      Use of questionnaires   246
      Summary   248
      References   249
      Recommended reading   249

23   Observation   250
      Philip J. Barker
      Introduction   250
      Direct (non-participant) and indirect (participant) observation   252
      The world of objective observation   253
      Observational targets   254
      Observational methods   257
      General considerations   261
      Summary   263
      References   264

24   The Critical Incident Technique   266
      Desmond F.S. Cormack
      Use of the critical incident technique in nursing   268

Application of the critical incident technique	268
Conclusion	272
References	274
Further reading	274

25 Physiological Measurement   275
Paul Fulbrook

Introduction	275
Measurement procedures	277
Measuring instruments	283
Data collection	285
Ethical issues	286
Summary	286
References	287

D: Data Handling   289

26 Data Storage   291
Desmond F.S. Cormack and *David C. Benton*

Storage in original form	292
Copeland Chatterson (Cope Chat) cards	293
Computers	295
Use of computers	298
State of the art solutions	300
Conclusions	301
References	301

27 Quantitative Analysis (Descriptive)   302
Peter T. Donnan

Good design = good statistics	302
Aids to the description of data	305
Normal distribution	309
Summary statistics	311
Summary	315
References	315

28 Quantitative Analysis (Inferential)   316
Peter T. Donnan

Inferential statistical methods	317
Parametric methods	318
Summary	327
References	327
Appendix 28.1: Formulae for confidence intervals	328

29 Qualitative Analysis   330
Sam Porter
What is qualitative analysis?   330
The place of analysis in qualitative research   330
The cycle of data collection and analysis   333
Triangulation   336
The practicalities of analysis during data collection   337
Reporting qualitative analysis   339
Conclusion   340
References   340

30 Computer Assisted Data Analysis   341
David C. Benton
Qualitative and quantitative data analysis   341
Computerized quantitative data analysis   341
Specialized quantitative computer analysis programs   342
Computerized qualitative research analysis   348
Software available for qualitative analysis   348
Teaching   350
Software analytical capabilities   350
Conclusion   353
References   354
Appendix 30.1: Qualitative software programs   355
Appendix 30.2: List of variable definitions, variable labels and value
    labels for research barrier questionnaire   355
Appendix 30.3: Sample of data list from barriers to research
    questionnaire   356

31 Data Presentation   357
Desmond F.S. Cormack and *David C. Benton*
Data presentation techniques – general issues   357
Presenting data as text, numbers, graphs and pictures   359
Conclusions   371
References   372

32 Reporting and Disseminating Research   373
Alison J. Tierney
Writing a research project   373
Publishing research   377
Writing for publication   380
Disseminating research   383
References   384
Further reading   384

Part III: The Use of Research Nursing   387

33   Research in Nursing Practice   389
Alison J. Tierney
Research use   389
Understanding research utilization   392
Improving research utilization   394
Conclusion   398
References   398

34   Research in Nursing Education   401
Patricia Osborne
The function of research in nursing education   401
Recent developments in nursing education research   402
The teacher experience: the role of the nurse-teacher   404
The student experience   406
Learning strategies   407
Future directions of nursing education research   408
Conclusion   410
References   410

35   Research in Nursing Management   413
James Connechen
Role of the manager in nursing management research   415
Applications of nursing management research   416
Future direction of nursing management research   420
Conclusion   422
References   423

Epilogue   425

Index   426

List of Contributors

F. Ian Atkinson BSc, PhD, RGN, RMN, Centre for HIV/AIDS and Drug Studies, Ward 14a, City Hospital, Greenbank Drive, Edinburgh EH10 5SB, Scotland.

Philip J. Barker RNMH, PhD, Professor of Psychiatric Nursing Practice, University of Newcastle-upon-Tyne, Royal Victoria Infirmary, Queen Victoria Road, Newcastle-upon-Tyne NE1 4LP, England.

David C. Benton RGN, RMN, BSc, MPhil, Regional Nurse Director, National Health Service Executive (Northern and Yorkshire), Benfield Road, Newcastle-upon-Tyne NE6 4PY, England.

Senga Bond RN, BA, MSc, PhD, FRCN, Professor of Nursing Research, Centre for Health Services Research, University of Newcastle-upon-Tyne, 21 Claremont Place, Newcastle-upon-Tyne NE2 4AA, England.

Diana E. Carter RGN, SCM, DiPNurs, RNT, BA, MSc, Senior Lecturer in Nursing Studies, Department of Nursing and Midwifery Studies, University of Glasgow, 68 Oakfield Avenue, Glasgow G12 8LS, Scotland.

James Connechen RGN, RMN, RNT, RCNT, BEd (Hons), MHSM, Associate Director, Scottish Hospital Advisory Service, Trinity Park House, South Trinity Road, Edinburgh EH5 3SE, Scotland.

Desmond F.S. Cormack RMN, RGN, DipNurs, MPhil, DipEd, PhD, Honorary Reader in Health and Nursing, Department of Health and Nursing, Queen Margaret College, Clerwood Terrace, Edinburgh EH12 8TS, Scotland.

Peter T. Donnan DCR, BA, BSc, MSc, PhD, FSS, Senior Statistician, Institute of Occupational Medicine, 8 Roxburgh Place, Edinburgh EH8 9SU, Scotland.

Robert J. Edelmann BSc, MPhil, PhD, FBPsS, CPsychol, Senior Lecturer in Clinical Psychology, Department of Psychology, University of Surrey, Guildford, Surrey GU2 5XH, England.

Paul Fulbrook MSc, BSc (Hons), PGDE, RGN, DPSN, Senior Lecturer, Critical Care Nursing, School of Health Studies, University of Portsmouth, Queen Alexandra Hospital, Portsmouth PO6 3LY, England.

Lisbeth Hockey OBE, SRN, SCM, HV, QNCert, RNT, FRCN, BSc (Econ), PhD, Visiting Professor, Buckinghamshire College of Brunel University; and Honorary Reader in Health and Nursing, Department of Health and Nursing, Queen Margaret College, Clerwood Terrace, Edinburgh EH12 8TS, Scotland.

Hazel E. McHaffie SRN, RM, PhD, Research Fellow, Institute of Medical Ethics, Department of Medicine, University of Edinburgh, Royal Infirmary, Lauriston Place, Edinburgh EH3 9YW, Scotland.

Patricia Osborne RGN, DipNurs, CertEd (FE), RNT, Senior Lecturer, School of Nursing and Midwifery, University of Glamorgan, Treforest, Pontypridd CF37 1DL, Wales.

Sam Porter RGN, DipNurs, BSSc, PhD, Lecturer in Sociology, Department of Sociology and Social Policy, The Queen's University of Belfast, Belfast BT7 1NN, Northern Ireland.

Allan S. Presly MA, DipPsych, PhD, FBPsS, CPsychol, Formerly: Head of Adult Psychology Services, Psychology Department, Fife Healthcare NHS Trust, Stratheden Hospital, Cupar, Fife KY15 5RR, Scotland.

Anne Marie Rafferty BSc (SocSc-Nurs), RGN, DN, MPhil, DPhil (Oxon), Director, Centre for Policy in Nursing Research, London School of Hygiene and Tropical Medicine, Keppel Street, London WC1E 7HT, England.

Alison J. Tierney BSc (SocSc-Nurs), PhD, RGN, Reader, Department of Nursing Studies, The University of Edinburgh, Adam Ferguson Building, 40 George Square, Edinburgh EH8 9LL, Scotland.

Christine Webb BA, MSc, PhD, SRN, RSCN, RNT, Professor of Nursing, The University of Manchester, Oxford Road, Manchester M13 9PL, England.

Preface

The general inspiration for this book came from the now widely accepted sense of the need for *all* nurses, midwives and related groups to become aware of, and knowledgeable about, the application of the research process to their specialist areas. All the teachers and colleagues from whom I have learned research skills are recognized as having sown the seeds of this work. These individuals, some of whom have contributed to this book, have made a unique contribution to the development of research.

Students to whom I have taught the subject and whose research I have supervised, have also contributed to this work. It might be argued that one of the best means of extending one's knowledge of a subject is to teach it – research is no exception.

Not all will carry out research work, although the potential for all professionals to do so exists. Many will choose to remain consumers of the research undertaken by others. A thorough understanding of the research process as outlined in this book, however, is essential to both researchers and consumers of research. Thus, *all* individuals in the professions for whom this book was written require an understanding of the research process; this text offers one means of doing so. This text has been prepared and designed so that it can be used to introduce the subject either during or after training.

Although the title and much of the terminology used in this text imply that it relates only to nurses and nursing, this is not so. The term *nurse* should be taken as 'shorthand' to also encompass other staff groups who are part of, or are in close relationship with, the nursing profession. Examples are midwives, health visitors, district nurses, occupational health nurses, and community mental health nurses. Indeed, because the research process is the same irrespective of the discipline being studied, other health care groups such as occupational therapists, psychologists, social workers, pharmacologists and chiropodists may find this book of value.

Although the contribution of both men *and* women in nursing, midwifery and so on to research is firmly recognized, they and researchers will be referred to as 'she' throughout this text. Where the subject of the research is referred to, for example the patient or client, the term 'he' will be used. Thus, the repeated use of the clumsy alternative 'he/she' or 'she or he' will be avoided.

Finally, those who contributed to this book have done so recognizing that no single text or experience can, of itself, provide all the answers relating to the research process or any of its parts. This book should be used as part of a planned programme of study for one of two purposes. First, by those who wish to read and understand research findings, examples of this group are all trained nurses and midwives and those in training. Second, as part of a programme of study which will enable reading and understanding of research, and which will then underpin further reading and *supervised* research being undertaken by some individuals.

Desmond F.S. Cormack
Edinburgh

Part I

Introduction to the Research Process

The purpose of Part I is to put the subsequent discussion of the research process into context and to 'set the scene' for the more detailed material which follows. The introduction is presented in the firm belief that this must precede a consideration of the detailed phases of the research process. Only with the initial more general introduction, will readers be able to optimize their understanding of research, and their potential contribution to the development of a research-based profession. Chapter 1 presents a clear description of what research is and why it is of importance. Not all readers will have a prior belief in the value of research; this chapter provides a persuasive argument which will reinforce the views of the converted, and convert the sceptic.

The use of specialist research terms may inhibit the use of published research and frustrate attempts to understand what the research process is, and how to make use of it. The selected common terms and concepts discussed in Chapter 2 are intended to introduce readers to the specialist language of research. Although over-use of technical terms or 'jargon' is to be strongly condemned, a number of terms and concepts must be understood by the reader of research reports. The purpose of this chapter is not to present a comprehensive list of such terms, rather it is intended to demonstrate the need to understand these, and the relative ease with which their meaning can be understood.

Chapter 3 is intended to reduce the potential isolation which many aspiring researchers experience or fear because they are unaware of the many and varied agencies which are available to give support. Some of these agencies may be unknown; some may be known but thought of as being only for the use of 'others'.

A full consideration of ethical issues pervades all aspects of research, particularly that which deals with human subjects as is often the case in health care. Chapter 4 considers these issues and offers guidelines which will direct both those who do and those who consume research.

Finally, Chapter 5 emphasizes the sequential nature of the research process and the interrelationship of each of its phases. This general overview of the research process should be seen as an introduction to the more detailed discussion of the steps in the process which are presented in Part II.

Chapter 1

The Nature and Purpose of Research

Lisbeth Hockey

The nature and purpose of research in general and nursing research in particular have not changed fundamentally since the second edition of this book in 1991. What has changed drastically in nursing research is the urgency to come to grips with both concepts and to recognize the increasing opportunities for nurses to become involved in research.

The nature of research

What is research?

The essential nature of research lies in its intent to create new knowledge in whatever field. It does this through a process of systematic enquiry governed by scientific principles. The principles vary according to the specific science or discipline in which the research is undertaken. Although the term *research* is now commonplace it still does not seem to be given its correct meaning by some people, both lay and professional. Definitions of research remain sparse, probably because authors of research texts continue to assume that the meaning of the term is self-evident. In my view this is an unwarranted assumption and misconceptions remain. In fact, it seems that increasing use of the term goes hand in hand with increasing misuse and abuse. There are still many people in all walks of life who believe that research connotes the kind of advanced scientific activity which is only undertaken by scientists in an academic setting, probably in a laboratory. Whilst such activity is likely to be research, the interpretation is narrow and does not include may other types of endeavour which are not necessarily undertaken by academic scientists in a laboratory. For others, it means little more than common sense, which is also a misguided belief. Common sense is extremely useful but not adequate. The essential characteristic of research is its scientific nature; research is a process which has to be undertaken according to certain scientific rules, the research process.

The research process can be learned and applied by people who are not necessarily academic scientists and it need not be confined to a laboratory. The research process consists of a sequence of steps which includes mental activities that are designed to increase the sum of what is known about certain phenomena in all types of disciplines.

Defining research

A definition, or rather an explanation of research was offered by Macleod Clark & Hockey (1989) as

> 'an attempt to increase the sum of what is known, usually referred to as "a body of knowledge", by the discovery of new facts or relationships through a process of systematic scientific enquiry, the research process.'

It is important to recognize that it is not only the discovery of new facts which adds to available knowledge, but also that of new relationships.

The variations in the research process between the various disciplines are due to their own specific modes of thought they bring to bear, their own paradigms and theories. Thus, the physical scientist's approach to the exploration of new knowledge will be different from that of the historian or the behaviourist. The basic principles of the systematic process will be observed by all.

The main types of research are fully explained in Chapters 11–19 inclusive. It remains here merely to draw attention to the differences which stem from the basic scientific roots of the discipline in which the research is undertaken. Nursing provides an ideal way of illustrating this point, it also demonstrates the need for nurses to familiarize themselves with the sciences underlying nursing.

Nursing research

What is nursing research? Is it different from other research and, if so, in what way? Many different definitions of nursing research have been advanced and there cannot be a totally right or wrong answer to the questions about its nature. Because nursing encompasses a wide range of activities, because it is interpreted differently in different parts of the world, and because it changes over time, a definition of the term nursing research and an explanation of its nature should make provision for these variations.

Nursing research is defined here as research into those aspects of professional activity which are predominantly and appropriately the concern and responsibility of nurses. Where nurses have little or no appropriate or predominant responsibility, nursing research makes little sense. Where nurses have responsibility for nursing education, for the administration of nursing services, and for all aspects of nursing practice, nursing research encompasses all these areas. At the time when nurses were not the appropriate personnel to monitor patients' vital signs, for example, blood pressure, nursing research would not have included studies of such monitoring procedures. Similarly in countries where nurses are not in control of nursing education, research in the field of nursing education would lie outside the scope of nursing research and the same is true for nursing administration.

In terms of the research process – the series of logical steps which have to be undertaken to develop further the available knowledge – nursing research is no different from any other. The same rules of the scientific method apply and, just as in any other research, the specific type, design and method of the research must be appropriate for the problems or questions to be investigated. Nursing represents a unique mix of several disciplines and any of the disciplines underlying nursing might be appropriate for research in nursing; for example, patients' anxiety can be viewed and studied from a psychological perspective, in which case psychological knowledge will be applied and psychological measurements might be utilized. Patients' anxiety can also be viewed and studied from a physiological perspective, in which case the biological sciences will be invoked to provide the necessary scientific guidelines. In time, nursing will develop more of its own nursing perspectives and nursing measures. It may be of interest to some to explore the development of nursing, which can be retrieved from documentary sources through systematic historical enquiry. Such historical research will also attempt to disentangle the events of the time, to explore primary and secondary sources in the hope of offering plausible explanations of events, and to throw new light on those events by the discovery of relationships.

The science of physiology has provided new knowledge about the relationship between skin integrity and pressure. However, it is possible that other variables, such as the action of certain drugs or mental state, may also play a part in causing skin sores.

In order to discover effective treatments, experimental research, that is the collection of data in rigorously controlled situations, will be appropriate. Organizational change might best be explored through action research (see Chapter 15) which deliberately rules out any control of the situation.

Nursing research is also explained by Montgomery Robinson *et al.* (1991), in a self-learning module. Clamp (1994) describes research in nursing as

> 'providing a link between practice, education and theory, thereby making it essential for all nurses to become knowledgeable consumers or for the minority research doers'.

It is important to recognize, therefore, that questions initiating research can and should originate in any field of nursing. Research must begin with a question and it invariably generates further questions. It is in this way that the knowledge underlying nursing grows like a spiral. There can be no end point as the universe will never be totally mastered (Fig. 1.1). It is this continuous never ending potential to create and use further knowledge, the opportunity for on-going learning, that not only enables nursing to develop its all important body of knowledge but also makes life exciting and worthwhile for us all.

The purpose of nursing research

Deductive and inductive research

Nursing research may set out to test theories developed in other settings: for example, organizational theories developed in industry have been tested in nursing. It may set out to test theories or models developed by other researchers in nursing.

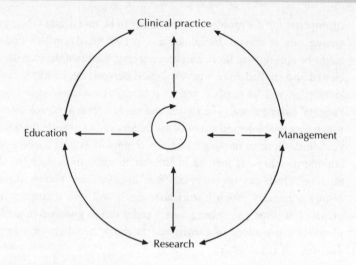

Fig. 1.1   The spiral of knowledge.

Research which is designed to test general theories in particular situations is referred to as deductive research. It is also possible to study nursing inductively. Here, the particular situation would be the starting point for study. Inductive research, which also has its own scientific rules, might result in the identification of certain patterns, eventually leading to the formulation of hypotheses or the advance of general theories which can then be tested deductively.

As suggested by the definitions of research advanced above, its purpose is to increase the body of knowledge, the sum of what is known. The purpose of research in nursing is, therefore, to increase the sum of what is known about the professional activity of nurses, which may be nursing education, nursing administration or nursing practice in its many forms and settings. Research in nursing is relatively new and a great deal of what nurses do and teach is based on tradition, convention, hunches and beliefs rather than on evidence. Research in nursing attempts to change this situation and to provide the professional discipline of nursing with a base which can be defended on grounds of scientifically established knowledge.

Research in nursing begins with questions about nursing. Questions may be generated by an intelligent curiosity, by a wish to find out more about the respective activity; they may also be generated by an urgent need to identify more effective and, probably also, less costly methods of providing nursing care, of educating nurses or of providing an effective administrative structure. There are many unanswered questions in nursing and there are even more questions which have not yet been asked.

The main purpose of nursing research may be summarized as:

(1) To establish scientifically defensible reasons for nursing activities.
(2) To provide nurses with an increased repertoire of scientifically defensible nursing intervention options.
(3) To find ways of increasing the cost-effectiveness of nursing activities.

(4) To provide a basis for standard setting and quality assurance.

(5) To provide evidence of weaknesses and strengths in nursing.

(6) To provide evidence in support of demands for resources in nursing.

(7) To satisfy the academic curiosity of thinking nurses.

(8) To facilitate inter-disciplinary collaboration in nursing and nursing research.

(9) To earn and defend a professional status for nursing.

At the first International Conference on Community Health Nursing Research in 1993, the purposes of community health nursing research embedded in 436 abstracts were distilled as shown in Fig. 1.2. At the same conference the overall purposes of community health nursing were stated as:

Purposes

- Targetting of services
- Curriculum content
- Instrument construction/testing
- Theory construction/testing
- Client assessment
- Direct care provision
- Others

Overall purpose – explicit/implicit

'Better' understanding of self and others

'Better' quality of:

- service
- care
- education

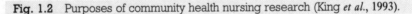

Fig. 1.2 Purposes of community health nursing research (King *et al.*, 1993).

'... an attempt to find means by which potential patients can be prevented from becoming actual patients and means by which the health and well being of both groups in the community can be promoted.' (King *et al.*, 1993).

This mode of thought concerning community health nursing research can easily be adapted to embrace nursing research in general.

Although the main purpose of nursing research in the current business orientated health service tends to be seen in terms of a direct *pay-off* for patient care, it is important not to lose sight of the other stated purposes.

The urgency of nursing research

In the opening paragraph of this chapter, the urgency of nursing research was stressed. The following section is intended to support this statement.

As early as 1972, the Committee on Nursing stressed the need to give nursing a research base, stating:

'... a sense of the need for research should become part of the mental equipment of every practising nurse or midwife.'

Cormack (1979) suggested that the nursing profession will be recognized as being 'research based' when the above situation is achieved *and* when research becomes an integral part of nursing practice.

From a paper by English (1994) it seems that the desired situation has not yet been achieved. He makes the point that

'in spite of an escalation of nursing research in the last 22 years, it has generally failed to influence clinical practice. Also, in spite of a considerable increase in nursing theory nursing still cannot claim to be a research based profession.'

Other authoritative statements point to the urgent need for nursing research.

The International Council of Nurses (ICN)

In 1985, the ICN published *Guidelines for Nursing Research Development*. The introduction states the commitment of the ICN to the development of nursing research worldwide.

'The International Council of Nurses is convinced of the importance of nursing research as a major contribution to meeting the health and welfare needs of people. The continuous and rapid scientific developments in a changing world highlight the need for research as a means of identifying new knowledge, improving professional education and practice, and effectively utilising resources.

The ICN believes that nursing research should be socially relevant. It should look towards the future while drawing on the past and being concerned with the present.'

and

'Nursing research should include what relates to a total research plan and what may be undertaken independently. In nursing research, available resources of different levels of sophistication should be utilized and research should comply with accepted ethical standards. Research findings should be widely disseminated and their utilization and implementation encouraged when appropriate.'

and

'ICN is aware that nursing research is at various stages of development in different countries, ... but efforts to promote it are made elsewhere.' (International Council of Nurses, 1985)

British nursing education

The educational reforms of nursing education in the United Kingdom support the move into higher education with its research ethos. This is true for first level education to the level of a registered practitioner as stated in Project 2000 (United Kingdom Central Council for Nursing, Midwifery and Health Visiting, 1986) and especially, for post registration education as set out in detail by the United Kingdom Central Council for Nursing Midwifery and Health Visiting in *The Future of Professional Practice: The Council's Handbook for Education and Practice following Registration* (UKCC, 1994).

Professional accountability for nurses is high on the agenda in all countries where nursing is moving toward true professional status. It is embedded in the Code of Professional Conduct (United Kingdom Central Council for Nursing, Midwifery and Health Visiting, 1984). The document states:

'Each registered nurse, midwife and health visitor shall act, at all times, in such a manner as to justify public trust and confidence, to uphold and enhance the good standing and reputation of the profession, to serve the interests of society and above all to safeguard the interests of individual patients and clients.'

and

'Each registered nurse, midwife and health visitor is accountable for his or her practice ...'

Research awareness is implicit in the above document. A nurse who is oblivious of the latest available knowledge relevant to his or her area of practice, using redundant methods, cannot expect public trust and confidence and such a nurse will *not* enhance the good standing and reputation of the profession. The interests of society will *not* be served and interests of individual patients and clients will *not* be safeguarded. Bassett (1992) suggested that nursing care should be based on a body of knowledge which gives an 'objective basis to justify nursing actions'.

Research involvement

Because nursing research is at different stages of development, the involvement of nurses must take different forms. First, there must be a research awareness, a recognition that questions can and should be asked, that reading of research articles and research based texts is essential, and that research findings should be assessed in terms of their usefulness, their relevance, and their potential for implementation. Research awareness must be cultivated by all nurses in all spheres of activity and at all levels. Such awareness should be inculcated early in the professional preparation of nurses and kept alive throughout it. Existing professional and academic education must continue to strengthen and refine research awareness and its application to nursing.

The systematic collection of information, in which most nurses are involved in one way or another, is another form of research involvement. For example, community nurses who keep records for their employing authority should be keenly aware of the purpose of the information they collect and record, and of its ultimate use in the formulation of policy.

Many nurses, knowingly – or, alas, sometimes unknowingly – become research assistants for their medical colleagues; they may collect specimens, for example, as part of medical research, or help in some other way. Such involvement can be helpful as a learning experience but it should be part of an official and fully understood contract. The nurse's part of the contract should be the contribution of the nursing dimension to the research in return for which she should be initiated into the scientific aspects of the research process and should be encouraged to participate as a colleague in the preparation of research papers.

An increasing number of nurses, especially those in first level management and teaching positions, find themselves with a research component as part of their job description. This aspect of their job should be clarified as soon as possible and jealously guarded. It is a precious jewel which gives opportunity for stimulating innovative activity. It should also provide legitimate time for thinking. Sometimes, nurses feel insecure in this research role and attempt to evade it by creating other 'more urgent' demands on their time. It is only too easy to do that but it may be a retrograde step in the long-term. There are opportunities for nurses to obtain advice and help with the research component of their role and they should strive to develop confidence in it. It is almost bound to add to job satisfaction, providing of course, that the thinking process is deemed to be both desirable and satisfying!

The research component of nursing may take many different forms: it may consist of initiating others in facilitating the creation of a research orientated environment, or it may consist of direct personal involvement. Finally, research may be undertaken by the nurse on a full-time basis as a member of a research team or as an individual. Several opportunities for such research exist.

In spite of the many positive aspects of research involvement and its acknowledged defensible and urgent purposes and aims, there are still many arguments in favour of leaving research in nursing well alone. Some of these arguments stress the urgency of other nursing activities at a time of scarce resources. It is considered that research activity cannot be defended when finance and manpower are not adequate to provide the necessary care and essential professional preparation for the basic licence to practise nursing. Managers with limited budgets feel reluctant to support research, the results of which are often unpredictable, when they could use the money for other, seemingly more urgent and certainly more easily defensible, purposes. Their views and hesitations must be respected and they must not be accused out of hand of being 'unprogressive'. Research does not always come up with results which can be utilized and, therefore, the type of research to be undertaken must be carefully considered.

However, some importance must be attached to the beneficial effects of continuing research within an organization, the dynamism it ensures, and the interest it generates. A recognition of possible long-term benefits rather than immediate results may change the outlook of understandably careful managers. In the long term, it may be possible to save either time or money or both on redundant equipment or practices by investing some of these resources in research in the short term.

Many members of the nursing profession fail to see, or do not wish to see, the importance of research and only perseverance and demonstration of its worth can be expected to change their attitude. Sometimes their lack of interest or enthusiasm is at least partially the fault of researchers who fail to communicate appropriately with their peer groups. The communication of research is as important as the research itself. This is discussed in Chapter 32.

There is also a body of opinion that holds that research in nursing should be the concern of trained researchers and that it should not infiltrate the profession as a whole. Some reasons for this view are worthy of thought; poor research by incompetent people can do a great deal of harm and so can thoughtless implementation of findings. More urgent attention must therefore be devoted to the appropriate education of nursing personnel for different levels of research involvement. An evasion of that responsibility can be expected to reverse any progress which has been made in advancing the sum of what is known in and about nursing.

Summary and speculation for the future

It is recognized that a substantial part of the professional activity of nurses at all levels and in all spheres is based on convention rather than substantive knowledge. The need to extend that knowledge cannot be denied and the responsibility for research support cannot be evaded.

Research activity requires knowledge of the scientific method; the research process consists of a series of steps which is subject to scientific rules. Knowledge of the scientific method can be acquired and need not be the province of individuals who work in academic settings. All nurses must develop an awareness of research and recognize its relevance to nursing.

More direct involvement in research at different levels should be encouraged and valued. Uncertainty should be overcome by seeking help rather than by escapism and avoidance. Qualified researchers can help a great deal by teaching, explaining and communicating intelligibly. The reservations about the investment of manpower and finance in research must be viewed sympathetically and the long-term benefits, as well as the immediate gains, of a research–orientated environment should be allowed to enter into the debate quite apart from the possibility of usable research results. The need for research is clearly indicated in the official documents relating to the future of professional practice following registration as a qualified nurse (United Kingdom Central Council for Nursing Midwifery and Health Visiting, 1994). This authoritative publication refers not merely to specific research training but also to the need for nurses to 'identify, apply and disseminate research findings' relating to clinical practice development. Health Service users are becoming increasingly aware of their rights and encouraged to ask questions about their care. Patient expectations have been raised through the media and also by the introduction of the Patient's Charter (Department of Health, 1993a).

The National Board for Nursing, Midwifery and Health Visiting for Scotland (1994) also commits itself to the provision of leadership and liaison for research in education and practice.

The future of nursing depends to no small extent on the development of nursing research. It is no coincidence that the terms *research* and *development* have been linked in official documents.

The report of the taskforce convened to consider the future of research in nursing points to the way forward (Department of Health, 1993b) in recognizing the contribution of the nursing profession to research and development (R and D) in the NHS as a whole. A strategy for nursing research is being pursued and augurs well for the future. In *Research for Health* such a strategy for England and Wales is described (Department of Health, 1991). Its declared primary objective is to see that R and D becomes an integral part of health care. Though not specifically addressed to the nursing profession, it clearly opens up new avenues for nursing involvement.

In Scotland, the Scottish Office published its own strategy document (Chief Scientist Office, 1993). In it, emphasis is given to better target R and D in value for money terms.

The crunch point seems to lie in attempts to identify the impact of nursing research on health care.

In Scotland, a multi-disciplinary conference was held in 1992 and reported by Watt (1993). Current problems in translating research findings into policy and practice were identified. Although health care research in general was the focus of discussion at that time, nursing research, being an integral part of it, must consider itself included.

Referring particularly to nursing research, Closs & Cheater (1994) stress the importance but also the complexity of appropriate utilization of nursing research and make a case for the development of a research culture in nursing which, as yet, has not been attained.

The challenges for nursing research permeate the totality of the nursing profession and its future. They are presented clearly and candidly by Tierney (1993). Whilst readily acknowledging the need for and the advantages of multi-disciplinary research, she makes a plea for preserving the identity of nursing research.

The current forces in the health care systems the world over must be taken seriously. Through the emphasis on cost containment nursing research can be either enlivened or annihilated. It is the professional responsibility of nurses to encourage the former and prevent the latter.

New opportunities for the development of nursing research abound and they must be grasped urgently.

If academic researchers can become more sensitive to professional needs and if professionals can become more sensitive to the need for scientific enquiry, the future for professional nursing – for the care of patients, for the education of nurses and for the management of nursing services – is exciting and justifies optimism.

References

Bassett, C. (1992) The integration of research in the clinical setting: Obstacles and solutions. A review of the literature. *Nursing Practise*, **6**, No 1, 4–8.

Chief Scientist Office (1993) *Health Service in Scotland*, Scottish Office, Home and Health Department.

Clamp, C.G.L. (1994) *Resources for Nursing Research*, 2 edn, an annotated bibliography. Library Association Publishing, London.

Closs, G.J. & Cheater, F.H. (1994) Utilization of nursing research: culture, interest and support. *Journal of Advanced Nursing*, **19**, No 4, 762–73.

Committee on Nursing (1972) *Report of the Committee on Nursing*. HMSO, London.

Cormack, D. (1979) Knowledge for What? Janforum. *Journal of Advanced Nursing*, **4**, 93–4.

Department of Health (1991) *Research for Health*. HMSO, London.

Department of Health (1993a) *The Patient's Charter*. HMSO, London.

Department of Health (1993b) *Report of the Taskforce on the Strategy for Research in Nursing, Midwifery and Health Visiting*. HMSO, London.

English, S. (1994) Nursing as a research-based profession: 22 years after Briggs. *British Journal of Nursing*, **3**, No 8, 402–40.

International Council of Nurses (1985) *Guidelines for Nursing Research Development*. ICN, Geneva.

King, M., Stinson, S.M. & Mills, K, (eds) (1993) *Proceedings of the First International Conference on Community Health Nursing Research*. Edmonton Health Board, Edmonton, Canada.

Macleod Clark, J. & Hockey, L. (1989) *Further Research for Nursing*. Scutari Press, London.

Montgomery Robinson, K.M., Montgomery Robinson, H.M., Hilton, A. & Clark, E. (1991) *What is Research? Research Awareness Module 3*. Distance Learning Centre, South Bank Polytechnic.

National Board for Nursing, Midwifery and Health Visiting for Scotland (1994) *Advancing Standards*. NBS, Edinburgh.

Tierney, A. (1993) Challenges for nursing research in an era dominated by Health Services reform and cost containment. *Clinical Nursing Research*, **2**, No 4, 382–95.

United Kingdom Central Council for Nursing, Midwifery and Health Visiting (1984) *Code of Professional Conduct for Nurse, Midwife and Health Visitor*. UKCC, London.

United Kingdom Central Council for Nursing, Midwifery and Health Visiting (1986) *Project 2000 a new preparation for practice*. UKCC, London.

United Kingdom Central Council for Nursing, Midwifery and Health Visiting (1994) The Future of Professional Practice: The Council's Standards for Education and Practice following Registration. UKCC, London.

Watt, G.C.M. (1993) Making research make a difference. *Health Bulletin*, 51 (3). Scottish Office, HMSO, London.

Chapter 2

Common Terms and Concepts in Nursing Research

Allan S. Presly

This chapter introduces and defines a number of commonly used terms and concepts likely to be encountered in a representative selection of research which is of interest to nurses. They will be introduced in the sequence in which they are likely to be met in a research report, but, obviously, by no means all of these terms will occur in any single research report.

Research

Research is a form of systematic inquiry. It sets out to answer questions through assessing, summarizing and drawing conclusions from what are often very large amounts of information. The intention is to reach as unambiguous conclusions as possible and to minimize the extent to which the reader has to interpret the results. Ideally, therefore, any two people studying the results of a piece of research should agree with the researcher's conclusions. It has to be said, however, that this is very difficult to achieve in practice! The research report must make clear the procedures used, the results obtained and the conclusions drawn. The golden rule should be that the report contains enough information to enable the research to be repeated exactly by someone else wishing to answer the same question in the same way. This repetition is called a *replication*.

Replication

In all sciences, replication serves at least two purposes. Each replication under the *same* conditions further establishes the reliability of previous results. Secondly, the same results might be replicated under *different* conditions. This would again increase confidence in the reliability of the original results, but it would also serve to establish their generality.

Retrospective and prospective research

Research may be *retrospective* or *prospective*. Retrospective research refers to the investigation of events which have already happened; for example, you might set out to discover, from an analysis of case records, factors which might identify which elderly patients are at risk of multiple falls (Gaebler, 1993). Prospective research sets out to investigate events which are yet to happen; in this case, you might set out to discover how may patients with urinary tract infections will be admitted to hospital in the coming year. The advantage of prospective research is that it can be planned in advance, for example, who and what is to be assessed and how the information is to be recorded. In retrospective research, the researcher has to depend on information which may have been recorded by a large variety of people who did not know it was likely to be needed for research purposes. The accuracy of such information can leave a lot to be desired! In either case, the results of the research will refer to some defined *population*.

Population

Population literally means 'all the people' and in research the term is most commonly used to refer to a specific group of people. However, in a research context, population refers to all members or objects of any defined group from which measurements might be taken or about which information might be collected.

A research population refers to the entire group to which the results of the research are to apply. A population could thus consist of all people of a specified age group whose blood pressure was to be measured, a whole series of laboratory animals on which a new drug was to be tested or all the items of equipment – for example, syringes, incontinence pads or lifting aids – whose efficiency was to be assessed. Membership of any given population should be specified clearly so that there is no doubt as to how widely the research findings can be generalized.

It is, of course, rarely possible to collect data concerning all the members of a given population. It might be possible to assess all known patients suffering from a rare condition, as was done in Scotland, for example, for babies who suffered damage due to their mothers being given the drug thalidomide. It would not, however, be possible to investigate all those patients with a diagnosis of, say, 'senile dementia'. Thus a *sample* of the population usually has to be taken.

Sampling

The sample must reflect, as far as possible, every aspect of the population from which it is selected. Suppose one wanted to study some aspect of patients with a common disease who were admitted to one hospital over a year. The population would be all the patients so defined, but if their number was very large, the researcher would probably decide to assess only a sample of them. The sample selected would, for example, have to show the same age range, the same proportion of males to females, the same proportion of urban to rural residents and the same proportions from each admission ward concerned.

Sometimes it may be appropriate to arrange things so that some characteristics of the sample are left to chance, while others are specifically selected. This is sometimes referred to as a *stratified sample*. One might want to ensure in advance that the sample contains the correct proportion of those aged 50 and over and the under-50s, or of males and females, if these factors – age and sex – were considered to have a particularly important bearing on the outcome of the research. Within each subgroup so selected, however – for example, those 50 and over and the under-50s – the subjects would still be chosen at random. Whatever type of sampling is used, the members of the sample are generally referred to as the *subjects* of the research. The study by Caruso *et al.* (1992), for example, used a stratified sample where groups were selected to represent four levels of body temperature.

Correlational research

Some research is of the *descriptive* or 'look and see' type. The research might, for example, investigate whether the amount of time spent in hospital following a particular operation is related to the age of the patients, that is: 'Do older people take longer to recover from this operation?'. A random sample of patients who had undergone the operation could be selected, their ages noted, and the length of time they stayed in hospital post-operatively calculated. A measure of the relationship between the two sets of figures is called a *correlation*. If there is a clear relationship, it can be concluded that age does have an apparent bearing on recovery time, older patients being more likely to stay longer in hospital.

Can it also be concluded that older people take longer to recover from the operation? It can not. All that can be said is that there is an association between the two things measured, referred to as *variables*, which needs to be explained. It cannot be concluded that one causes the other, that is, that increasing age is a cause of longer stays in hospital. The difficulty with this type of research is that both the variables being measured may be connected to a third factor which may account for the relationship between them. In this example, older people are more likely to be widowed or to live alone. As a result, staff may be more reluctant to discharge older patients as quickly where there is no support at home, even though their physical conditions may be as good as that of younger people. Here, living alone is a possible explanation of the connection between age and longer stays in hospital. It cannot simply be said that older people take longer to recover from the operation, although, as seen above, there is a correlation between age and length of stay in hospital.

Gennero and Stringer (1991), for example, found a correlation between various stress factors and low birth weight. The study could not demonstrate, however, that the stress factors caused the low birth weight.

Experimental research and testing hypotheses

Another type of research is often referred to as *experimental research* where the researcher sets out to test a *hypothesis*. A hypothesis is a type of prediction which is usually derived from a survey and analysis of previous published research. It is a statement of the kind: 'If X is done to this sample, then Y will follow' (or, more correctly, if X was not done Y would not have happened). It can then be concluded that X caused Y to happen. This is the main advantage of experimental research over the descriptive type in that it makes *causal relationships* much clearer. The researcher in this case does not simply observe what happens or has happened, she introduces some form of *control* into the situation.

Dependent and independent variables

The experimenter, for example, might set out to test the hypothesis: if a new method of teaching physiology is introduced into the School of Nursing, then nurses' exam marks will improve. Here, an experiment is set up where the researcher deliberately manipulates or controls one major factor or variable, the type of teaching, referred to as an *independent variable*, in order to assess its effects on another factor, exam marks, referred to as the *dependent variable*. This type of research is frequently used in the evaluation of new drugs or methods of treatment as it is more likely to allow the researcher to say that one thing causes another than does the correlation type. It makes it less likely that alternative explanations of the kind noted in the previous example regarding recovery from operations can be put forward to explain the results. Research of this type generally follows one of a number of plans which are decided in advance. Such a plan is called the *design* of the experiment (see Chapter 14). In the study by Caruso *et al.* (1992), for example, the independent variable was the temperature of cooling blankets which was set at four different levels. The dependent variable was a measure of the cooling effect of each temperature level on patients with fever.

Pilot study

Before the research proper, a *pilot study* may be carried out. This takes the form of a small-scale trial of the research method, to ensure that the design is feasible. A pilot study may be on a small number of subjects only, but might help to determine a variety of practical questions: Can the subjects understand what is being asked of them? Does the nurse understand the new procedure which is to be tested? Are a large enough number of the type of subjects required likely to appear within the time available? Is the information needed always available from case records? How long is the new procedure likely to take? Does a new drug have undesirable side-effects?

Measurement

Scales of measurement

Following selection of subjects, some kind of assessment or *measurement* will usually be carried out on each one. Such measurement may be *qualitative*. Subjects of the research are differentiated only by possessing or not possessing a given characteristic, for example, pass/fail, recovered/died, single/married/widowed/ divorced. The subjects are divided into a number of categories, but the differences between these categories are not measurable in any real sense. This is referred to as a *nominal scale*. A more informative measurement is an *ordinal scale*. Here, subjects can be categorized more precisely, at least in terms of rank order from greatest to least, or best to worst. Examples might be the grading of essays on a scale of A–E, or grading according to social class. Again, however, there is no precisely measurable difference between any two grades.

If the temperatures of a group of subjects are taken, however, measurement becomes genuinely *quantitative* in the sense that any level between the known upper and lower extremes is possible. Precise statements of difference can now be made: the difference or interval between 10° and 11° is the same as the difference between 11° and 12°. Where this is so, the scale is an *interval scale*. Where, additionally, a scale has a true zero point, the scale becomes a *ratio scale*. This would be the case for measures of height and weight, but not for temperature, where the zero point is arbitrary.

Reliability

Measurement must give a *reliable* result whether done by observation and recorded on a simple rating scale (for example, the patient looks 'more cheerful'), by checking or counting such as in recording the number of times a patient is incontinent, or by technical means as in the case of blood pressure or temperature. The same results must be achieved, as far as possible, regardless of who is doing the measuring, so that several nurses weighing the same patient on the same set of scales in quick succession should get the same result each time, or very nearly so. *Inter-rater* or *inter-observer reliability* should thus exist.

With an accurate or reliable method of measurement, any influence or bias on the part of the person(s) doing the measuring is reduced to a minimum. This is relatively easy with measures such as height, weight, temperature, and so on because of the technical means available for such measurement. However, research frequently involves assessing or measuring variables which are much harder to quantify. It may be necessary for a nurse to assess how depressed a patient is, whether his colour is better, whether he can move more easily, or the degree of pain he has experienced. There are no absolute standards or technical aids for measuring these parameters, and eliminating inter-observer influences or inaccuracy due to different raters can be very difficult.

Operational definitions

Reasonably reliable judgements, however, can still be made if precise definitions of what is meant by such things as degrees of depression or mobility are provided. These precise definitions are sometimes referred to as *operational definitions*. These are necessary because the same term can often have different meanings for different researchers. 'Intelligence' is a good example. Although it is a concept of great value, there are many varied and even contradictory definitions of it. For a particular research project, therefore, an operational definition usually has to be arrived at. This might be 'intelligence as measured on Test A'. This does not mean this is the exact or only definition. It does mean that for the purposes of this research, this definition can be conveniently agreed upon.

A second sense in which measurements must be accurate (reliable) is that, given an unchanging condition, the measurement should give constant results over time. It might be known that a given dose of a drug should show up as a given concentration in a urine specimen. If the treatment is not changed, the estimates of this concentration should remain the same. If not, then explanations for this would have to be sought, and an obvious one might be that the method chosen to measure the concentration is unreliable. Whatever the type of measurement used, the research report ought to include an assessment of how reliable the measurements quoted are, and this is one area where statistical methods might well be used (see Section D, Chapters 27 and 28).

Validity

Another essential feature of all measurement used in research is that it must be *valid* – researchers should be able to predict accurately on the basis of the measures taken. Given that a reliable method of measuring blood pressure exists, such information will only be of value if it allows predictions to be made. Measurement of blood pressure is only valid to the extent that it allows identification of what treatment is necessary if blood pressure is too high or too low and what will happen if the treatment is applied. Measurement of intelligence is only valid to the extent that it will allow predictions to be made about the research subjects, for example, what type of school class they are best suited to, what type of job to try for, and so on. A good example of the question of *predictive validity* can be found in the article by Lothian (1989) where he considers the value of a number of scales which claim to assess the risk of developing pressure sores.

Two other studies which deal with some of the issues of reliability and validity are those of Weiss (1992) and Stager (1993).

Procedure

Having selected subjects and decided upon measures, a research report should describe accurately the *procedure* followed. The reported procedures should include when the measures were taken and by whom, under what conditions, and how the results were recorded. This is of considerable importance, because it will enable the research to be repeated in precisely the same way by others, if necessary. If more than one sample is involved in the research, it is also essential to know that exactly the same procedure was followed in each case. Research frequently involves a comparison of one group with another, where, for example, a new drug is applied to one group and compared with the effects of an established one applied to another similar group. Clearly, if it is to be claimed that the new treatment is superior to the old, the treatment procedure must be identical for each group except for the single difference of the drug given.

Results

A research report will then present *results* based on analysis of the *data* collected (see Part II, Section D). Data are the raw materials from which conclusions will be drawn and will often consist of lists of tables or information, in quantified form, containing such things as heights, weights, ratings, scores, test results or percentages. To make sense of these data, especially if the research project is on a large scale, it will often be necessary to make some use of *statistical methods*. First of all, these will enable the researcher to summarize and present a large quantity of results by means such as easily understood averages, graphs and histograms. Second, they will help the researcher to arrive at legitimate conclusions and reduce the element of subjective bias which anyone analysing the research findings will inevitably bring to them.

In most cases, the results of research projects do not work out in such a way as to allow clear-cut or definite conclusions to be drawn. Although not often phrased as if this were so, most research findings are simply statements of *probability* and should, strictly speaking, be stated as such; for example, 'the probability is less than one in 20 that this result could have occurred by chance'. That is, the researcher should state what degree of *confidence* can be placed in the results. It would mean, in effect, that if the same research were repeated 20 times under exactly the same conditions, the same result would be expected in at least 19 of them (or if repeated 100 times in at least 95). Thus it is evident that the higher the level of confidence which the statistical analysis will allow to be stated, the more certain one can be that the results could not have occurred by chance.

Generalization

The purpose of nearly all research is to allow general statements about whole populations to be made. The extent to which the researcher can *generalize* on the basis of one piece of research will depend on the large number of factors outlined above and the extent to which they have been taken into account. Thus if a research project claims to have proved that treatment A is superior to treatment B for condition X, then before this is accepted, there are a number of questions which must be asked.

(1)   Were the samples of patients given treatment A and B representative of all patients for whom treatments A and B might be appropriate? Were they selected at random? If the treatment could potentially be applied to all adults,

then a research sample not quite representative of all the adult population – for example, on average older, or with more males than females – would not invalidate the research altogether. It would be necessary, however, to be more cautious about the claims of the researchers that the results apply to all adults.

(2) Were all the factors which might affect the results controlled for? That is, were all the research patients treated under the same conditions by the same people, applying the same procedure?

(3) Were the measures of the treatment's effects reliable and valid? Does the research report give enough information on this to be able to judge?

(4) Were the results of the research presented in full? Were appropriate statistical methods used? Researchers unfamiliar with statistical methods should seek expert advice on this subject.

(5) Were the results stated with a high level of confidence?

(6) Possibly most important of all, does the research report give enough information for others to be able to repeat the research if they wish to?

The same questions, suitably modified, can be applied to any research report, and only if these conditions are met can the conclusions be accepted. It will also be evident that, given the above, research is a difficult exercise. No one ever performed the perfect piece of research, nor is anyone ever likely to!

References

Caruso, C., Hadly, B., Rakesh, S., Frame, P. & Khoury, J. (1992) Cooling effects and comfort of 4 cooling blanket temperatures in humans with fever. *Nursing Research* **41**, No 2, 68–72.

Gaebler, S. (1993) Predicting which patients will fall again . . . and again. *Journal of Advanced Nursing*, **18**, 1895–902.

Gennero, S. & Stringer, M. (1991) Stress and health in low birthweight infants: a longitudinal study. *Nursing Research*, **40**, No 5, 308–10.

Lothian, P. (1989) Identifying and protecting patients who may get pressure sores. *Nursing Standard*, 4(4), 26–9.

Stager, J.L. (1993) The comprehensive breast cancer knowledge test: validity and reliability. *Journal of Advanced Nursing*, **18**, 1133–40.

Weiss, S. (1992) Measurement of the sensory qualities in tactile interaction. *Nursing Research*, **41** No 2, 82–6.

Chapter 3

Agencies Supportive to Nursing Research

Senga Bond

This chapter is devoted to sources of support for nurses who wish to carry out research. Of course, research efforts extend from large-scale, multi-disciplinary, multi-centre projects involving major financial and manpower resources, to those which can be done by an individual requiring little more resources than a notebook and pencil and lots of time. It is well nigh impossible to carry out good research without support. Different forms of assistance are appropriate for all types of research, and all research workers, whatever the stage of their research career. However for those at the earlier stages of wishing to do research, it is of the utmost importance to obtain advice as well as the means to support the research.

Let us assume you have the motivation, interest and a bright idea and want to embark on research but lack the knowledge of where to begin. The fact that you are reading this book would suggest that you are on the right track! Books like this are a useful source of ideas but because they are not interactive in the same way as people, they are at best only a partial answer. If we posed the question, 'What kind of help do I need?' it might be answered in a number of ways including:

- Education for research
- Supervision
- Specific advice
- Kindred spirits
- Financial support
- Information resources.

Education for research

Some aspects of research are generally included as a small component of most nursing courses and there are many short 'research appreciation' courses as well as longer forms of research preparation at diploma and masters level. While you may have had some introduction to research ideas and to research studies, it may be worth considering more extended research training through one of the full, or part-time courses. Such courses in research methods are available in many higher educational institutions. It is generally easier to obtain time off work for a part-time day/evening course, while it is often easier to appreciate the benefits of being able to concentrate on full-time study if it can be arranged. The calendars of universities and colleges should provide full details of whether suitable courses are available, and of entry requirements. It may be that research does not feature in the course title and so course content needs to be examined carefully. Such courses may be found in nursing departments or in social sciences or in health services research in medical faculties. Some provide an option which permits progress from diploma to higher degree level.

Should an appropriate course not be available locally it is well worth considering doing the Open University 3rd Level Research Methods Course, Principles of Social and Educational Research (DEH313). As its title suggests, this course is orientated generally towards the social, rather than the biological sciences. It also forms part of an MSc which may be taken subsequently through the Open University.

Another way of obtaining research education is to apply for one of the research studentships awarded annually by government Health Departments in Scotland, England and Wales and Northern Ireland, as well as the increasing number being made available through the National Health Service in the regions. These are usually for diplomas or higher research degrees. In Scotland, traditional research training has given way to include different kinds of award. Some involve the development of proposals between the individual and the employing authority to increase the service value of the research and research training; some involve short term secondments into on-going research programmes and some involve joint appointments between service and academic institutions. These studentships are generally advertised in the press at around the turn of the year for commencement at the beginning of the next academic year, while National Health Service opportunities are advertised internally, often in the newsletters produced by each Research and Development director. The appropriate liaison person for the government departments in each country from whom information can be obtained is given at the end of this chapter.

Glancing through the appointments sections of the nursing press indicates that there are nurses with research appointments in many National Health Service Trusts as well as a few remaining in the National Health Service Executive regional offices. One of their responsibilities is likely to be maintaining a list of research courses available locally. Research orientated courses are not for those about to do research, they are orientated more for 'consumers' and 'participants' in research rather than 'doers'. One advantage of doing a formal research methods course is to assist beginners in deciding whether they really have the motivation and ability to proceed to carry out research. While taking a course may delay the start of a project, it does lay down a good foundation from which to proceed as well as opportunities to obtain supervision. It is for this reason that students embarking on a higher degree by research are advised to participate in a general methods course first, so that as well as learning through a project using a particular method, they extend their knowledge to other methods and techniques used in research.

Supervision

Those who embark on a formal research course will be allocated a supervisor or find one for themselves. It is very important that supervision relates to the methodological aspects of the study as well as to the practical aspects of planning and conducting the research. There may also be need for supervision in the substantive topic – from a nutritionist or a psychologist or nurse expert in the subject of the study. Supervisors are there to discuss, guide and offer advice, not to do the project. They need to be asked for help and are encouraged when students have done preparation and thinking through the problems of conducting the research at theoretical, methodological and practical levels. Most supervisors, especially if they are good, will have heavy demands on their time. However if they are faced with a keen student who is well prepared, then demands are more likely to be met. Most higher educational institutions now prepare guidance for students and supervisors in managing projects and the supervision process.

Specific advice

Of course the need for advice could be at any stage of the research process, but in general terms the earlier advice is sought the better. Recognizing the need for advice could be in working up a project that inspires you but you are not sure what to do next. As a formal supportive agency, this is the kind of work for which nursing personnel with a research remit in the health service would be the first port of call. This person should have a sufficiently broad overview of research to enable you to refine your ideas and begin to formulate possible directions for the project. It is important to bear in mind that it is not possible for any one individual to have detailed knowledge of every research problem with which they are faced, but nurses in research appointments should be able to assist you sufficiently to enable you to prepare to consult with some more specialist interest if this is warranted. While the Nursing and Health Services Research Units in universities as well as the Daphne Heald Unit at the Royal College of Nursing will be able to provide assistance in a few cases, they could be inundated with requests for help and their purpose is, first and foremost, to carry out their own research. It is important, therefore, to obtain help locally whenever this is possible. The increased emphasis on health services research within the National Health Service has resulted in staff being available in the regions in England and Wales, or supported by them, but placed in university departments with the specific remit of providing a tutorial or advisory service. In Scotland five research networks have been created to cover the whole of the country and to offer advice to those wishing to conduct health related research.

There are often local resources besides nurses who are able to give advice on specific aspects of research. These include research workers in related fields: medical colleagues or social or biomedical scientists and statisticians. Ask your colleagues whether they know of anyone and watch out for local names in publications. Personal recommendation of someone who is helpful is by far the best way of securing useful contacts. Research interests are certainly one way of bridging professional boundaries as well as drawing service matters into closer communication with academic departments in universities. The message is to begin where you are and to use whatever talent is available locally before proceeding further.

Kindred spirits

Another type of support, which is rather different from specific advice or supervision for your project, is to find like-minded individuals who are carrying out research and facing similar problems. It is probably a universal finding that research workers at some point in developing or carrying out a project feel isolated, dejected and ready to give up. At such times it is useful to share your experience with someone who may have gone through, or be in the process of facing the same distress. This is when membership of an informal or formal research group may be useful. All local research interest groups serve several functions, one of their strengths is a bringing together of people who have a general interest in learning about and supporting research. On the whole you are likely to find others with research interests very willing to help and listen, and offer support of different kinds. In this regard the Research Networks in Scotland serve a useful function in bringing together people from a range of backgrounds and interests.

Other benefits to be gained from membership of a local research group are in hearing of current developments in research, internationally, nationally as well as locally, learning how others have gone about research and how they have attempted to overcome their particular difficulties. By providing an informal setting to discuss research issues generally, research meetings can be very positive occasions for those planning to begin, or already engaged in, research. Less formal get-togethers of nurses involved in research are also useful. Sometimes an informal lunch time gathering is sufficient to air a difficulty and regain vital energies which may be dwindling.

At a national level the conferences organized by nursing organizations including the annual conference of the RCN Research Advisory Group provide occasions for hearing research workers talk about their work. This is most effectively done at residential conferences where there are opportunities for networking as well as hearing about recent developments, and special interest groups can meet to discuss particular issues.

The other kind of non-nursing groups and associations worth considering joining are those with a more specific focus of interest; examples would be the Society for Tissue Viability, the British Society of Gerontology and the Society for Research in Rehabilitation and the Society for Social Medicine. While some of these are not specifically research groups, a major interest is the discussion of current research and methods in their respective fields. These groups would be of major importance in keeping abreast of developments which are broader than nursing and maintaining current awareness of findings and methods. Membership of such a group would bring you into contact with others who share an interest in a narrower substantive field. In time, it is to be hoped that professional nursing groups like the RCN societies and forums may develop more research-orientated opportunities in their conferences and professional meetings to enable them to become a focal point for researchers.

Financial support

Financial assistance may be sought for research education or for funding a specific project. The opportunities available for research education described above also carry remuneration with them. The funds apportioned to research education within the health service are highly variable. While all R and D directors are committed to supporting the research infrastructure, how they do so is highly variable and obtaining funding is generally in open competition, with nurses competing with other disciplines. National Health Service Trusts vary widely in the amount of funding made available for research training with some regarding funding of research training as appropriate, while others do not. With training budgets now devolved into clinical directorates, some say it is increasingly difficult to obtain research training. Employing authorities also have the discretion of paying Open University fees but on this, as in all educational matters, views and policies differ widely.

In financial terms, far more money is available for funding individual projects than for research training. In nursing the problem is not that there is not the funding but that there is a shortfall in the number of nurses with the experience to attract funding. Grant awarding bodies are unlikely to finance research proposed by an inexperienced researcher with no evidence of their capability of managing a research project. It is naive to expect funding without a track record, so how does one get into the game?

There are no short answers. Traditionally individuals build up research credibility by working with experienced researchers and learning the craft from them. By so doing one gradually develops a reputation sufficient to enable grants to be awarded on the basis of sound proposals. Research budgets are available to nurses in all of the health related charities as well as central government research funds, the National Health Service Research and Development budget and the Medical and Economic and Social Research Councils. Funds are not earmarked for nurses but are open to competition on the basis of the quality of the proposal. In some ways nurses are disadvantaged by the membership of many funding bodies being medically rather than health orientated and with a preference for particular methods.

Many research funding sources operate in 'response mode' – that is they will respond to proposals originating from the applicants. However, increasingly, priority areas are being identified and proposals invited in line with specified topics. This is not a bar to nurses applying for funding so long as their proposals are in line with what is requested. It is important, therefore, to know what are the priorities of different funding agencies and to ensure that proposals are appropriately targeted.

To assist novices some National Health Service Research and Development offices make small amounts of money available which do not have to go through the usual peer review process. Intermediate level grants then are pitched at £25K– £50K over one to two years, while larger grants are also available. In Scotland there are two schemes. Project grants provide support over a three-year period for sums up to about £100K, and there are about 50 such projects at any one time. Applicants for this funding should tailor their research to meet the customer needs of a specific commission. The Mini-project Scheme aims to provide support up to £5K for small health services research projects, and pilot studies, which might lead to the development of applications for larger project grants. The purpose of this scheme is to encourage newcomers to health services research from any health profession or academic discipline.

Research grants may be obtained from the Medical Research Council (MRC) or the Economic and Social Research Council (ESRC) to which appropriate submissions may be made. Nurses are likely to apply to the Health Services Research Board of the MRC and a Small Grants Scheme for projects costing less than £30K and another with the National Health Service up to £60K exist. All projects are submitted to peer review and must be of a very high standard to be funded.

A directory of grant-giving bodies specifically for nursing is provided in the *Directory of Nursing Charities* (Loxton, 1993). Many of these provide small amounts of money for educational purposes but some also indicate a willingness to finance research projects. Other charitable sources are described in publications by the Association of Medical Research Charities (1994/95) and the Charities Aid Foundation (1993/94).

Finance for research may also be attracted from industry and commerce, particularly the pharmaceutical companies and those devoted to other health products. Some companies like 3M, Smith and Nephew and Maws annual award scholarships, but ad hoc projects may also be funded. Commercial concerns could probably be more widely used than they are but sometimes ethical considerations intervene with taking research moneys from companies like Nestle which sells milk powders to third world countries or the tobacco industry's conscience-salving research fund The Health Promotion Research Trust. Parahoo (1988) provides another view of funding nursing research.

Chapter 9 in this volume deals with writing a proposal which is only one facet of attracting research money. The proposal, irrespective of its scientific merits, must prove sufficiently appealing to attract sponsorship and there is an art in preparing such a submission.

Information resources

While information resources have been placed last, they are by no means least in importance. Anyone wishing to carry out research will need to know what has already been published on the topic. For this reason libraries and information services are integral to research development. Chapter 7 describes major libraries, indexing and abstracting resources and the increasing accessibility of information on CD-ROM and on-line computer facilities. Clamp *et al.* (1991) offer a helpful resource.

While using abstracting and indexing journals is important for individual researchers to keep abreast of current literature, group efforts to share knowledge and reading can be most useful. In some clinical and academic departments, journal clubs meet on a monthly basis to discuss recent important publications and to inform participants of useful papers and books which have been identified. By allocating particular journals to members and sharing the reading, an enormous amount of scanning can be shared and useful items located which might otherwise have been missed. Journal clubs have the added advantage of encouraging discussion, learning how others regard methods and findings and generally sharpening research awareness. An active journal club demonstrates to others the importance placed on knowing what is happening nationally and internationally. They are, therefore, as important for 'users' as for 'doers' of research.

Conclusion

No matter who it is, or the degree of development in their research career, some forms of support are necessary to carry out research. This chapter has done little more than indicate some of the sources of such support. It would be easy to consider support purely in financial terms, for research education or to fund a project to buy staff or materials. This is only part of the story. Just as important are sources of support which are sustaining in intellectual and emotional terms. One has only to read the acknowledgements section of any thesis to find reference to the assistance given by supervisors and colleagues, not to mention long-suffering spouses. Often it is the generosity of others in terms of their time, intellectual application and listening ability, as well as their skills in motivating and encouraging the writing of proposals and reports, which enable research to succeed.

The research community itself is perhaps the most important supportive agency. Researchers, by their willingness to give the same encouragement and assistance to others which they themselves have received, are an important source of mutual support. Used wisely they are of incalculable benefit.

Useful addresses

Deputy Chief Nursing Officer, Department of Health, Dundonald House, Upper New-townards Road, Belfast, BT4 3SF.
Deputy Chief Nursing Officer, Welsh Office, Cathays Park, Cardiff, CF1 3NQ.
Nursing Officer (Research), Chief Scientist Office, Scottish Home and Health Department, St Andrew's House, Edinburgh, EH1 3DE.
Principal Nursing Officer (Research), National Health Service Executive, Quarry House, Quarry Hill, Leeds, LS2 7UE.

References

Association of Medical Research Charities (1994/95) *Handbook of the Association of Medical Research Charities*, British Heart Foundation, London.

Charities Aid Foundation (1993/94) *Directory of Grant Making Trusts*. Charities Aid Foundation, London.

Clamp, C.G.L., Ballard, M.P. & Gough, S. (1991) *Resources for Nursing Research: an annotated bibliography*. Library Association Publishing, London.

Loxton, D. (1993) *Directory of Nursing Charities*. Queens Nursing Institute, London.

Parahoo, K. (1988) Funding nursing research. *Senior Nurse*, 8(9/10), 12–14.

Chapter 4

Ethical Issues in Nursing Research

Hazel E. McHaffie

Consider, if you will, two scenarios.

> Joseph Lyons is struggling. He is an inpatient on a medical ward following a stroke. For some time he has had difficulty with bladder control largely because of his slowness in movement. The nurse seeing him struggling will instinctively come to his aid, attend to his needs and prevent unhappiness. The researcher observing Mr Lyons may well simply watch, wait to see how long it will take someone to respond to his needs, note his distress, record the nurses' reaction to another wet bed, and analyse the possible causes and effects of the various components of this experience. For the researcher who is also a nurse a dilemma will present. What are the boundaries of her responsibility?

> Robin Allen is a nurse working as a clinical specialist in a busy intensive care unit. He agrees to participate in a study looking at the impact of personal experience of loss and bereavement on professional attitudes and behaviours. During the course of his interview he discloses that he has lost three partners who died from AIDS- related illnesses. He further admits that none of his colleagues know he is HIV positive. What should the researcher do with this information?

In nursing, research depends for its success on careful observation, contemplation, recording and analysis. But this may involve hearing and seeing what others do not know about. The contract a researcher has with a participant allows confidences to be given which would compel clinicians to act. Respondents are not unaware of the opportunities: sharing troubling thoughts and experiences can be therapeutic. Thus, for example, if a safe and confiding atmosphere is provided, a mother may well tell a researcher that she has harmed her baby. To divulge that information to a health visitor or a social worker has obvious ramifications and possible penalties.

A range of ethical problems present themselves not only to those actively engaged in research but to clinicians whose patients are involved in projects, to educators and to managers. By definition, where a dilemma presents there are no easy answers. It may be necessary to weigh up present safety, long term benefit, or the conflicting interests of different parties against the integrity of the research. Simply because there are few concrete points of reference the decisions can be difficult and worrying.

Ethics is a branch of philosophy which deals with thinking about morality. In assessing the morality of a person's conduct we make a judgement about whether something is right or wrong. Each of use has our own values, beliefs and standards and this very diversity complicates matters. Codes and official guidelines only take us so far. We are each individually accountable for our practice and must be able to justify the decisions we make.

Responsibilities of all nurses

Nursing has made enormous strides in scientific, technological and social developments in recent years. Emerging ethical dilemmas have exercised the minds of many. Fundamentally the biomedical ethical principles underpinning practice remain unchanged: respect for autonomy, and the principles of doing no harm, doing good and acting justly (Beauchamp & Childress, 1989). Professional advice has become more expansive but is consistent with these basic tenets (British Medical Association, 1993; Royal College of Nursing, 1993).

The United Kingdom Central Council for Nursing, Midwifery and Health Visiting (1992), in its Code of Conduct, requires all its practitioners to 'safeguard and promote the interests of individual patients and clients'. In its 16 items it clearly places responsibility with the individual: it is no defence that someone else gave the instruction, or that one was an innocent bystander. Acts and omissions alike can incur censure. The professional bodies reinforce this responsibility, applying it to research as well as clinical practice (Royal College of Nursing, 1993; Royal College of Midwives, 1989; International Confederation of Midwives, 1993). Indeed the Royal College of Nursing document, *Ethics Related to Research in Nursing*, spells out the issues clearly and comprehensively.

Individual professional accountability

Nurses can be caught up in the ethical issues around research without ever being actively involved in the process itself. Simply because their patients become participants, they can inherit a special responsibility. Research can be detrimental and the nurse has a specific obligation to ensure that nothing jeopardizes the well-being of patients.

Good nursing practice should be based wherever possible on sound evidence. It is not ethically acceptable to follow tradition or received wisdom without question. In order to practise safely and well, nurses need to be aware of the research in their field of practice and able to use it effectively. But not all research is valuable and usable. Being personally accountable involves discrimination. This means being able to read, critically evaluate and effectively utilize reports of studies.

A fundamental requirement in any endeavour is to possess the knowledge and skills which are compatible with the demands of the task. It is important to recognize the limits of one's competence and not to take on tasks unless they can be carried out in a safe and skilled manner. Research is a skilled occupation just as clinical practice and education are. It should not be thought that it can just be 'picked up' without the advice and help of experts.

Where nurses are asked to be actively involved, at even a minimal level, in the research process they must be acquainted with what the procedures involve. Thus, if they are asked to witness the signing of a document giving informed consent, they should satisfy themselves that the patient has fully understood the risks involved and understands that he has the right to withdraw at any point without influencing in any way his therapeutic management.

Nurses are not infrequently employed as data collectors. Given the clinical load they already carry, it is vital that this additional role is not detrimental to the well-being of their patients. They are obliged to state if this is the case. As at all other levels of involvement, if they undertake data collection, they are bound by the same ethical principles incumbent upon all researchers. Integrity and accuracy are mandatory. Clearly the success of the research is dependent on the willingness, accuracy and conscientiousness of such data collectors.

Particular tensions may present with this dual role. Confidential information may be acquired as part of being a clinician or in the course of data collection. Such information must not be divulged outside the sphere in which it was collected except with the express permission of the respondent himself. As we have already seen, conflicts of interests can place the nurse researcher in an unenviable position.

Responsibilities of the researcher

Personal integrity

Researchers are bound by their professional codes as well as the guidance provided for the conduct of research in general. Intellectual honesty and integrity are required at each level of the enquiry.

There is an initial obligation to ensure that the work they are proposing is appropriate. It is not appropriate, for example, to conduct a study which does nothing to contribute to further knowledge; to do it for the wrong reasons; or to carry out tasks for which one is inadequately prepared. This may sound perfectly straightforward. In reality conflicts may arise even here. Sometimes the requirements of an academic institution may not concur with those of clinical practice. On occasion it is not possible to afford expert methodological, computing or statistical advice and a researcher falls back on books and secondhand advice. These are compromises and force uneasy decisions.

Recognizing one's personal limitations is essential at every level: few researchers are expects in all methods and in all aspects of the research process. In addition, every individual brings some personal history to research. Where this might prejudice the work in any way, it should be declared. Even very eminent researchers have taken a subject on board because of their personal agendas: this is not of necessity a bad thing, but it is a potential bias. The reader must calculate its effect. Such honesty is part of the requirement for personal integrity and accuracy. By the same token, the effect the researcher may have had on the subjects should be openly acknowledged (Hunt, 1989). If such matters are not made explicit, doubt may be cast on the integrity of other parts of the enquiry.

Conducting research and then allowing the results to gather dust on a shelf is unethical. If the study was needed in the first place, its results should be published and disseminated appropriately. Many subjects as well as data collectors over the years have lamented the lack of availability of findings (Hicks, 1994). It is unethical to 'use' people in this way. Where they have contributed time, energy and emotions, they are entitled to some feedback. Funding bodies who resource the enquiries are entitled to some tangible return for their investment too.

Actual examples of researchers falsifying their results are few. More common is the practice of 'doctoring' the reporting to omit those aspects of the project which were less than successful. Not only is this intellectually dishonest, but it carries the grave risk that others will subsequently repeat the errors in judgement. No research project carried out in the natural world can be perfect. It is far better to acknowledge the limitations, delays, unexpected hitches and inappropriate use of tools or ambiguous questions, than to pretend the exercise was perfectly planned and executed and risk losing credibility and integrity. A conflict may, however, present where the results would be unwelcome to the host organization. If, for example, the research uncovers undesirable practices amongst some of its nurses, reporting them may offend the hosts. It is important in these circumstances to balance the value of the information, the context and nature of the reporting and the overall message against the damage which may result from the disclosure.

Another aspect of intellectual honesty relates to the extent of the reporting. It is important to present findings which do not support one's hypothesis or hunch as well as those which do. Researchers are scientifically accountable to their peers: the advancement of theory and methods for the profession depends upon their integrity (Clark, 1991; Sandelowski, 1993). Widespread peer review, competent scrutiny and constructive criticism from within the research community as well as from without, can do much to promote good quality at all stages of any enquiry. Building in such advice is advisable.

Responsibility to participants

Informed consent

In any research which involves human subjects in the United Kingdom, there must be safeguards for their protection. The hazards of radioactive substances or of aggressive drug treatments are obvious. Less well recognized are the emotional, psychological and social harms which might accrue. It can be damaging to be asked insensitive questions. Confidence can be undermined if a subject is left feeling ignorant about a topic. Where a participant is assigned to a control group he can feel disadvantaged if the experimental intervention appears more beneficial.

It is imperative that potential subjects are warned of the potential risks of involvement before they agree to participate. Of course, it is perfectly possible technically to spell out these drawbacks but not to truly inform. If the researcher is to behave ethically, she should give the individual every opportunity to question, to receive accurate information and to reflect on the matter or consult others before committing himself in any way. Wherever possible it is wise to supply written material to accompany verbal information. It should also be made perfectly clear that a patient has an absolute right to decline to participate or to withdraw at any time. No risk of less effective or kindly nursing treatment should ever be a result of such a refusal: a fact which should be spelled out plainly. Ill people are very vulnerable and feel disempowered. It is imperative that this vulnerability is not exploited in any way.

How and when such consent is obtained matters. To approach a patient minutes before they go to theatre for major surgery, or when they are under the influence of sedatives or preoccupied with other anxieties is unacceptable. Simple reflection will demonstrate the truth of this statement. Less clear is the issue of how much to tell. For some studies, it is not possible to divulge all the information known about the subject. In other cases it would be detrimental to the study for the subjects to know everything about the aims of the project. Take, for example, an investigation of non-accidental injury in children in an Accident and Emergency Department; or a study of the effects of intramuscular vitamin K for newborns; or the behaviours of married men who have sex with men. In all these areas of interest, the quality of data produced might well be jeopardized if too much information is divulged to potential respondents. If the parents think the researcher suspects them of deliberately harming their child, they are not likely to want to talk about the 'accident'. Mothers will be reluctant to expose their babies to possible danger, no matter how remote. Married men might view with dismay the prospect of someone studying homosexuality appearing on their marital doorstep. Where does society's right to accurate information or the funding agency's right to good quality data, or the individual's right to be informed begin and end?

A fundamental respect for other people should be the guiding principle. Their right to be autonomous should be respected. In the field of HIV and AIDS the need for a partnership between researchers and subjects has been clearly demonstrated. People with the virus have gone to extreme lengths to ensure that participation in clinical trials does not unfairly discriminate between patients or potentially damage the health of any individual person (Institute of Medical Ethics, 1992). Not all patients have been as articulate or well informed. But again, their very vulnerability should make the researcher more vigilant in protecting their interests.

It is sometimes assumed that information collected during the course of providing nursing care is available for research purposes. This should not be assumed. If clinical data are to be used for research, permission needs to be sought from the patients and in some cases the person who is in clinical charge of the patient and the authorities by whom the records are held (Dimond, 1990).

The identity of the researcher

Researchers can undertake projects for many and various reasons. Some of these reasons may be questionable. A person with strong negative homophobic prejudices is probably not an appropriate person to research attitudes to patients who are HIV positive. Someone employed by a drug company may not be able to declare all his findings if they demonstrate that a particular product has unwelcome side-effects. A lay person may not fully comprehend the nuances and culture of a specialized paediatric intensive care unit: interpretation of what she sees may be inaccurate. The identity of the researcher can influence the quality of the design, conduct and recommendations of the study.

It can sometimes seem important to conceal the identity of the researcher. Examples of such disguise can be found in the literature and include researchers pretending to be criminals, police, homosexuals and nursing auxiliaries. Extremely rich data can be obtained in some circumstances where respondents see the incomer as 'one of them'. Indeed such data might be unobtainable in any other way. But serious attention must be given to the rights of those people who disclose information unwittingly for research purposes (Johnson, 1992). Many people have strong moral objections to such deception.

In health care enquiries, the research may well overlap with clinical management. Where the researcher is not involved in delivering the treatment, it is important that the clinicians are aware of their patients' participation. Naturally if an intervention is necessary which includes a new or altered form of treatment, close liaison will be imperative. But the courtesy of informing clinical colleagues should apply even when their permission is not necessary.

Confidentiality and anonymity

During the course of data collection, researchers may be told much that is confidential. They are required to give assurances of confidentiality and anonymity in almost all cases. Indeed the rich quality of data obtained in many studies has only been possible because of such assurances. These confidences must be respected. Where it appears imperative to disclose any such information the explicit permission of the respondent is required. On the surface, this seems beyond question. In practice, conflicts may arise. Information may be disclosed which puts emotional well-being at risk as well as lives. It is very burdensome to be told that a respondent is contemplating suicide; feels she may do violence to her infant; is living off money acquired by immoral or illegal means; or is putting others' safety in danger. Conflicting interests and risks must be balanced and judgements made by the researcher which sometimes weigh heavily.

Where there is any possibility that information will be obtained relating to safety, well-being or clinical problems, it is important to establish accepted lines of communication before the event. Who will the researcher tell? Who else will be informed or contacted? How much will be disclosed? Roles and responsibilities will then be clear. Appropriate action can be instigated promptly.

Preserving the anonymity of respondents or of participating institutions or organizations is another requirement. Individuals may very well not wish to admit that they supported the administration of drugs to end a life peacefully and in a dignified way if such information could be traced back to them. Junior nurses may be reluctant to disclose their views on the management of the wards they work on if they fear identification. Respondents have a right to such protection.

Ethics Committee approval

As part of the protection of people's rights and interests, Local Research Ethics Committees exist for the scrutiny of proposed projects. Each Health Authority (Health Board in Scotland) has a requirement to set up appropriately constituted committees (Royal College of Physicians, 1990; Department of Health, 1991; Scottish Office Home and Health Department, 1992). Some academic institutions also operate their own systems of vigilance. The modus operandi of each committee varies, and intending researchers must obtain the necessary information and documentation from the relevant body. Contact information can usually be obtained through the headquarters of the relevant Health Authority/Board. With the advent of Trusts there is a potential for additional problems in accessing subjects and in collaborating between organizations. Commercial and professional sensitivities have added a competitive dimension to the provision of health care and for a variety of reasons managers may be less open with information about their services in the future.

Nevertheless, irrespective of whether the researcher is or is not an employee in the National Health Service, projects involving patients must be scrutinized by ethics committees. Where research subjects are the health care professionals themselves, different areas have differing policies about whether such approval is necessary. Advice from the Health Authority/Board or the Local Research Ethics Committee should be sought.

Ethics committees are made up of representatives from the health professions, individuals with various interests such as law or theology and members of the lay community. Each committee has boundaries relating to the geographical or subject area it will review. Problems do arise, and with the increasing complexity and range of research projects, there is some concern that these ethics committees may withhold approval less to protect potential respondents than to demonstrate their power or because they are unfamiliar with the nature of the enquiry (Pollock & Tilley, 1988; Neuberger, 1991).

Responsibilities of the educator

Research is no longer a tiny component of a course tagged on at the end to fill in a Friday afternoon slot. It is something which underpins all of nursing to a greater or lesser extent depending on the evidence available. Part of the preparation of its practitioners is to equip them to care well. The quality of the care offered depends on an understanding of what research has shown to be good practice.

If individual clinicians are to be professionally accountable they require the skills accurately and critically to assess the evidence. Educators have a specific responsibility to give them such equipment. But using research to inform one's practice can be difficult. Resistance, resentment and jealousy can all present barriers to change. It is unacceptable to provide nurses with the knowledge of what needs to be done without the skills to do it. They require skills of negotiation and assertiveness to practise in a world which has a long way still to go in its striving to be research aware and research based.

The increasing inclusion of research components in nursing courses at both basic and post basic levels is to be applauded. However, the requirement that students undertake a small project as part of their course raises problems. To begin with such endeavours are necessarily time limited. They usually have fairly tight geographical limits which carries the threat of overloading respondents in their area. Resources are inevitably constrained. The inexperience of the students may seriously compromise entry to the field for senior researchers subsequently. Since many of the fundamental principles and skills may be taught in the classroom, it is debatable whether the practice of requiring practical experience in the field is appropriate.

Responsibilities of the manager

Entering an institution or community to carry out research is a privilege not a right. There are costs and risks to the organization acting as host to such an endeavour. Managers will require to assess the psychological as well as the financial costs, both direct and indirect. Researchers can impede work, distract staff, create unrest and expose undesirable, unethical and questionable practices.

Those with the authority to sanction or commission research carry a heavy obligation. In negotiating with researchers, clinicians, educators and sponsors they will require great tact and diplomacy. They have a duty to encourage the conduct of good research in their area of responsibility. It is imperative, therefore, that they understand what is worthwhile and achievable, and what is feasible given service demands. With the strong pressures on resources and time, it is easy for managers to expect too much too quickly. In the furtherance of sound knowledge, studies must be well conducted, with rigorous checks on reliability and validity. It is just as harmful to support all research attempts indiscriminately as to resist research. Some studies simply should not be encouraged. Good communication and liaison with expert researchers will enable managers to make such judgements effectively.

Where managers commission research, they have an obligation to respect the right of any individual to refuse to undertake a project if they consider it to be outside their range of competence. There may well be ways of negotiating the involvement of others with the necessary skills. Reservations relating to the feasibility of carrying out the study within the time and resource limits must also be heard.

There are special duties attending those who simultaneously manage health services and commission research. Data collected for the research must not be used for purposes outside the research endeavour, for example in disciplinary proceedings. Such material is confidential with specific boundaries. Neither should there be any attempt to probe for identifying information which the researcher has deliberately concealed. Where results call for changes these will need to be assessed in the light of wider knowledge and implemented carefully. Managers have a weighty responsibility to ensure such changes are recommended by expert reviewers in addition to the researchers who might have a vested interest in their own project.

Special protection should be ensured for the vulnerable. This applies at the level of conducting the enquiry as well as reporting the results. The interests of patients, the staff and the service must not be compromised by the demands of the research undertaken.

The effect of research on the community

Participants in research are part of a wider community. Their involvement in enquiries can cause problems. Managers need to be alive to the possibility of complications.

Where the health care professionals themselves are involved as participants there may be implications if they are withdrawn from the service temporarily or required to take on additional work or given specific opportunities not available to all. Frustrations and resentments may result.

Feelings of envy or resistance can quickly accumulate if specific groups are frequently targeted for research. The enormous sums of money projected into research relating to HIV and AIDS represent a case in point. Provision of resources in various forms is seen to be discriminating in favour of a select group and at the expense of other specialities who feel they are at least equally deserving. For the communities so over-researched there can be negative as well as positive results. A sense of elitism can be counteracted by a tendency to self criticism, introspection and doubt, as well as fatigue and lack of enthusiasm.

Conclusion

Ethical dilemmas result from conflicting values. They can relate to whether or not to do the research, the subject to be studied and the actual conduct of the enquiry. Difficulties can present at both a personal and a professional level.

Judgements about what is right conduct lie on a continuum ranging from the clearly unethical to the clearly ethical. Individual tolerances vary, and people's values and attitudes change over time. The issues are not often all black or all white.

Nurses involved at the level of protecting the patients in their care as well as those conducting the research, require to be sensitive to these issues. They must be prepared to defend what is ethical, renounce the indefensible and support each other in the move towards sound knowledge-based practice.

References

Beauchamp, T.L. & Childress, J.F. (1989) *Principles of Biomedical Ethics*, 3rd edn. Oxford University Press, Oxford.

British Medical Association (1993) *Medical Ethics Today. Its Practice and Philosophy*. British Medical Journal Publishing Group, London.

Clark, E. (1991) *Evaluating Research*. Module 10 in Research Awareness programme. Distance Learning Centre, South Bank Polytechnic, London.

Department of Health (1991) *Local Research Ethics Committees*. HMSO, London.

Dimond, B (1990) Legal aspects of research. *Nursing Standard*, **4**, 39, 44-6.

Hicks, C. (1994) Bridging the gap between research and practice: An assessment of the value of a study day in developing critical research reading skills in midwives. *Midwifery*, **10**, 18–25.

Hunt, J.C. (1989) *Psychoanalytic Aspects of Fieldwork*. Sage Publications, London.

Institute of Medical Ethics (1992) AIDS, ethics, and clinical trials. *British Medical Journal*, **305**, 699–701.

International Confederation of Midwives (1993) *International Code of Ethics for Midwives*. International Confederation of Midwives, London.

Johnson, M. (1992) A silent conspiracy? Some ethical issues of participant observation in nursing research. *International Journal of Nursing Studies*, **29**, 2, 213–23.

Neuberger, J. (1991) *Ethics and Health Care*. King's Fund, London.

Pollock, L. & Tilley, S. (1988) Submitting for approval. *Senior Nurse*, **8**, 5, 24–5.

Royal College of Midwives (1989) *Practical Guidance for Midwives Facing Ethical or Moral Dilemmas*. Royal College of Midwives, London.

Royal College of Nursing (1993) *Ethics Related to Research in Nursing*. Royal College of Nursing, London.

Royal College of Physicians (1990) *Guidelines on the Practice of Ethics Committees in Medical Research involving Human Subjects*. Royal College of Physicians, London.

Sandelowski, M. (1993) Rigor or rigor mortis: the problem of rigor in qualitative research revisited. *Advances in Nursing Science*, **16**, 2, 1–8.

Scottish Office Home and Health Department (1992) *Local Research Ethics Committees*. HMSO, Scotland.

United Kingdom Central Council for Nursing, Midwifery and Health Visiting (1992) *Code of Conduct for Nurses, Midwives and Health Visitors*. United Kingdom Central Council, London.

Chapter 5

An Overview of the Research Process

Desmond F.S. Cormack

Irrespective of the discipline in which research is undertaken, the series and sequence of steps are essentially the same. What will differ between disciplines such as nursing and psychology for example, will be the subject of the research rather than its structure or process. The research process discussed in Part II of this book is a description of what is commonly referred to as 'the scientific method'. The strength of the scientific method as an approach to problem solving is that it optimizes the possibility of arriving at the most 'correct', although rarely perfect, solution. Thus, subjectivity is reduced and objectivity increased in the examination of a particular issue or the asking of a specific question.

An understanding of the research process is not, of itself, sufficient to enable its application. The topics discussed in the first five chapters of the book, for example, are each important in the development of research skills. Similarly, the subjects described in the final three chapters are of importance in relation to undertaking, participating in, and using research. Part II cannot be seen in isolation from other parts of this book, it is merely one distinct phase in a number of interrelated parts of understanding the nature, purpose and structure of research. A knowledge of research principles will not, of itself, make a skilled researcher. The need for appropriate guidance and supervision during all stages of research experience is of considerable importance. As with many activities, including nursing which requires a high level of knowledge and skill, the knowledge and skill required to undertake nursing research can be learned. They are learned in a number of ways: being told by others, discussing the subject with others, reading about the subject and by doing a piece of research. Although all educational methods are of value, the ability to undertake research – like riding a bicycle – is never fully developed until practical experience is obtained.

To some extent, the phases of the research process are sequential, each study tending to follow the same series of steps in a similar order. Part II of this book presents the sequence of steps in the order in which they are normally undertaken. However, as will be demonstrated in this chapter, there is considerable overlap, interrelationship and possibly some variation in the sequence of events. Figure 5.1 shows the outline of the research process in terms of each of the phases to be considered and also identifies the chapter(s) dealing with each phase.

The interrelationships of the various phases of research are many and complex. Figure 5.1 is not intended to demonstrate all these possible relationships; rather it is

Phase	Interrelationship of phases of the research process	Chapter number(s)
(i)	Asking the research question See Fig.	6
(ii)	Searching the literature 5.2	7
(iii)	Reviewing the literature	8
(iv)	Preparing a research proposal	9
(v)	Gaining access to the research site	10
(vi)	*Research design*	11–19
	Qualitative research	11
	Grounded theory	12
	Quantitative research	13
	Experimental research	14
	Action research	15
	Historical research	16
	Descriptive research	17
	Evaluation research	18
	Survey	19
(vii)	*Data collection*	20–25
	Attitude measurement	20
	Interview	21
	Questionnaire	22
	Observation	23
	The critical incident technique	24
	Physiological measurement	25
(viii)	*Data handling*	26–31
	Data storage	26
	Quantitative analysis (descriptive)	27
	Quantitative analysis (inferential)	28
	Qualitative analysis	29
	Computer assisted data analysis	30
	Data presentation	31
(ix)	Reporting and disseminating research	32
(x)	Ethical issues in nursing research	4
	Preparing a research proposal	9

Fig. 5.1   Phases in the research process.

intended to show the existence of some of these. Although Chapters 11–32 may appear to present the process as a series of relatively isolated phases, in practice these overlap.

Asking the research question

Although phase (i) is often regarded as the first formal part of the research process, a number of factors and experiences precede it. It is unlikely, for example, that a potential nurse researcher will suddenly decide that a particular subject should become the focus of a research-based study. It is more probable that, in the course of professional experience and activity, a problem area will slowly emerge as a possibility for a research project. For example, a nurse may have suspected for a long time that the design and height of hospital beds prevent nurses from lifting patients 'properly', thus placing the patient and nurse at risk. Similarly, an experienced nurse may suspect that all is not well with the methods used to teach learners how best to develop and use interpersonal skills. These examples, in themselves, are not formal research questions, they need to be developed, refined and made specific, as described in Chapter 6. Every trained nurse, therefore, has the experience with which to start to participate in the nursing research process, an advantage which is not available to those without a nursing background.

It may well be that the ability to think in this enquiring and constructive manner is one of the most important features of potential nurse researchers. Although such individuals may be considered strange, difficult or over-critical by their colleagues, there is no doubt that they are a vital part of the development of research in nursing.

Asking the research question (phase i) will almost certainly overlap with the next two phases of the process, that is searching and reviewing the literature, in the following way. Before having formally identified the research question, and before having undertaken a systematic search and review of the literature, published materials are likely to be read in order to help decide exactly what to research. Figure 5.2 demonstrates this relationship.

It can be seen that formulation of the research question comes between a general and relatively unstructured literature search and review (from which it is partly derived) and a more structured and specific search and review (to which it gives direction).

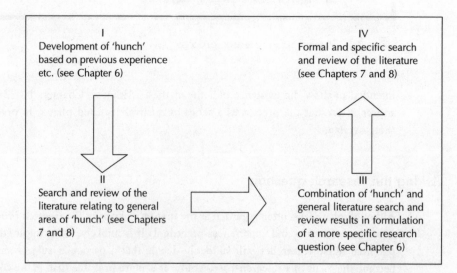

Fig. 5.2 Relationship between research question and literature search and review.

Searching the literature

The relationship between the literature search and other early stages of the research process has been outlined above. Its relationship between other stages throughout the research is also important and considerable in that it is related to all stages and continues throughout. Although the intensive and formal search will occur at the early stages of the work, literature continues to be published throughout the time it takes to undertake the study. Similarly, some aspects of the literature may be of particular relevance to the latter part of the study, for example to data analysis.

Chapter 7 describes and discusses the means of and the facilities available for searching the literature, and shows that a knowledge of this aspect of the research process can make the difference between finding a wealth of appropriate literature and wrongly concluding that 'nothing has been published relating to the subject'. As with all aspects of research, there are rules and guidelines which will make the task easier. There are also an increasingly large range of facilities, aids, organizations and resource people who can be of assistance. 'Practice will make perfect' if the potential nurse researcher is motivated to learn and is willing to invest time and effort.

Reviewing the literature

The literature review, although described in a different chapter from that dealing with searching the literature, is closely related to the search in that both occur virtually simultaneously. Indeed, the review of material found early in the search often gives direction to subsequent parts of the search. However, because the search and review require very different skills, these two closely related phases are dealt with in two chapters rather than in one. The major feature of the literature *review*, and one which differentiates it from the literature search, is that the review consists of a critical evaluation of the literature obtained as a result of the search.

The value of acquiring the skills required to undertake a literature search and review is by no means restricted to their use in the research process. These skills are also central to the notion of professionalism in nursing in that all nurses require to be familiar with the literature in their subject area. Without skills in literature search and review it is difficult, if not impossible, to have a firm understanding of the nursing literature.

Preparing a research proposal

Figure 5.1 places 'Preparing a research proposal' towards the beginning *and* at the end of the outline of phases of the research process; this is done for the following reasons. The researcher uses a knowledge of the entire research process in constructing a research proposal. The proposal, when constructed, will include some detail of all phases of the research process. Finally, having constructed a research plan which is contained in the proposal, you then implement that plan and thereby carry out the piece of research. It is necessary to prepare a proposal before undertaking a piece of research, but it is only after the first time researcher is familiar with the research process, that a proposal can be prepared. Thus, you first learn the theory relating to the research process, prepare a practical research proposal, then, if submission of the research proposal is successful, carry out the research.

In Chapter 9 there are general and specific guidelines available to those undertaking a research study and who have to prepare a research proposal. Whatever the local regulations relating to gaining permission, failure to prepare and present the proposal to the appropriate persons and committees may cause long delays or, still worse, damage an otherwise excellent research project.

Gaining access to the research site

The research site refers to the place where research data are collected; it can vary in size from a single ward to a sample of hospitals. In some instances the researcher will be part of the organization in which the data are to be collected, and may consequently find entry to the research site relatively easy. When the nature of the study is more complex and involved, entry into facilities which are not part of the organization in which the researcher is employed, or associated with, may be considerably more difficult. In the absence of guidelines to the means of gaining entry, this part of the research process can present considerable difficulty. Surprisingly, it is a topic which receives very little attention in discussions of the research process, or in many research reports. It is intended that Chapter 10 will provide a number of suggestions which will minimize this potential difficulty.

Research design

A considerable range of research designs are available, with Chapters 11 to 19 dealing with a *selection* of those which are in relatively common use. The research design is not to be confused with the data collection method(s) which are used in a study. The former, research design, is used to describe the overall research approach which is to be used. The latter, data collection method(s), describe the means by which data for a study will be collected. Thus, the data collection method is part of the research design.

Many data collection methods such as interview or observation can be used as part of a number of different research designs. For example, interviews or observation might be used as part of quantitative, qualitative, experimental, action, descriptive or evaluation research.

Decisions regarding research design precede selection of data collection methods. First, the design is selected on the grounds that it is the most suitable to answer the research question; the most suitable data collection method(s) is then selected.

Although some research designs are mutually exclusive in that they cannot occur simultaneously, others are less so. For example, experimental and descriptive designs are quite different. Experimental design will include *descriptions* of phenomena before variables are changed and/or introduced as part of the experiment. However, a descriptive research design will not include such a change to, or introduction of, variables. Another example of 'overlap' is the relationship between action research and qualitative and quantitative research designs. For example, action research may include qualitative or quantitative design, or both.

Grounded theory is both a form of research design *and* a data collection method; discussion of it is equally appropriate in the section titled Research Design *and* the one titled Data Collection. Grounded theory is presented in the Research Design section as an example of qualitative research design, although it is a method of collecting qualitative data.

Data collection

Choice of a data collection instrument, followed by actual collection of data, is a phase which offers the researcher considerable scope and choice. Researchers have a wide range of means of collecting data available to them, and need to consider which of these are best suited to their needs. If you wish to collect respondents' opinions, an interview or questionnaire may be chosen. Alternatively, if you wish to establish what a particular work group does, observation, or the critical incident technique may be used. The purpose of this book is not to present the entire range of data collection techniques which are available, but to introduce six commonly used ones in Chapters 20–25, and provide references to suitable publications where more may be learned about the use of each. It is important to realize that, when using an existing method of collecting data, you must judge whether or not it is exactly suitable to your needs and, if not, adapt it to meet personal requirements. Finally, bear in mind that no method of collecting data is perfect; each has its own limitations and strengths. The job of the researcher in this respect is to select or adapt a method which is as near perfect as possible, and to discuss fully the strengths and weaknesses of this chosen method.

Data handling

Having collected data, they need to be handled in a way which will enable the aims and objectives of the research to be met. The major elements of data handling are storage, analysis and presentation. Although these three topics have considerable overlap, they do require different skills and considerations.

Data storage

Having collected research data, these are stored in a way which will allow easy access. If very small quantities of data are collected, for example ten questionnaires, then no special storage techniques may be required. However, if larger quantities of data are collected, for example 1000 questionnaires, some form of storage which will assist counting and sorting must be used.

At present, nurses store large amounts of data in the form of information about patient care and features of nursing practice. However, the researcher often finds difficulty in retrieving the data in order to examine some aspects of patient care or nursing practice. This difficulty relates to the means by which information is stored – on charts, graphs and in books – these being the storage techniques with which all nurses are familiar. Chapter 26 describes data storage techniques which are commonly used by researchers and which enable easy retrieval and analysis.

Data analysis

Chapters 27 and 28 describe two approaches to quantitative analysis: the use and manipulation of numbers to describe and make inferences from the data. These chapters introduce two types of data analysis: descriptive and inferential statistics. They are not designed to teach you how to understand fully the statistical techniques but to help you understand what statistics are, what they can and cannot do, and how to further knowledge of the subject. In dealing with data analysis, the researcher, as in all phases of the research process, recognizes and takes full account of personal limitations and seeks expert assistance at an early stage.

Data can be analysed by other than statistical techniques; they can also be analysed by means of the researchers' thought processes and the subsequent use of words to describe and discuss the data, that is by using qualitative analysis. Indeed, many important pieces of nursing research have used qualitative, rather than quantitative (statistical) data analysis. Chapter 29 deals with qualitative analysis of data and demonstrates how conclusions from the data can be arrived at without necessarily applying either descriptive or inferential statistical techniques. However, as with other phases of the research process, the applications of quantitative or qualitative data analysis techniques are not necessarily mutually exclusive. For example, in some circumstances it may be necessary to apply quantitative techniques to qualitative data.

Data presentation

The presentation of data following its analysis and as part of writing a research report offers a variety of techniques from which to choose. Choice will obviously depend on the nature of the data and what one hopes to achieve with its presentation. Whilst the use of words is a crucial part of data presentation, and one with which nurses are familiar, alternative forms of presentation can add considerably to its impact and meaning.

Reporting and disseminating research

Reporting and disseminating findings, including the preparation of a written report, is a feature of all pieces of successfully completed research. There can be no doubt that this phase of the process presents real challenges. However, there is also no doubt that, with the help of an experienced supervisor, the beginner can develop the skills required to successfully report and disseminate research.

Whilst the structure and form of almost all research reports is invariably similar, the same cannot be said of the means chosen to disseminate findings. The word 'disseminate' in this book refers to any means used to present the research findings to others. Examples include the preparation of a research-based thesis, writing articles, and speaking at conferences. As will be seen in Chapter 32, researchers use a range of means available to them for reporting and disseminating their findings, and the research methods used to obtain them.

Throughout this book, the need for full, continuous and complete documentation in relation to all phases of the research process is shown to be essential. Beginners frequently assume (wrongly) that report writing begins at the stage of the research process entitled 'Reporting and disseminating research'. In reality, nothing could be further from the truth in that the written report will include material documented during *all* phases of the process. This documentation, appropriate supervision and systematic application of the phases of the research process will not, of course, guarantee success. However, it will maximize that possibility.

Ethical issues in nursing research

Although Fig. 5.1 concludes with reference to ethical issues in nursing research, it is not being implied that the subject is either of less importance than the others or that it occurs as an afterthought. Ethical issues are integral to *all* phases of the research process, as well as to the use and application of nursing research. All phases of the research process, therefore, include a full consideration of appropriate ethical issues.

Part II

The Research Process

Although the phases of the research process are presented in sequential and separate chapters, it is essential to see these as being interrelated and, in some circumstances, occurring in a differing sequence. In preparing these chapters, decisions were made about what to include and exclude. Although all major steps in the process are included, not all research designs, or all possible means of collecting, storing or handling data are discussed. However, those topics chosen for inclusion are in relatively common use in most research studies.

The four major sections of the research process are Preparatory Work, see Chapters 6 to 10, Research Design, see Chapters 11 to 19, Data Collection, see Chapters 20 to 25 and Data Handling, see Chapters 26 to 32.

In this Third Edition, the opportunity has been taken to revise and update all chapters, and to extend the text by including a number of additional subjects. In particular, attitude measurement, physiological measurement and computer assisted data analysis have been added.

An understanding of the elements of the research process does not, in itself, equip the beginner to undertake a research study. All beginners must undertake further extensive reading, and subsequently work under the supervision of others who have appropriate research skills.

A: Preparatory Work

As with all complex activity, and research is no exception, it is necessary to do a considerable amount of preparatory work prior to undertaking the main task. Time so invested will maximize the possibility of the research being of high quality. The preparatory work described in this section also includes making decisions regarding all of the topics dealt with in Chapters 11 to 32. Thus, a knowledge of the subjects dealt with in those chapters is necessary before the preparatory work can be completed, and decisions regarding research design, data collection, and data handling, made.

This preparatory stage of the research study is more time consuming than is often realized; it might use as much as one third of a total 'time budget'.

The elements of preparatory work, although presented in sequence and separately, are closely related. 'Asking The Research Question' for example (see Chapter 6) is a basis for, and an integral part of, all other aspects of preparatory work, and of the research process generally.

The research question gives direction to the search and review of the literature (see Chapters 7 and 8) which in turn influence the developing research question.

Once the research question has been finalized, and the preliminary literature search and review has been undertaken, all aspects of the proposed study are encapsulated in the form of a research proposal (see Chapter 9). The proposal has a number of functions, one of which is to obtain funding, obtain permission to collect data and gain access to the research site (see Chapter 10).

Chapter 6

Asking the Research Question

Desmond F.S. Cormack and David C. Benton

Excitement and wonder are emotions that are commonly experienced by those who undertake a piece of research. However, we have observed that these emotions are often replaced with feelings of uncertainty when the inexperienced researcher attempts to ask a research question. This uncertainty can be easily rectified if a number of guiding principles are followed.

In this chapter, it is intended to identify and address those issues which often cause inexperienced researchers concern when attempting to formulate a research question. This initial stage of the research process can not only be difficult, but is crucial to the success of the remaining parts of the study.

The process of asking a research question is very rarely a once and for all event. It is highly unlikely that, all of a sudden, you will scream 'Eureka' and be satisfied with the first question that comes into your head. More often the process entails days, weeks or even months of thought and effort to refine and sharpen the question that you will eventually feel happy and confident about researching. The development of the research question can best be seen as a process of systematic refinement and can be schematically represented by Fig. 6.1.

It has been our experience that attempting to ask a research question generates a large number of associated queries to which the neophyte researcher often finds difficulty in obtaining answers. In this chapter, those questions most frequently expressed about asking the research question are identified, and by providing solutions, will assist in the process of asking your research question.

What is a research question?

This may seem a rather obvious question, but for those who are embarking upon the research process for the first time, it is often asked. It is perhaps important for us to make explicit at this point that we are using the term 'research question' as shorthand for 'research question/statement/topic/subject/hypothesis/problem/issue'.

A research question occurs in one of two forms, that is either as an interrogative or declarative statement. A research question in the interrogative format is a statement, in question form, which identifies a gap in nursing knowledge. 'What is the relationship between the provision of post-registration education and the

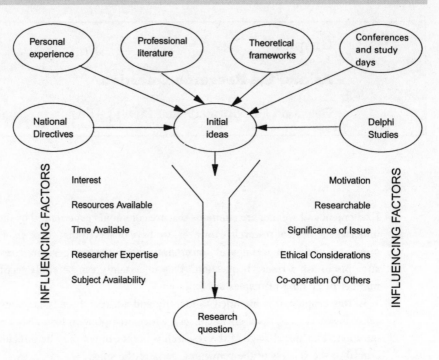

Fig. 6.1   Development of a research question.

retention of staff?', for example. A declarative research question is a statement that defines the purpose of the study by declaring the intention to investigate a particular event, phenomenon or situation. 'The purpose of this research is to investigate the relationship between the provision of post-registration education and the retention of staff', for example. The research question (or questions) is often translated into the aims of the study. However, the question comes first.

A 'good' research question, in the case of experimental research, is one that is short, sharp, specific and clearly states or implies a relationship between two or more variables. In the above example, the variables are post-registration courses and staff retention. The variables identified must be capable of observation and measurement. Furthermore, the phrasing of the question should be free from value judgements and bias, since it is the prime objective of any research study to investigate the problem identified from a scientific and objective stance. However, in the case of qualitative or descriptive studies specific variables will not be identified but clarity should still be sought. For example, 'An ethnographic study of the role of newly qualified midwives'.

Do I need a research question?

Research is a scientific and logical process of investigation and requires that you follow a particular direction of enquiry. Unless you have a clearly defined research question, you will be unable to progress your study in a planned and efficient manner.

In essence, the research question identifies and describes a gap in nursing's knowledge base which the research study seeks to fill. It helps to focus thoughts and efforts, assisting in developing a framework which will guide you through the entire research process. You cannot undertake a research study without identifying a research question.

Most research studies will have one specific, or primary, research question but some may have a number of secondary, or subsidiary questions. Secondary questions must relate to the primary question. For example, the primary research question, 'what is the relationship between the provision of post-registration education and the retention of staff?' may have the following secondary question:

- Which post-registration courses are available?
- Who provides the funding for post-registration courses?

How do I find a research question?

Inexperienced researchers often find difficulty in identifying the research question. Nevertheless, you will find that no sooner have you thought of one topic to investigate when another will come to mind. This experience is often confusing, since with so many valuable topics to investigate, how can you decide which is the most important. In addition, you may be unfamiliar with the existing literature, a fact that often compounds uncertainty and confusion. If this is not bad enough, lack of familiarity with the research process may also cause additional perplexity. However, do not let all the initial uncertainty put you off. If you are interested and motivated towards conducting research, you will identify, in time, a specific topic which you will find suitable for investigation. To assist you in identifying a research question, you may wish to consider a number of sources which will help identify a gap in nursing's existing knowledge base.

Your own experience

Turn to your own experience. How often have you questioned, either in your mind or with your colleagues, a situation, treatment or outcome, wondering what has happened, why it should be that way or how you can improve it. In seeking to identify a research question various sources can be consulted or used to stimulate ideas (Fig. 6.2).

Professional literature

Professional literature often triggers further research. You may note the findings of a study and consider whether such an approach can be applied in your own area of practice or to the particular client group you work with. The deliberate use of methodology already reported, but used in a different setting and with another subject group, is termed replication. Such an approach is extremely valuable since

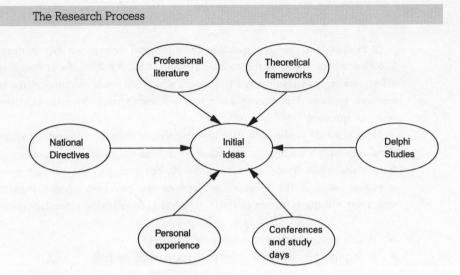

Fig. 6.2 Getting ideas for a research question.

far too few nursing studies have been conducted with more than one client group or in different locations (Chapman, 1989). It is perhaps appropriate to note at this point that the research question does not have to be novel to be worthwhile. However, if you choose to repeat a study that has already been carried out, it is important that you examine the previous study carefully and avoid methodological or conceptual flaws.

Alternatively, if you read a number of research reports about a topic, you may notice inconsistencies in findings which can stimulate further research. You may wonder why the results obtained with one group, or at one location, or using a particular method, are different from those reported elsewhere.

Yet another means by which research questions can be derived from literature is when a gap in the existing knowledge base is observed. For example, increased commitment to the use of computer technology as a tool in health care provision or monitoring has been advocated by a national education body (English National Board for Nursing; Midwifery and Health Visiting, 1994). Despite the fact that few studies have investigated the effectiveness of this approach to the provision of care, many hospitals have allocated considerable resources to the purchase of equipment.

Theoretical frameworks

In the past 40 years, a number of theoretical frameworks have been proposed: Peplau's (1952) interpersonal relations model, Roy's (1980) adaption model and Rogers' (1970) unitary man model, to name but three. Each of these models can be used as the basis for the development of a research question. The model can be tested to determine whether it can predict the outcome of treatment (McKenna, 1994). To date, few studies have been developed to test the available theoretical models, and as yet, most remain inadequately validated. Cormack & Reynolds (1992) propose 13 criteria for evaluating the clinical and practical utility of models used by nurses. Each of the criteria are well suited to forming the basis of a research question.

Conferences and study days

When you attend a conference or a study day it is often the discussion that occurs during coffee and meal breaks that proves to be the most valuable element of the day. Such interactions can result in the discovery of a wide variety of means of treating a particular client, often prompting thoughts which can be developed into a research question.

National Directives and Delphi Studies

From time to time the government or a national body will identify specific topics which they feel require investigation. Such topics are usually of major national concern and have significant implications for the health of the nation. For example, the English National Board for Nursing, Midwifery and Health Visiting (1994) recently published their research and development priorities which could be used to steer the formulation of research questions.

Another means of identifying topics of concern to a large number of individuals is the use of a Delphi survey. A Delphi survey is a technique where subjects are asked to respond to a series of questionnaires. The first questionnaire usually attempts to elicit views on a specific topic. Subsequent questionnaires feed back the original comments made by the subjects who are then asked to rank the statements in order of importance. In the case of a study by Macmillan *et al.* (1989), nursing staff in three Health Boards in Scotland were asked to identify those topics which they felt required to be researched. This approach may yield a number of topics that can then form the basis for further investigation.

How can I decide which question to study?

Often you will have a number of ideas which you may wish to investigate. The tentative question identified may be related, or may be on completely different subject areas. The problem is how to decide which one of a number of topics to investigate first. There are a number of guiding principles which will assist the choice.

Interest and motivation

The research process can be simultaneously exciting, stimulating, arduous and depressing. When things are going well, nothing seems to be too much of a problem, but there are those times when you will confront difficulties. Unless the research question focuses on a problem about which you feel strongly, it is likely that during difficult times you will be unable to sustain enthusiasm for the study.

Any research questions considered for investigation must therefore be of sufficient interest to keep you motivated through the 'bad' as well as the 'good' times.

A researchable question

Not all questions are amenable to investigation. Any question which poses a philosophical or ethical question is not directly answerable by research. For example, 'is it ethical for foetal tissue be used for cerebral implantation?' poses an ethical question, and although it is possible to debate this issue, no amount of research will give you an answer. The question is not researchable.

It is often possible to change the focus of the question which addresses an ethical or philosophical dilemma to one that is researchable, 'does the implantation of foetal tissue alleviate symptoms of Parkinson's Disease?', for example. Although it is possible to answer this question by research, it does not address the original ethical question; it may, however, provide evidence which will influence your viewpoint on the issue.

Problem significance

Any problems selected should be of significance to the client group you care for and/or to nursing's knowledge base. The significance of a problem can be best judged by assessing the question's worth in terms of a number of criteria. First, does the question address a problem which affects large numbers of patients? Second, will the outcome of the research significantly improve the quality of life of individuals or groups? Third, does the question address a nursing problem? Finally, will the results be suitable for use in a (non-research) practice environment?

Feasibility

Many potentially interesting and researchable questions have to be discarded because they are not feasible. If you are to assess the feasibility of a research question, you must consider a number of issues. These would include time available, researcher expertise, ethical considerations, resources available, subject availability and cooperation of others.

Time available

If you are undertaking a piece of research for the first time, it is likely that you will have difficulty in trying to assess how much work is involved and how long it will take. You can, however, make a more accurate assessment of the feasibility of undertaking a particular study by drawing up a detailed timetable. It is also important to note that for certain elements of a study, you will be able to arrange a schedule to suit your own pace, but alas some will be determined by those individuals or agencies providing support and information. A good starting point for attempting to assess the length of time the study will take is to use a framework for steps in the research process (see Chapter 5). Each step in the process can be broken down into as much detail as possible, then time allocated appropriately. The total length of time required can then be calculated and an appropriate decision taken. That is, either to proceed with the study, try and negotiate time from your employer, redefine the study in such a way as to 'effect' the time available or reject the study as being unfeasible. Remember, if you have a detailed breakdown of time required, you are in a stronger position to argue for the appropriate study time.

If you are aware of anyone who has conducted some research, seek their advice. Valuable information about how long literature searches will take and more importantly how long it will take to locate and access literature, can also be obtained from librarians.

If ethical committee approval is required, studies may often be delayed for considerable periods of time. It is not uncommon for such a committee to meet on a bi-monthly or even quarterly basis. If delays are to be avoided, it is important that you make contact with the committee at an early stage.

Resources available

Closely associated with the requirements for sufficient time, is the need for appropriate and adequate resources. The resource requirements for any study can vary considerably. A study undertaken as part of a course may need only nominal resources, whereas some research will require vast quantities of both material and money.

When attempting to assess feasibility, it is important to clearly identify all the resources you will require to enable you to complete the study. Obviously the design of your study will influence the amount of resources required. By starting with a detailed timetable, you are less likely to omit items. Always consider literature search charges, photocopying, telephone, postage, computer access, and any specialized equipment, travel costs, office space (often a premium), document typing and report production. The more detailed the list you can produce, the better prepared you are to assess the feasibility of the study.

Researcher expertise

It is important that you examine closely the level of expertise required to undertake and successfully complete the study you have identified. Unless such an assessment is undertaken, it is likely that you will end up attempting a study which you are unqualified to carry out. A timetable of events can be particularly useful. If there are a few elements about which you have little or even no knowledge, you can seek assistance and support at an early stage. With appropriate advice and supervision, what would have been unfeasible can become possible.

Ethical consideration

When assessing the feasibility of a particular study, you should always consider the ethics of undertaking the research. Research should cause no harm or distress and it is important that any proposals should be reviewed by an unbiased individual or a group. If patients are involved, or if your research involves any invasive procedure, it is normal practice to seek the approval of the District's or Health Board's ethics committee. Research that is undertaken and which does not have the potential to advance our knowledge should not take place. Similarly, any piece of work that does not offer subjects' confidentiality and anonymity, should on most occasions be considered inappropriate. Only if a study can be shown to be ethically acceptable should it be considered feasible (see Chapter 4).

Subject availability

If you intend to investigate a very rare phenomenon, it is likely that either you will be unable to recruit enough subjects to your study, or you will have to travel considerable distances to do so. Consequently, it is important to identify and assess the availability of subjects, for without subjects you have no study. Furthermore, it is important to recognize that potential subjects may not be as enthusiastic about the research study as you are. It is likely that some may refuse to participate and this is a point well worth consideration.

Cooperation of others

When you plan a study, identify those individuals and groups who will come in contact with your work. It is always worth investing time, at an early stage, gaining their support. Any individuals who will be directly involved should be contacted personally and given the opportunity to discuss issues of concern. Only after obtaining the cooperation of all those involved in the study should it be undertaken. More specific information on the closely associated issues of gaining access to research sites is provided in Chapter 10.

How can the research question best be described?

Research questions, despite being short, clear and specific, will still require to be explained in some detail to those who read the final report. In addition to being implicit in the title of the study, an explanation of the rationale for undertaking the study should appear very early in any publication. The fact that a gap exists in the knowledge base, and that the research question has relevance to nursing, should be clearly established and stated.

A common difficulty experienced by novice and expert researchers alike is the imprecise nature of language. Words often have more than one meaning and hence if your research question is to be described in absolute terms there is a need to offer

precise definitions of any words, terms or procedures central to your research. The
normal definition which is given in the dictionary is frequently inadequate. It is
therefore necessary to state the operational definition of terms, that is, the definition
given to words by the researcher, that is by you. For example, a dictionary might
define a patient as 'a person who is receiving medical care', whereas you may choose
to operationally define the term patients as 'any male, who is hospitalized in a
surgical ward, who has undergone surgery in the previous 24 hours, and who is
aged between 16 and 65 years'.

Does the research question influence the research process?

It should be evident that the research question has total influence on all aspects of
the research process. Having asked the research question, all other aspects of the
study are designed to answer it. For example, the question determines the scope
and content of the literature review. A methodological approach will be selected
that is capable of answering the question. All collected data will be destined for
analysis and this will provide results. The results will present an answer to the
question which when compared and contrasted with previous research will
determine any recommendations. The research question is the thread which unifies
the entire study.

Relating the research question to the research process

It is common for inexperienced researchers to have difficulty in defining the exact
relationship between the research question and other components of the study.

How do the title of the study and the research question relate?

The research question should be formulated first and subsequently the title of the
study should be derived from it. Often there is little difference between the two. A
suitable and appropriate title for the research question posed earlier might be 'A
study of the relationship between the provision of post-registration education and
the retention of staff'.

Is the aim of the study the same as the research question?

Although they are not identical in expression, they are identical in meaning. Some
researchers decide to pose a number of questions which the research seeks to
answer. Others convert the question to a series of aims which, when achieved,
provide a solution to the research question. In the example used in this chapter, the
question may generate the following aim: 'To describe the relationship between the
provision of post-registration education and the retention of staff'.

Is the research question the same as a hypothesis?

Despite the fact that a hypothesis can be derived from a research question, if that question seeks to establish whether or not there is a relationship between two or more variables, the research question and the hypothesis are not the same. The hypothesis for the study suggested above might state: 'The retention of staff is increased by the provision of post-registration education'.

It is not always possible to derive a hypothesis from a research question. The hypothesis can only be stated for those studies suitable for investigation at the outset by quantitative methods, and which predict a relationship between two variables. For example, if the research question had asked 'Which factors influence staff's decision to remain with a Health Authority for more than five years?', then a hypothesis could not be formulated until the factors had been identified.

How does a research question relate to literature review?

It has been suggested that the research literature itself may stimulate the formulation of a research question. Irrespective of whether the question was, or was not, stimulated by a publication, the literature review should cover two main domains which support the question's formulation. First, the question should be derived from a specific theoretical perspective so as to ensure that any findings can be appropriately integrated into the knowledge base. Secondly, the literature review should identify any previous research carried out and provide an objective critique of the work. It is common for the literature review to move from a general description of the topic to a more focused evaluation. The move from the general to the specific is a means of identifying surrounding issues so as to place the research question in context.

The literature review should be considered fundamental to the development of any research question. The literature presented to the reader should cogently argue that there is a need for the study to take place and that the findings will have potential significance to nursing or those cared for.

Can the original research question be changed?

Having conducted preliminary work, it is not uncommon for the research question to be modified or even abandoned completely. If it is to be modified, this is done prior to the specific literature review. The research question cannot be changed or modified at a subsequent stage. If this is done, the research process must be restarted.

A change or modification may take place following a pilot study if the pilot study indicates that such a change is necessary. In that case, the pilot study is repeated until the research question is found to be appropriate. Furthermore, it is not uncommon for researchers to be tempted to add secondary questions at the pilot study stage. However, this temptation should be avoided if possible. Any addition will result in extra work and may require further resources which may not be available. If the research question is to be modified or secondary questions added, a full assessment of the implications of such a change requires to be made.

Conclusions

The process of asking the research question is, in part, simply the logical application of a number of guidelines. However, those questions which identify a significant issue are often the result of inspired curiosity. All professional nurses who take a critical and questioning view of nursing practice, management and education have the ability to identify such issues and generate a research question. This chapter has summarized the common sources of research ideas and considered the process by which those initial ideas are moulded into a final research question by the influence of various factors. Asking the research question is central to the entire research process. Once you have identified a research question, you are well on the way to completing the study. It is now up to you to decide whether you wish to pursue the opportunity.

References

Chapman, C. (1989) Research for action: the way forward. *Senior Nurse*, 9(6), 16–18.

Cormack, D.F.S. & Reynolds, W. (1992) Criteria for evaluating the clinical and practical utility of models used by nurses. *Journal of Advanced Nursing*, 17(10), 1472–1478.

English National Board For Nursing, Midwifery and Health Visiting (1994) *The Board's Response to the Strategy For Research in Nursing Midwifery and Health Visiting*. English National Board For Nursing Midwifery and Health Visiting, London.

Macmillan, M., Atkinson, F.I., Prophit, P. & Clark, M.O. (1989) *A Delphi survey of priorities for nursing research in Scotland*. Department of Nursing Studies, University of Edinburgh.

McKenna, H.P. (1994) *Nursing Theories and Quality of Care*. Ashgate Publishing Limited, Avebury.

Peplau, H. (1952) *Interpersonal Relations in Nursing*. Putman, New York.

Rogers, M.E. (1970) *An Introduction to the Theoretical Basis of Nursing*. F.A. Davies, Philadelphia.

Roy, C. (1980) The Roy adaption model. In *Conceptual Models for Nursing Practice* (eds J.P. Riehl & C. Roy), 2nd edn. Appleton Century Crofts, New York.

Chapter 7

Searching the Literature

David C. Benton and Desmond F.S. Cormack

The ability to conduct a literature search is essential to any type of research. Indeed, it has been argued that the skills associated with literature searching should be considered a fundamental skill requirement of all professional nurses (Department of Health and Social Security, 1972; McSweeney, 1990). Whether from a research or a professional perspective, the ability to conduct a literature search is essential if nurses are to question their practice, management or education in a structured and meaningful way.

Without reference to the past, we are unable to learn from mistakes. The techniques discussed in this chapter help empower the reader with skills that enable the discovery, location and unlocking of the wealth of material which constitutes our profession's knowledge base.

The research literature

Every day we come into contact with a wide variety of research literature, the volume of which seems to be ever increasing. By research literature we mean any form of information, either paper or electronic that relates to nursing research, irrespective of source, format or quality. Chapter 8 deals with how to review and evaluate the quality of literature.

Research literature can originate from many sources such as individuals, groups, academic institutions, professional organizations or manufacturers and suppliers of products. Clearly, the volume of material available is unmanageable unless you are selective in the material which you consult. Depending on the research topic, certain types of literature may be of greater value to the enquiring nurse than others. Research literature can come in many forms, each of which have particular characteristics which, if known, can assist you in deciding the likely value of the material prior to obtaining access. Figure 7.1, for example, lists common formats used to convey information to the nursing profession.

Journals

Journals are frequently used by researchers who wish to obtain information on a specific topic. However, not all journals publish original research. Journals such as

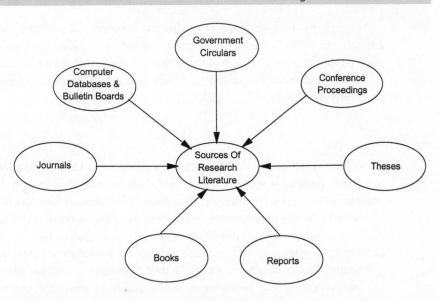

Fig. 7.1 Sources of literature used in conveying research information.

the *Journal of Advanced Nursing*, *Nursing Research* and the *Western Journal of Nursing Research*, which publish original material, are termed primary journals. Invariably, papers published by these journals are refereed, that is, all papers are examined by an independent external expert prior to publication: this tends to ensure that only papers that are of the highest quality are published.

Secondary journals are another valuable source of information and, although they do not usually publish original papers, they do serve an important function. That is, articles published in secondary journals could be described as a means of providing a 'taster' of the full paper. Articles often consist of a brief synopsis of research published in a primary journal, often written in less technical terms so as to appeal to a wider audience. Hence, secondary journals are an ideal means of ensuring that a piece of work is disseminated more widely than would be possible otherwise.

There are a number of specific types of secondary journal. First, there is the limited circulation journals which are distributed free to members of an organization or specialist interest groups. *Reflections* is an example of a limited circulation journal which is distributed to all Sigma Theta Tau members – an international nursing honour society. It contains brief, often opinion based, articles specific to Sigma Theta Tau members or gives snippets of information about work specific members are undertaking. Second, there are review journals, which provide information on pre-selected topics. Articles are frequently written by subject experts who, in the course of the article, will debate the findings of a particular piece of research. *Advances in Nursing Science* is an example of such a journal. Third, there are professional journals, for example *Health Visitor*, which are aimed to cater for the needs of the practitioner as opposed to the academic. This type of secondary journal will often focus on the aspects of utilization of research rather than on pure findings.

Although we have drawn a clear division between primary and secondary journals, the reality is somewhat different. Secondary journals, for instance, will often publish original work – something that can confuse an informed researcher and mislead them into discounting an article prematurely simply as a result of its apparently poor 'pedigree'.

Books

Books are a major source of information for researchers. Unlike journal articles, which are limited by space, material published in book form usually has the opportunity to develop arguments in more detail, provide a more extensive literature review and generally provide a more substantive treatment of the subject. However, books take longer to get into print and are generally published to make money for a publishing company, two factors which may detract from their academic value.

Another point to consider is whether a book has single or multiple authors, for this can sometimes lead to variations in the quality of individual chapters and problems with the flow and development of arguments. It is fair to say that this should be the exception rather than the rule, if the book has an experienced editor.

Reports

Many research studies are published in report form and unfortunately, as a consequence, only reach a limited audience. Authors can take steps to avoid this by submitting their work to abstracting services such as *Nursing Research Abstracts*. Some health authorities also endeavour to increase the availability of reports produced by encouraging authors to submit copies of their work to a local collection. Despite such undertakings, reports are notoriously difficult to obtain, can be of extremely variable quality and come in all manner of shapes and format. Nevertheless it is often useful to obtain original reports as opposed to journal articles since the report will often give fine detail which, by necessity of space limitation, are frequently omitted from the published work. It is common to find included within the appendices of reports, copies of data collection instruments, or other such valuable materials.

Theses

Theses, sometimes referred to as dissertations, are usually the product of higher academic study. Accordingly they can be a veritable goldmine of information since they include in-depth literature reviews, detailed methods sections, as well as findings and learned debate. Usually no more than three or four copies of a thesis are produced and this can cause difficulties for those who wish to read them. However, most universities send copies of all doctoral and master of philosophy theses to the British Lending Library where they are microfilmed and can then be made available on request. In addition, those nurses who live within travelling distance of London can consult the Steinberg collection at the RCN library. This collection contains copies of a large number of theses and dissertations, either written by nurses or of interest to the nursing profession.

Conference proceedings

It is not always possible to attend a conference in person, and although we would argue that there is no real substitute for being there and getting involved in the debate, conference proceedings can provide a valuable source of information. Papers appearing in conference proceedings usually consist of the latest, most up-to-date, state-of-the-art material. Papers are then often rewritten in light of comments made by the audience and then submitted for publication to primary journals. Conference proceedings can thus provide researchers with access to materials at an early stage. Although for the more prestigious conference proceedings, papers often go through a rigorous review procedure, this is not always the case, hence material gleaned from such sources can be of variable quality.

Government circulars

The Department of Health issues a wide variety of documents each year, many of which can be of interest to the nurse researcher. However, the distribution and access to these documents is often limited in the first instance to senior officers of a Health Authority. Researchers who think that the Department of Health may have published material on a specific topic can pursue the current edition of *The Hospital and Health Services Year Book*, (Chaplin, 1994) which, amongst other things, lists all current governmental circulars.

Computer databases and electronic bulletin boards

With the advent of relatively inexpensive computer equipment, increasing amounts of information are being held on computer database. You can often obtain the most up-to-date information from this type of source. Unfortunately use of these systems is often expensive – you require the correct equipment and you usually have to use a telephone line – and the organization running the service can charge quite high fees for the privilege of access. Another disadvantage of these systems is that the amount of information stored on any one item is often limited to essential details and a brief abstract. A relatively recent development is the electronic bulletin board which enables researchers or anyone with the right equipment to 'post' material to an electronic board which can then be read by others. Researchers from across the world can therefore exchange or stimulate ideas with like-minded colleagues who have the correct computer equipment.

Choosing a library

Irrespective of your topic of interest, it is highly unlikely that you will have all the literature you require immediately to hand. For most of us, it is necessary to use a library as the main source of our research literature, whether it be in journal, book or any of the formats previously discussed.

Not all libraries are the same and some offer far more in the way of services than others (Cheung, 1988). Make a point of exploring all local libraries so as to discover the strengths and weaknesses. Some will allow access to all their facilities but some, such as those attached to universities and colleges, may restrict users who are neither students nor staff of the institution to reading rights only. There are a number of features which are particularly useful and will make the task of literature searching far easier. Many of these will depend on the size of the library.

First, if the library is large, it may have subject specialist librarians who will be able to greatly assist you in a search for material. Conversely, in smaller specialist libraries such as those attached to colleges of nursing or health studies institutions, it is usual for the librarian to have extensive knowledge of health care literature. If you are to make the most efficient use of your time, endeavour to contact the librarian at the onset of the search and engage their assistance. Librarians are specialist in literature storage and its retrieval; seek their advice and save time.

Second, it is important to familiarize yourself with the cataloguing system of the library. Unless you know how materials are catalogued, you will be unable to retrieve them. Again, seek the assistance of the librarian and read any guides that may be available. Most libraries publish a short guide that will show the layout of the stock and tell how it is catalogued. Recently, some libraries have started to employ the use of personal stereos for this purpose and these can be hired or borrowed. These walk you round through a guided tour of the layout and give instructions on how to find material.

There are a number of methods of cataloguing materials, but the two most commonly used for health care literature are the *Dewey Decimal Classification Scheme* and the *National Library of Medicine Classification Scheme*. The former uses a series of numeric digits to break down subjects from the general to the specific, while the latter uses a combination of letters and numbers. Although manual card index systems are still quite common, larger libraries are now tending to install computer systems for cataloguing their material. Whichever approach is being used, become familiar with the system so as to maximize the chances of finding the material you wish to find when conducting a literature search.

Third, some libraries offer a far more comprehensive range of textbooks and journals than others. If a library is to be of value, then a wide variety of stock that covers both major and minor nursing specialities is required. Textbooks should be up to date, but, perhaps more important for a researcher, the journal holdings should be extensive and ideally should have been subscribed to for as long a period as possible. Back issues of journals are a valuable literature source and since nursing research often addresses diverse health care themes, access to nursing, medical, general sciences, social sciences, education and professional journals allied to medicine is desirable.

Fourth, a range of reference texts, including indexes, research abstracts and bibliographies, is essential. These may be available in a variety of forms. For example, they may exist as books, or they may be accessible by means of on-line or compact disk based computer systems.

Fifth, even the most comprehensive library will not stock everything that its subscribers could possibly want. Accordingly, access to an inter-library loan service is very important for a researcher who is attempting to achieve an in-depth coverage of a topic. Inter-library loan requests can be expensive, but a good library will often offer a subsidized (or even free) service which is prompt to respond to reasonable requests.

Sixth, most researchers will require access to photocopying facilities which are reasonably priced. However, it is essential that copyright laws are not infringed; this does limit the use that can be made of copies and the amount of material which can be reproduced from any one book or journal.

Seventh, microfiche or microfilm readers can be useful, particularly if you require access to theses. In addition, some libraries stock microfilm of back issues of their journals to save space; if this is the case, some means of obtaining a printed copy of an individual article should be available.

Finally, some libraries will have a special reference collection which can be of great assistance to a researcher. The Royal College of Nursing, for example, holds the Steinberg collection which includes copies of many masters and doctoral theses relating to nursing and conducted both in the United Kingdom and overseas. Details of the Royal College of Nursing and other national libraries (see Appendix 7.1).

How to search the literature

Anyone who has attempted to look for literature related to a particular subject, quickly discovers that there is usually a wealth of material available. Of course, not all literature provides exactly what you require, hence it is necessary to systematically identify only those items which relate directly to the subject under study. A literature search can be defined as the process of systematically identifying published materials which meet set pre-determined criteria. For example the subject of the search might be 'worldwide literature, published between 1985 and 1995, relating to the role of the community psychiatric nurse treating patients with medical diagnosis of paranoid schizophrenia'. Literature searching, which is a critical component of any research study, can be conducted either manually or with the aid of computer technology.

You will often need to consult the literature at various stages of the research process. First, it will assist in the definition of the topic to be studied. Second, it will provide substantive material for both the theoretical and methodological frameworks. Third, it will enable you to contrast findings with previously reported studies. The ability to efficiently and accurately search the literature is clearly central to the development, conduct and completion of any research study. Without a specific strategy, a literature search will not only prove time-consuming, but will also yield an incomplete coverage of the topic. Try to have a rough idea of an area of interest before you walk into a library. If you simply browse along the shelves you may or may not, depending on the size of the library, find some material on your topic of interest. Such an approach is clearly unacceptable for it will waste valuable time and is no way of ensuring that all the material available on the subject will be found. Although serendipity is a wonderful and even joyous experience, it is neither scientific nor time-efficient and for these reasons make use of tools such as the subject index, the author catalogue, classification catalogue, indexes, abstracts and bibliographies.

Subject index, author and classification catalogues

All libraries will have author and classification catalogues as well as a subject index of their book stock so as to enable material of interest to be found. Author catalogues are simply a listing of all stock organized in alphabetical order by author. Joint authors, series entries as well as the chairpersons of government committees, are usually included. Classification catalogues list all stock as they appear on the shelves in the library. The order of the stock is determined by the particular classification system in use. By examining the classification catalogue you can identify all books on a particular subject stocked by the library, irrespective of whether they are out on loan. The subject index, for those who are not fully conversant with the classification system, can be considered as a key to enable access to the library's book stock. All major (and minor) subjects are listed along with the corresponding classification code thus enabling researchers to go to the appropriate part of the classification catalogue and identify the material held. For libraries that still use manual systems, the index and catalogues often consist of a series of card indexes. If, however, a computerized system is in use, material is stored in a relational database. The term 'relational', although a computer jargon term, effectively emphasizes the fact that although the material in the catalogues and index are separate, they are closely related.

Both journal holdings and audio-visual material are usually catalogued and indexed separately from book stock. Audio-visual catalogues are usually indexed in the same manner as books. However, access to journal articles is usually obtained, in the first instance, by indexes, abstracts and bibliographies.

Indexes, abstracts and bibliographies

The stock held by any one library will be limited by a number of factors such as the needs of the population the library serves, the means by which and by whom new stock is added to the collection, the budget and the physical space available. The examination of stock held locally on any one topic will, on most occasions, result in the identification of only a small part of the literature available on the topic. What is required is some means of knowing what material is available, not just locally but nationally and internationally if a complete and detailed literature search is required. Examination of indexing, abstracting and bibliographic tools can all be used to achieve far greater coverage of the topic.

Indexes

Indexes are used to list all material published in a specified list of journals. The material is indexed by both subject heading(s) and by author(s). Indexes are generally produced monthly, bi-monthly or quarterly and cumulated annually. There is a wide selection of indexes available, but not all extensively cover nursing journals. For example, *Index Medicus*, although listing well over 3000 journals includes only 25 nursing titles, whereas the *Cumulative Index to Nursing and Allied Health Literature* covers just over 300, the predominant number of which are nursing and allied health periodicals. The *International Nursing Index* and, despite its name *Nursing Bibliography*, are two further examples of indexes commonly available in this country. The choice of index or indexes that should be consulted to achieve optimum coverage of the literature available will be dependent on the specific topic. There is a degree of duplication between the various indexes hence, if time is at a premium, and it usually is, go to the librarian for advice as to which indexes are likely to be the most appropriate.

The amount of detail given in an index about a particular article is limited to that likely to be found in any reference that is:

- Name of author(s) [but not always all of them]
- Year of publication
- Title of article
- Name of journal
- Volume and part numbers
- Page numbers of article.

The drawbacks of such a brief description are obvious and often what sounds like a valuable reference turns out to be only of peripheral or no value.

Abstracts

The major drawback with indexes is that no detailed information about the content of an article is given. Only by retrieving the article, sometimes by means of an inter-library loan, can you be sure of the content. Abstracting journals, however, circumvent this problem since, in addition to all the general reference data, a short abstract is also given which gives a succinct synopsis of the article. The quality of the abstract given can, however, vary considerably from, on one hand, the simple outline to a detailed summary of the entire study giving all the major points.

As with indexes, there are a wide selection of abstracting journals available, all of which have different criteria for material inclusion. Perhaps the best known abstracting journal in the United Kingdom to deal with nursing research is *Nursing Research Abstracts*; valuable material, however, can often be obtained from those sources that have a wider coverage. These include *Hospital Abstracts*, *Health Service Abstracts*, *Social Service Abstracts* and *Excerpta Medica*.

Bibliographies

Bibliographies can be a useful starting point for any researcher. They are, essentially, a reference list of books, periodical articles and reports on some particular subject. A number of national libraries, professional organizations, and many colleges of nursing libraries, produce such bibliographies. For example, the Royal College of Nursing has published a bibliography of nursing literature in two series, and the Scottish Health Service Centre library regularly publishes specialist bibliographies. Furthermore, the Royal College of Midwives, the Health Visitors Association and in addition many colleges of nursing, produce a 'current awareness service'. This is a particular type of bibliography that regularly covers a (usually pre-set) number of topics listing all the articles, reports or newly published books on the topic since the publication of the previous current awareness bulletin.

Citation indexes

Indexes, bibliographies and abstracts simply list all the material published irrespective of its quality. However, citation indexes only list those articles that have been cited by other authors in their work. It is assumed that only those articles that are of value or significance will be cited by other authors. The *Nursing Citation Index*, which is a tandem publication of the *International Nursing Index*, records the number of times a particular article has been cited, listing in which publication it was referenced, the volume, part and page numbers, and by whom it was cited. The entries are listed by author.

By examining the number of times an article has been cited, it is possible to speculate as to the quality of the work. Generally speaking, the more frequently cited, the more significant the material. Authors of articles can also use the citation index as a means of identifying colleagues with a similar interest. For example, authors can identify and contact those who have cited their work, thus extending their professional network.

The *Nursing Citation Index* can be used to identify work that is closely related to earlier published material. If you are aware of a particular article that has been written about a specific topic, you can, by referring to that article in the index, identify more recent work that has cited the original material. Such an approach ensures that you are aware of any debate stimulated by the publication of an author's work.

Manual or computerized searching

Until the advent of relatively inexpensive compact personal computers, most libraries had only manual systems for accessing literature. Researchers would have to thumb through card after card of the subject index, classification or author catalogues, until they found the material they sought. This could take considerable time and effort, particularly since there is no way of knowing from a card system whether a book is available or out on loan.

Modern computer controlled library stock management systems hold their information on a database. A database can be thought of as a form of electronic card index system which is extremely efficient and flexible in the manner in which information can be stored and retrieved. Not only will a database hold all the usual information about a book, it will also record whether the book is in stock, out on loan, or reserved for a subscriber. Users of such systems can, by the use of a limited number of commands, search the library catalogue for books on a subject or subjects, ascertain whether they are in stock, print a list of the books on the topics and request that those out on loan be reserved on their return to the library, all without leaving the computer terminal.

Similarly, indexes, abstracts and bibliographies are now available via computer systems. Until recently, the only way to access the databases containing this information was via the telephone line (on-line searching). Databases were located some distance from the library and were maintained by commercial companies (hosts). Although there are a number of databases maintained in the UK, the most popular and largest host organizations are located in Europe and the USA. However, the introduction of compact disk read-only memory (CD-ROM) technology, has meant that the entire database for major indexes such as Medline or CINHAL can be stored on a single 4.5 inch compact disk.

The storage capacity of a compact disk is truly phenomenal since the equivalent information contained in the books on 20 feet of library shelves or the entire 12 volumes of the original *Oxford English Dictionary* can be held on one single-sided disk (Edwards *et al.*, 1989; Green, 1990).

Both on-line and CD-ROM systems are more expensive than their manual counterparts. Libraries have to pay a subscription to use the database as well as possess the appropriate computer equipment and, in the case of an on-line system, have to pay telephone line rental and connect charges in addition to a payment for all data accessed. These additional costs have resulted in most libraries not allowing individuals to use on-line systems themselves. Instead, you explain the search that is required to the librarian who then conducts the search on your behalf. Databases held on CD-ROM are, however, usually accessible to the researcher since there is no telephone, connect or access charges. On-line databases are nevertheless more up to date (by a month or two) than either the CD-ROM or manual base systems and if this is an important consideration then the additional cost may be justified.

On-line and CD-ROM searching has a number of distinct advantages over manual systems. Specifically, they can save you a tremendous amount of time, are far more flexible in the manner in which literature can be retrieved and can produce printed lists of references on request. Conversely, there are a few minor disadvantages: for example, cost and the fact that users do require a minimal degree of computer literacy; keyboard skills and the knowledge of the commands, are also required.

Conducting a search

Conducting a literature search, if given detailed thought, is relatively straightforward. The process should be systematic and unhurried if optimum results are to be obtained.

The first step in the process is to think around the research topic. Authors may use different terms for the topic that you are interested in. If you are to successfully retrieve material, time is needed to consider all key words and their synonyms or associated terms that can be used to describe the topic to be researched. To achieve this, a number of approaches can be used. For example, it is often helpful to 'brainstorm' your thoughts and commit them to paper, all thoughts should be noted and none dismissed prematurely. Having done this, consult a good thesaurus and write down all synonyms. Now start to group them together and form logical links between the topics.

Next, decide whether to conduct a manual or computer search. If a computer system is available, then a considerable amount of time can be saved; a computer will also allow you to use search strategies based upon what are known as logical operators. The two most common logical operators are 'AND' and 'OR'. By use of 'AND' and 'OR' you can search for a combination of key words simultaneously. For example, if you were interested in finding material on the treatment of alcohol abuse, a search using the word treatment would yield many references as would a search using alcohol abuse. However, by stipulating that you are requiring material that refers to both treatment AND alcohol abuse, you could obtain a smaller but more specific result. Use of the logical operator 'OR' will yield a result that includes all those references that include either treatment OR alcohol abuse (or both).

Irrespective of whether a computer or manual search is to be conducted, great care should be taken on deciding which catalogues, indexes, abstracting journals and bibliographies should be consulted. An appropriate choice may result in few references being found (Fox and Ventura, 1984; Schoones, 1990).

Throughout the literature search, the help and assistance of a subject specialist librarian, or an experienced researcher, can be invaluable. Both can often help to focus thinking, offer advice and assist in the selection of appropriate sources. Having selected the sources, it is now necessary to examine the subject and key word headings, those used by the index, for example, so as to enable you to finalize the search strategy. Computer systems will allow entries to be searched word on word, but often this rules out references that are inappropriate to the research topic. The use of key word fields will increase the number of usable references. Bear in mind that the more specifically defined and exacting your search criteria, the fewer references you will retrieve. Figure 7.2 illustrates how a seemingly unmanageable number of references can be searched to produce a useful bibliography. The search was conducted using a CD-ROM based product, a version of the ERIC (Education Resources Information Centre) database. As currently seen, the commands issued (in block capitals) are easy to use and simple to recall. The complete list of 41 references, including abstracts, can be reviewed on screen before deciding whether

Command	References found
FIND Research	101 222
FIND Utilization	4 839
FIND Nursing	1 661
FIND Research AND Utilization AND Nursing	41

Fig. 7.2 Sample dialogue of CD-ROM literature search.

to widen or restrict the search further or to print the entire or selected portion of the list for future use.

Literature searching is a simple process, but it does take time. Even when computer technology is used it is not always possible to be absolutely sure that a reference is exactly what is required. Only once an article is read can you be sure of its value and significance to the study. The process of accessing articles is invariably the most time consuming. Often articles are not available locally and it is necessary to request them on inter-library loan. The process of requesting an inter-library loan for material can add considerably to the time required to conduct the literature search. However, when the literature search and retrieval is complete, it is then necessary to read and critically appraise the articles obtained. These and subsequent steps, such as the coherent synthesis of material, are dealt with in the following chapter (Chapter 8).

References

Chaplin, N.W. (ed.) (1994) *The Hospital and Health Services Year Book 1994*. The Institute of Health Services Management, London.

Cheung, P. (1988) Library and information services in a Health Authority. *Nurse Education Today*, 8,6 364–5.

Department of Health and Social Security (1972) *Report of the Committee on Nursing*. [Briggs Report]. CMMD 5115. HMSO, London.

Edwards, A., Heap, N., Loxton, R. & Pimm, D. (1989) *Information Technology in Education and Training, DT 200, Block 4, Part 4, Satellite and Optical Storage*. The Open University Press, Milton Keynes.

Fox, R.N. & Ventura, M.R. (1984) Efficiency and automated literature search mechanisms. *Nursing Research*, 33(3), 174–7.

Green, T. (1990) CD-ROM going for a song. *What Personal Computer*. 1(7), 78–80.

McSweeney, P. (1990) How to conduct a literature search. *Nursing*, 4(3) 19, 22.

Schoones, J.W. (1990) Searching publication databases. *The Lancet*, 335(8687), 481.

Appendix 7.1: List of national libraries

Department of Health
Alexander Fleming House
Elephant and Castle
London SE1 6BY
Tel 0171-407 5522 (ext 6363/6415)

Open to all NHS employees but appointment is required. Holds an extensive international collection of material relating to health services. Photocopying available.

Health Education Authority
Health Promotion and Information Service
78 New Oxford Street
London WC1A 1AH
Tel 0171-631 0930

Open to the public. Wide selection of health education material. Photocopying and selective literature searching service available.

King's Fund Centre
Library
126 Albert Street
London NW1 7NF
Tel 0171-267 6111

Open to the public without appointment. Extensive collection of material on health care, equipment and practice. Photocopying and literature search service.

Northern Ireland Health & Social Services
Library
Queen's University
Institute of Clinical Sciences
Grosvenor Road
Belfast BT12 6BJ
Tel 01232-322043

Open to students and staff of Queen's University and all health and social services staff throughout Northern Ireland. Comprehensive collection of material on all aspects of health and social services.

Royal College Of Midwives
Library
15 Mansfield Street
London W1M 0BE
Tel 0171-580 6523

Open to RCM members, and members of the public on request to the librarian. Extensive collection of material on midwifery and computer search services available.

Royal College of Nursing
Library
20 Cavendish Square
London W1M 0AB
Tel 0171-409 3333 (ext 345)

Open to RCN members, non-members should contact the librarian. Holds the Steinberg collection of nursing research and material on nursing and allied health literature. Photocopying and literature search available.

Scottish Office Home and Health Service
Centre Library
Crewe Road South
Edinburgh EH4 2LF
Tel 0131-332 2335

Open to all Scottish health service employees. Comprehensive collection of material relating to all areas of health and practice

Welsh National School of Medicine
Library
University of Wales
School of Medicine
Heathpark
Cardiff CF4 4XN
Tel 01222-755944

Open to all students and staff of the university and for reference to all nurses. Collects material mainly on medicine, dentistry and nursing.

Wellcome Institute for the History of Medicine
Library
183 Euston Road
London NW1 2BP
Tel 0171-387 4477

Open to the public for research and reference only. Collection of material relating to the history of medicine and allied subjects.

Chapter 8

Reviewing and Evaluating the Literature

David C. Benton and Desmond F.S. Cormack

Reviewing and evaluating the literature is central to the research process. However, many neophyte researchers have some difficulty in mastering the skills required to systematically read, critically appraise, then synthesize their views into a coherent, structured and logical review of the literature. Unfortunately, not all published articles are of the same quality or scientific integrity, and all research papers have both strengths and weaknesses. By being able to identify these strengths and weaknesses, the researcher is able to make sound judgements regarding the adequacy, appropriateness and reliability of the material presented, the validity of the conclusions drawn and the applicability of the recommendations made.

Although this chapter cannot hope to fully teach these skills, it does set out to identify a number of points as to how they can best be developed. Whilst it is important to be able to critically appraise and make judgements as to the content of a single article, so as to enable the researcher to assess the worth of the material under consideration, it is the integration of the literature base into a well structured, tightly argued and succinctly written review that challenges most of us. However, the researcher should not underestimate the importance of conducting a critical and systematic review of individual articles for it is these that form the basic building block of a scholarly evaluation of the literature.

A place to read

How often have you sat down to read an article only to be interrupted by the telephone or a request for assistance? Although this may be acceptable when reading material for pleasure, such interruptions can cause the researcher to waste a great deal of time reading and re-reading the same article unproductively. If you are going to critique a research paper, more commonly papers, find a quiet, comfortable, well lit spot with plenty of room to spread out the material. Try and choose an area which you can, over time, associate as the place where you go to work on your research study. Ensure, at the outset, that you have at hand adequate supplies of pencils, highlighting pens and papers for taking notes. One final point: set yourself a time limit, or better still, decide to complete certain tasks before you stop for a break.

Identifying the structure of a research publication

Most research publications, whether qualitative or quantitative, follow a recognized structure. A knowledge of the structure of a research report gives clues as to where to look for certain facts or details and thus enables the researcher to scan an article rapidly so as to assess whether the article is of value and worth the investment of time in detailed reading (Avis, 1994a, b).

The process of scanning an article should be systematic and thorough. Examine a full page at a time with a left to right movement of the eyes while simultaneously 'panning' down the page. Inspect the start of each paragraph for clues to its content. Pick out headings, enlarged, bold, underlined or italic print as well as perusing all illustrations, graphs and tables. For books, monographs, theses, or longer research reports, use the contents list or index for initial clues as to the content. Always stop and read any phrases that signal conclusions or recommendations. For example, 'it has been demonstrated . . .', 'the outcome of the investigations is . . .', 'it is suggested . . .', 'in conclusion . . .', 'therefore . . .', 'hence . . .', and 'it is recommended . . .'.

Certain types of article, for example the research report, consistently follow a standard format. By being aware of the format you can turn in the first instance to those parts of the report that are most likely to yield valuable information. Furthermore, by being aware of the form and function of the various parts of a research article, readers are in a position to evaluate the worth of the material presented. The left hand column of Fig. 8.1 details the possible component parts of a research paper.

Having scanned an article and concluded that it is worthy of more detailed review, each of the areas identified in Fig. 8.1 can be critically examined. To enable the researcher to assess the worth of a particular research paper a series of questions should be asked. The format used in Fig. 8.1 is designed to assist in identifying where the strengths and weaknesses of the paper being assessed lie. As a general point the greater the number of 'No' and 'Don't know' responses checked the more ambiguity there will be and hence the greater care that will need to be taken in drawing any conclusions from the paper.

Recording of critical evaluation

Once the detailed appraisal of an article is complete, it is essential that all relevant information gleaned is recorded in a manner that will facilitate recall at a later date. Without any such documentation, it would be necessary to read, re-read and perhaps even search for articles time and time again.

There are several approaches that can be used to store the information necessary to record the essential facts. Emerson & Jackson (1982) argue that the use of a marginal punch card system is particularly useful since such a system is inexpensive, readily available, and it is possible to devise quite flexible means of recalling information stored. These cards are approximately 4 inches × 6 inches

Heading	Questions To Be Asked	Yes	No	Don't know
Title	• Is the title concise?	✓		
	• Is the title informative?	✓		
	• Does the title clearly indicate the content?	✓		
	• Does the title clearly indicate the research approach used?		✓	
Author(s)	• Does the author(s) have appropriate academic qualifications?	✓		
	• Does the author(s) have appropriate professional qualifications and experience?	✓		
Abstract	• Is there an abstract included?	✓		
	• Does the abstract identify the research problem?		✓	
	• Does the abstract state the hypotheses (if appropriate)?	–	–	–
	• Does the abstract outline the methodology?	✓		
	• Does the abstract give details of the sample subjects?	✓		
	• Does the abstract report major findings?	✓		
Introduction	• Is the problem clearly identified?	✓		
	• Is a rationale for the study stated?	✓		
	• Are limitations of the study clearly stated?		✓	
Literature review	• Is the literature review up-to-date?	✓		
	• Does the literature review identify the underlying theoretical framework(s).		✓	
	• Does the literature review present a balanced evaluation of material both supporting and challenging the position being proposed?			✓
	• Does the literature clearly identify the need for the research proposed?			✓
	• Are important references omitted?			✓
The hypothesis	• Does the study use an experimental approach?		✓	
	• Is the hypothesis capable of testing?	–	–	–
	• Is the hypothesis unambiguous?	–	–	–
Operational definitions	• Are all terms used in the research question/problem clearly defined?	✓		
Methodology	• Does the methodology section clearly state the research approach to be used?	✓		
	• Is the method appropriate to the research problem?	✓		
	• Are the strengths and weaknesses of the chosen approach stated?		✓	
Subjects	• Are the subjects clearly identified?	✓		
Sample selection	• Is the sample selection approach congruent with the method to be used?	✓		
	• Is the approach to sample selection clearly stated?	✓		
	• Is the sample size clearly stated?	✓		

Heading	Questions To Be Asked	Yes	No	Don't know
Data collection	• Are any data collection procedures adequately described?	✓		
	• Have the validity and reliability of any instruments or questionnaires been clearly stated?		✓	
Ethical considerations	• If the study involves human subjects has the study ethical committee approval?			✓
	• Is informed consent sought?			✓
	• Is confidentiality assured?			✓
	• Is anonymity guaranteed?			✓
Results	• Are results presented clearly?	✓		
	• Are the results internally consistent?	–	–	–
	• Is sufficient detail given to enable the reader to judge how much confidence can be placed in the findings?	✓		
	• Does graphic material enhance the clarity of the results being presented?	✓		
Data analysis	• Is the approach appropriate to the type of data collected?	✓		
	• Is any statistical analysis correctly performed?			✓
	• Is there sufficient analysis to determine whether 'significant differences' are not attributable to variationis in other relevant variables?			✓
	• Is complete information (test value, df and p) reported?		✓	
Discussion	• Is the discussion balanced?	✓		
	• Does the discussion draw upon previous research?	✓		
	• Are the weaknesses of the study acknowledged?	✓		
	• Are clinical implications discussed?	✓		
Conclusions	• Are conclusions supported by the results obtained?	✓		
	• Are the implications of the study identified	✓		
Recommendations	• Do the recommendations suggest further areas for research?	✓		
	• Do the recommendations identify how any weaknesses in the study design could be avoided in future research?		✓	

Fig. 8.1   Questions to be asked of various sections of a research report.

and have a series of holes cut into the margins and are also referred to as Copeland Chatterson cards (for a fuller description see Chapter 26). Each hole represents a specified subject. By extracting all the cards on a particular topic, for example care of the elderly, then extracting those relating to the treatment of incontinence, all articles relating to the treatment of incontinence in elderly patients can be identified.

Tyznik (1983) suggests that by using the international classification of disease coding system, literature can be indexed in such a way thus to facilitate recall on a disease orientated basis. Whilst this may provide a well established, international classification framework, we would suggest that the use of subject classification systems used by indexes such as the *Cumulative Index of Nursing and Allied Health Literature* or *The International Nursing Index* is more applicable to those conducting nursing research. In addition, using one of the nursing index classification systems has the advantage that references identified from such sources will already be classified. The use of existing subject classification will accordingly save the researcher time and will also ensure that personally held references will be consistent with their internationally classified source.

With the advent of inexpensive and powerful personal computers, the reference material can be stored by means of database software packages (Cormack & Benton, 1990). The database package enables references to be recalled in a fast, efficient and flexible manner. References can be searched simultaneously on a number of criteria, and those identified can be displayed on a screen or printed for subsequent use. Irrespective of the type of approach chosen to store the information, it is necessary to ensure that a minimum amount of data in addition to the critique are recorded. For example, in the case of journal articles, it is necessary to record the author(s), publication date, article title, journal title, volume and part number and page numbers. In the case of books, additional information such as book title, editor(s), publication place and publisher is required. In the case of a card based system the information needed to access the article can be recorded on the front of the card and the critique written on the back. In the case of a computer based system, two screens can be used, with the first equating to the front of the card, the second to the back.

Writing a literature review

It has already been stated that the ability to critique an individual article is essential to the writing of a literature review. However, it is the manner in which these individual reviews are integrated that often presents the greatest challenge to both the experienced and inexperienced researcher.

A review of the literature should be written objectively, with criticism based on factual material and supported by appropriate evidence and argument. In addition, any review should be balanced with both the positive and negative aspects of material being discussed. Furthermore, the implications of any flaws identified in previous work must be highlighted. A good literature review will provide far more than the critical appraisal of a series of articles, it should create a structure upon which further research can be based. Gaps in the knowledge base will be identified, as well as strengths and weaknesses of the previous work. The issue of structure is central to the production of a sound review and warrants further detailed discussion.

Structure of a literature review

Having spent hours, days or even months reviewing individual articles, it is essential that equal emphasis be placed on how these individual appraisals will be woven into a structured, coherent review. Just as with all other component parts of the research process, unless this activity is planned, then time and effort are likely to be wasted. By spending some time on the development of an outline, the researcher will have a guiding framework for the production of the review. Figure 8.2 identifies the component parts of such an outline.

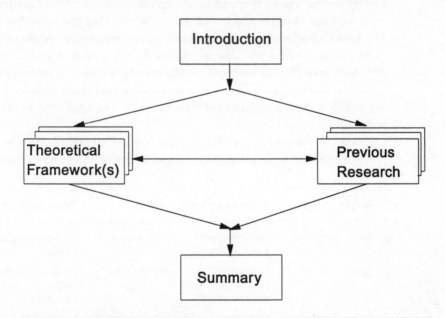

Fig. 8.2 Literature review outline.

As can be seen from Fig. 8.2, the literature review should start with an introduction. This introduction should contain some reference to the sources consulted as well as an indication of the amount of previous work established. The rationale for any constraints should be clearly stated. For example, in the case of a review of the literature on HIV and AIDS it would be reasonable to limit the search from 1980 onward since before that time there is little literature available. In addition, the introduction should (briefly) describe the structure and purpose of the review so as to guide the reader and help place all evidence in context.

The main body of the review will consist of the critique of previous work addressing both theoretical and previous research dimensions. The author should paraphrase previous work whenever possible. Direct quotes can be used to emphasize central issues, but when these are taken out of context of a document, their significance may be lost, or worse still, they may be interpreted differently by the reader. Furthermore, long quotes may interrupt the flow in the development of an argument.

Figure 8.2 attempts to convey that when reviewing the literature on any topic, a number of competing theoretical frameworks may exist, as well as any number of previous research articles that provide conflicting research results. A well organized review will clearly identify the various theoretical perspectives identified, detail strengths and weaknesses of each, and compare similarities and differences between them. Research findings should be related to the appropriate framework and any anomalies explored and explained (if possible) in terms of the theoretical models available. Any gaps in the research or inconsistencies should be clearly identified. Articles central to the development of arguments should be dealt with in depth. Researchers may choose to set out, in summary form, a figure of the major findings along with any strengths and weaknesses of the individual articles reviewed (see Fig. 8.3). Such a figure can assist in identifying common findings or discrepancies in the results as well as providing an opportunity to collate in an easily accessible form both strengths and weaknesses in the existing literature. A summary under each of the headings can be made if the quantity of literature being considered is not too extensive. Such summaries can then be readily expanded upon in the main body of the literature review.

Unless the literature is analysed in detail, and the interrelationships between previous publications identified, the quality of the review will be poor. Inadequate

Author(s) and date	Methodology issues	Results	Recommendations
Brown, A. (1994)	Qualitative; poor sampling method	Inconclusive	Implement practice change
Green, A. (1994)	Quantitative; random control trial; small sample size	Inconclusive	Replicate with larger sample
Red, A. (1994)	Qualitative; grounded theory study	Categories seem saturated; theory seems robust	Test predictive power of theory
Summary			
Range of authors, but all recent publications	Variety of research approaches but some weaknesses in design	Theory has been developed but no conclusive quantitative results reported	Further research required before practice change is advised

Fig. 8.3   Previously published literature (fictitious).

analysis and synthesis of literature results in a review that may only present a series of disjointed paragraphs that echo the findings of previous studies. By planning the review, a logical, structured and coherent argument for further research, or an appraisal of the current state of our knowledge can be presented.

The review should conclude with a summary of the synthesized findings of the previous work which should clearly describe the extent of the current knowledge base. Gaps in the knowledge base or inconsistencies both in terms of the research results and in the theoretical frameworks should be restated succinctly, thus forming the rationale for conducting further research.

Presentational issues

When the researcher is considering a number of research papers, it is essential that the material is presented in a way that facilitates understanding. Great care should be taken to use the most appropriate referencing system so as to ensure the flow of any argument is not disrupted. It is, however, often the case that researchers are restricted by the requirements of the journal or institution for which they are preparing the work. Nevertheless, if you have a choice be conscious of the impact that a poorly referenced review can have on the reader. We would argue that either the Harvard or Vancouver (numerical) methods of reference citation significantly add to the clarity of the argument.

Harvard system

This is perhaps the most widely used system for citing references within scientific publications. In essence it requires that the research cite the surname of the author followed by date of publication of the work being cited from within the text. It is usual that both are included within parentheses unless the author's name forms an integral part of the sentence. For example two fictitious references are cited to illustrate the format that is normally used.

> Research methods are being increasingly taught as part of the pre-registration curricula (Black, 1995). However, Brown (1995) has argued that this is not enough and specialist post-basic courses need also to be offered.

As can be seen from the above example full reference details are not included within the text for this would interrupt the flow of the sentence. Cited material is detailed in a section headed 'References' at the end of the article. All cited material is listed in alphabetical order. If two articles are cited from the same author then they are placed in chronological order. If however two articles are cited by the same author and published in the same year then it is necessary to add 'a' and 'b' within the year descriptor. For example:

> Brown, J. (1995a) The first paper cited in the text. *Journal of Tomorrow's Science*, **99**(1), 230–32.

Brown, J. (1995b) The second paper cited in the text. *Journal of Tomorrow's Science*, **99**(3), 145–63.

When the Harvard system is used and there are multiple authors it is usual to cite only two in the text. Three or more are cited by use of the first author's name followed by *et al.* So Brown & Black (1995) would appear but in the case of Brown, Black, White & Green (1995) only Brown *et al.* (1995) would appear. Although each journal may have different rules about giving the details of multiple authors it is usual to give the names and initials of all authors in the reference list.

Vancouver or numerical citation system

The other citation system in common use is the Vancouver or numerical system. This is where a number (1) appears in the text. At the end of the paper all cited material appears in the order referenced. In the case of books, and when the researcher is referring to a particular section of the cited work a page number may also be added (1, p. 22).

Irrespective of which system is used, both book and journal sources are handled the same when being cited in the text. However, slight differences do appear in the reference list.

Journal and book references

In the case of journal references it is usual to give the author's surname and initial(s) followed by the date, the article title and the journal title followed by both the volume and part numbers as well as the page numbers. The journal title appears in italics. For example *Nursing Research*, *Journal of Advanced Nursing* or *Nursing Management*.

When a book is cited slightly different information appears in the reference list, in this case the author's surname and initial(s), date of publication, title of the book, place of publication and publisher. For example, Black, D. (1995) *The Basis of Life*. Fast & Accurate Publishers, London. In this case it is the book title that is printed in italics. For further information on more complex material such as unpublished reports further details can be found in specific texts on publication (Cormack, 1994).

Identifying the anatomy of a published review

To conclude this chapter and to reinforce the various points made, a published review of literature on 'learning to care' by Smith (1985) is reviewed using the Harvard reference citation system.

First, the title of the work clearly informs the reader of its content. Specifically, it states that the article is a literature review and that the topic is learning to care. The author is identified as being a senior nurse (research) and is both academically and professionally well qualified.

Second, an abstract is provided. Although it has no title, it is enclosed in a box at the start of the article, and separated from the main text. It clearly outlines the content of the article, identifying that the author intends to review the literature and the relationship between the provision of care and learning to nurse. Furthermore, it is identified that the principal means of evaluating this relationship is by examining the quality of care, and this is identified by the use of reference to dependency studies, quality assurance instruments and the nursing process.

Third, the introduction informs the reader of the extent and nature of the literature review conducted as well as providing a succinct statement on the purpose of the article.

Fourth, major headings are used throughout the publication and these conform with the principal elements reported in the abstract. This consistency assists the reader in comprehending the logical progression of the arguments presented. Various themes are well integrated throughout the article with the relevance of the material being frequently stated in terms of the relationship between learning to nurse and the giving of patient care.

Fifth, throughout the article the author does not simply report the findings of previous studies, but examines the material in terms of content, method and theoretical perspective. In short, a comparative analysis both in terms of theory and research results has been undertaken resulting in a review that compares and contrasts the findings of previous work.

Finally, although the author does not include a heading in the article, a summary is presented. This final paragraph draws together all the various threads presented, but, unfortunately, an additional element is also introduced. The introduction of Donabedian's (1966) 'structure, process, outcome' model at this late stage without the inclusion of appropriate debate detracts from what is otherwise a well written critique of the literature.

The article by Smith (1985) demonstrates many of the points that have been discussed in this chapter. Writing a critical review of the literature is a skill that requires to be learned. If you are to become a nurse researcher, or you are to practise from a research base, it is essential that you are able to proficiently conduct a critical review of the literature; learning from the past you can change the future and increase the quality of care delivered.

References

Avis, M. (1994a) Reading research critically I: An introduction to appraisal: design and objectives. *Journal of Clinical Nursing*, 3(4), 227–34.

Avis, M. (1994b) Reading research critically II: An introduction to appraisal: assessing the evidence. *Journal of Clinical Nursing*, 3(5), 271–7.

Cormack, D.F.S. (1994) *Writing for Health Care Professions*. Blackwell Science Ltd, Oxford.

Cormack, D.F.S. & Benton, D.C. (1990) Reading the professional literature. In *Developing your Career in Nursing*, (ed. D.F.S. Cormack) Chapman and Hall, London.

Donabedian, A. (1966) Evaluating the quality of medical care. *Millbank Memorial Fund Quarterly*, **44**(2), 166–206.

Emerson, S.C. & Jackson, M.M. (1982) Organize your references. *Nursing Administration Quarterly*, **13**(6), 33–7.

Smith, P. (1985) Learning to care: a review of the literature. *Nurse Education Today*, **5**(5), 178–82.

Tyznik, J.W. (1983) Taming the medical literature 'monster'. *Postgraduate Medicine*, **74**(1), 77–80.

Chapter 9

Preparing a Research Proposal

Senga Bond

Research proposals may be written for a number of reasons: to obtain funding, to present to a higher degrees committee in a university, for ethical approval or as an academic exercise as part of a research course. This chapter focuses on the first of these since this is the most frequent and in some ways the most important reason for writing a proposal. However, features of proposal writing apply to all of the situations mentioned.

Preparing a research proposal will be addressed in two ways. First to provide researchers with some straightforward guidance about possible structure and content. The second is to suggest some ways of making a proposal more appealing and thus more likely to be funded.

The most important function of research proposals is to make explicit a reasoned argument about the need for the proposed study on practical and theoretical grounds and how it will be carried out. The very act of writing a proposal assists in identifying the strengths and weaknesses of a study. This is achieved through the process of setting down a clear statement of the question that the study proposes to answer, the methods that will be used to find the answer and the resources required to do it. Information should also be provided about how the results will be disseminated and any products likely to arise. The particular form that a proposal takes will depend on the requirements of the organization to which it is being submitted and some produce special forms giving guidance about the different sections within which information should be provided. However, what follows is general guidance about preparing a proposal which may be amended to suit the requirements of a particular case.

The content of a research proposal

It is useful to have a checklist of the main topics to be included. Such a list would contain the following:

(1) Title of project
(2) Summary
(3) Justification for the study
(4) Related research

(5) Aims and objectives
(6) Plan of investigation
(7) Ethical considerations
(8) Expected end products
(9) Dissemination of results
(10) Resources
(11) Budget
(12) Curriculum vitae.

Let us consider each of these headings in turn and give some pointers to the kind of information within each one.

Title of project

Research projects become known by their title so it is important to make the title explicit and relatively brief while describing the proposed study. Sometimes studies change in direction during their evolution while the subject matter remains essentially the same. An experiment may collapse or the nature of the variables being considered in a survey may be altered on the basis of pilot work. The title should be able to override these changes while still conveying the essence of the study. The use of words like 'evaluation' and 'survey' in titles are helpful in alerting readers to the approach the study will take. It is more informative to call a study 'An evaluation of a counselling scheme for patients who have had a mastectomy' than to call it 'Caring for mastectomy patients' even if the design or counselling methods change over time.

Summary

Most research award applications ask for a brief summary. In practice this is usually written after the main body of the proposal has been put together since it requires to be succinct yet state clearly the objectives of the study and how it will be carried out. It should contain only the most relevant information. The space allocated to it or word length specified means that every word is important and it is an art to describe a major project in a paragraph.

Because it appears early, the summary again alerts the reader to what to expect in the subsequent text. The summary is an important indication of the quality of the remainder of the proposal and so it requires careful consideration and probably several drafts to ensure all of the main points are included.

Justification for the study

The statement of the problem which opens the main body of the proposal must convince the reader that the proposed study is important. It must introduce the research questions and put them into a context which indicates the importance of the problem, its size, costs and consequences. It should identify how the proposed study will add to previous work and build on theory. In nursing studies there are likely to be practical implications of the research so that, as well as having value in contributing to knowledge, its utility value needs to be stressed. There may be methodological gains, for example in developing a new research instrument, which would have future applications, as well as gains in education or practice.

In developing the problem statement the researcher needs to keep a careful balance between putting forward claims for the study which are either too grandiose or too general or that the study is no more than the whim of the researcher based on some closely held belief. Novices often express research as setting out to *prove* something, for example that parents prefer booked visits from health visitors, rather than an open question of their response to different systems of visiting, or a formal hypothesis of preference. There is also a tendency to be over ambitious, and this applies even to quite experienced research workers when the enthusiasm for the topic overrides their judgement about delivering the goods. A key piece of advice therefore is *to focus on the manageable.*

When writing this section it is sometimes helpful to underline or type in a bold face a succinct statement of the problem to draw the reviewer's attention and to foreshadow the remainder of the proposal. Sketch out a couple of sentences indicating the broad approach that the study proposes to take.

Related research

Next, it is important for the researcher to demonstrate his/her command of the current state of the field and how this study would move it forward. To achieve this, those few key studies which provide the basis for the proposed project should be included. Indicate in language for non-specialists how they are relevant to the proposed study and how this study moves beyond them. This review should relate both to substantive concerns and methods, and be provided in sufficient detail to inform the reader of its relevance. It may also be useful to include knowledge of studies under way as a reflection of the author's competence in keeping abreast of developments.

At this point competence can also be demonstrated in making explicit the theoretical aspects of the study and the firmness of the theoretical base. This information can be extremely influential in demonstrating the researcher's grasp of complex issues and in showing that the study has more than practical implications.

The development of the literature base is a major feature of the research process described in Chapters 7 and 8 and it is equally an important feature of the research proposal. If the literature search and the literature section of the proposal is an afterthought, it will shine through by virtue of its unrelatedness to the remainder of the proposal.

Aims and objectives

Any reviewer of proposals likes to see clear, specific and concrete objectives which are achievable. List and number them in order of importance in a clear sequence, taking only a sentence or two for each.

The remainder of the proposal will be judged in relation to what you have told the reader about what this study aims to do. To achieve this, avoid vague terminology and generalities; define criteria as specifically as possible. Do not leave it up to the reader to have to do the guesswork about what the objectives are or their order of priority. You will stand more chance of being clearly understood by listing them than by leaving the reader to abstract objectives out of a prosaic statement.

The objectives of the study may take the form of questions, when research is exploratory, or a survey where specific facts are being sought. It may be possible to state objectives in the form of testable hypotheses where this is a basis for predicting results. It is more enlightening, as well as more convincing, if hypotheses are stated whenever possible. However, these need to be precise and relationships clearly specified.

Plan of investigation

This section could be called 'Plan of Investigation, 'Procedure' or 'Method' and is likely to be the section most carefully read by both funding and ethical committees. Up to this point, the researcher has been able to present a picture of the positive implications of the research and what it hopes to achieve. It is when procedures are spelled out that those reading the proposal gauge the researcher's capacity both to undertake and complete the proposed work.

The specific format of this section will depend on the methods adopted. Different emphases will be required depending on whether the study takes a survey, an experimental or field study approach. Irrespective of method there are several important matters to convey and these are best written in discrete sections.

Method/design

The method to be adopted and the precise design of the study should be clear. Simple descriptions are more readily available for particular types of experiment and for survey research than other types of research, and can be specified in advance. Equally it is straightforward to indicate whether the study is prospective or retrospective, cross-sectional or longitudinal. For exploratory studies, case studies or ethnographic research, equally the basic method should be made clear and this section will often require appropriate adaptation when application forms issued are set out as if for trials. Sandelowski *et al.* (1989) and Cohen *et al.* (1993) offer particular guidance for qualitative studies.

For experimental studies details will be required about which variables are controlled and how control is to be achieved. In some instances, there may be complete randomization while in others, subjects may be matched on known relevant variables, or included in a factorial design. What is important here is showing awareness of as many relevant variables as possible and how control can be realistically managed. In health services research, control of all variables is virtually impossible and the challenge is to make the best use of available situations and be sophisticated in designs which offer the closest approximation to experimental proof.

When compromises have to be made to facilitate experimental design in the 'real world' of patient care, then the reasons for such compromises should be made clear. For example, if patients are to be allowed some degree of choice of treatment (Brewin & Bradley, 1989) or randomization is by ward or general practice rather than patient, the reasons for doing so need to be made explicit. The general point is that often the reasons for not adhering to the 'gold standard' of the randomized controlled trial expected by some research bodies needs to be spelled out.

Specification of design in observation studies, survey research using case notes or other forms of data should make clear that this is the intended method.

Population and sample

The initial literature review will have indicated the nature of the population relevant to the study as well as giving a clue to the generalizability of the study findings. This section will include a clear statement of the population from which study samples will be drawn, and details of the characteristics of the sample. When particular sampling techniques are used, for example, stratified or cluster sampling, as described in Chapter 19, this choice should be justified. Should a whole population be used rather than a sample, the reader will want to know why this is so.

Evidence should be provided that the sample is available and can be recruited and that, where appropriate, a sampling frame exists. Clear criteria for inclusion and exclusion should be included, or variables by which individual subjects will be matched. Again clarity is the essence.

Critical also are questions of sample size. What reviewers will be looking for are indications that the sample size will be big enough to detect differences or carry out other appropriate statistical manipulations so as to come up with a clear answer. It is generally expected that proposals include a statement of the expected and acceptable size of effects, at what degree of power, and the sample size required to detect them.

It is equally important to specify the sampling intended in field studies. Case studies or individuals will be selected on some criteria and sometimes these can be specified in advance, for example to include a gender, ethnic or geographical mix or other theoretically relevant variable. When these can only be specified on the basis of ongoing theory development then this should be made clear.

Data collection

In this section measures and procedures to be used in data collection are described. These should reflect back to the variables included, show that the measures to be used represent acceptable operational definitions of them, and that they have appropriate measurement or psychometric characteristics. In many topics of relevance to nursing research, well validated scales exist and it would be foolish to develop a new scale. Where proposed measurements have been used in other relevant studies it is helpful to indicate this. When methods of measurements do not already exist and new methods are proposed, these are best described in detail as an appendix to the proposal. In some cases proposal reviewers wish to see copies of instrumentation, test items, questionnaires or interview guides. It makes sense to find out if this is required. However, for some studies, a substantial part of the work entails such methodological developments.

While data collection techniques may involve conventional methods like questionnaires and interviews, they may also involve invasive biochemical or physical measures or assessment of observed behaviour. Only if novel techniques are involved should mention be made of the apparatus to be used to obtain these data and whether any special conditions are required for their use. If the data to be collected or the methods used to collect them are likely to be controversial, then plans indicating how problems would be dealt with should be included.

Pilot study

It is extremely useful if some of the above are based on the results of a pilot study to provide evidence of likely recruitment, response rates, size of effect and so on. Indeed many proposals are submitted to enable pilot work to be carried out as a preliminary to a larger, more expensive study. If no pilot work has been carried out prior to submitting the proposal then the objectives of doing so and how it would be done should be stated. This will tell reviewers what steps will be taken to ensure that the proposed methods are workable, are acceptable to subjects and manageable. The pilot study is worth specifying in some detail. For example, to conduct a postal sample survey from first principles would involve going through several stages to arrive at a questionnaire before going on to a postal pilot study to gauge its acceptability and response rate. If an already validated instrument was to be used again then obviously the amount of development and pilot work would be that much less. When new methods are to be used, such as lap-top computers to collect interview data or new scales have to be developed, then the pilot or development work will be much more time-consuming and important to the eventual quality of the study. It is always worth investing time and effort to ensure that the development, feasibility or pilot work for a study is thorough, and stressing this in the proposal.

Analysis

It is essential to have considered data analysis in the development of any study even though it may be some way off from becoming actuality. Most important is to show that the methods of analysis are consistent with the objectives and design of the study. Again, in some ways this is easier to specify in advance for quantitative studies. It is less easy to describe details of the analytic procedures used in qualitative studies. In cases where complete specification is not possible, the stages of data analysis can be outlined indicating an appreciation of the kinds of methods likely to be used. If studies rely on multivariate or discriminant techniques or longitudinal analyses, then this should be specified even if it has to be at a general level. It should be indicated that sufficient statistical expertise is available to inform and, if necessary, carry out statistical analysis. Knowing what techniques to apply to the analysis of data is more important than indicating that a statistical package like SPSSx or Mini-Tab or qualitative data software like Nudist or Ethnograph is to be used (see Chapter 30). Access to computers and appropriate packages are almost taken as universally available. What is important is to convince the reviewers that you know what analysis is appropriate and have the appropriate personnel, hardware and software to achieve it.

Work plan

Details of the time scale and plan of work should be included to show the anticipated duration of each stage of the study. The complexity of the plan of work would reflect the complexity of the study. It need be no more than an indication of the time allocated with each major stage of the study/pilot study, main subject recruitment and data collection, data analysis, report writing. When the study is more complex and different activities are happening simultaneously, then more sophisticated flow charts or critical paths may be necessary to identify the anticipated progress of work. Often a diagram says more than words (see Chapter 31).

Generally, the time taken to complete each part of a study is underestimated, particularly data collection which depends on a prospective series. The tendency is to be over-optimistic. This can also apply to the time it takes to negotiate entry and gain ethical approval to collect data. Formal project planning activities should be undertaken to determine the time scale required in relation to critical events as well as resources and books (for example, Hayes, 1989; Weiss & Wysocki, 1992); a number of software applications (such as Microsoft Project) are available to assist in achieving this (see Microsoft Corporation, 1994). A clear and realistic time schedule is another indication of the researcher's competence and the likelihood of a successful project.

Ethical considerations

The reviewer of a research proposal will have been alerted to any ethical issues while reading the methods section. The proposal may be reviewed by a committee whose primary objective is to assess the scientific methods of a study but they will not be unaware of ethical issues and they are likely to assess whether 'the ends justify the means'. Many grant awarding bodies require that a study has approval from an ethical committee prior to being reviewed.

A proposal viewed by an ethics committee, however, will take an entirely different perspective and, while considering the science of the proposal, will be giving most attention to the protection of human and animal subjects from undue distress. When submitting a proposal for ethical clearance it is wise to show how informed written consent (if at all possible) will be obtained from adults or from parents, guardians or advocates when the subjects themselves cannot give approval. Permission forms as well as the tools used to collect data should be sent in with the forms. Ethical matters may also be relevant to describing the protection of subjects from any negative consequences of a study, and protection of staff can equally apply when they may be involved in handling noxious substances or administering procedures as well as when they are themselves the subject of research. How data will be stored and measures taken to protect the identities of subjects or participating institutions should be included. A helpful article on the subject of obtaining ethical approval is provided by Ayer (1994).

Expected end products

The end product of most research studies is a final report to the funding or commissioning body, or a thesis. However, products may also be new research instruments or methods of data collection as well as teaching or clinical aids. If the study is likely to yield a product of value, then ownership of the intellectual property rights and the patents to the products need to be made clear. Also it may be appropriate to include costs for product development.

Dissemination of results

Increasingly, attention must be paid to the dissemination of the results of research. Reports and published papers are taken for granted but they are not the only way to present results. Videos, presentations and the like may be equally if not more relevant in some instances as a means of disseminating findings to particular audiences. It may be appropriate to make specific suggestions about how this is to be achieved, especially through executive summaries of findings targeted to specific audiences. Some grant-awarding bodies are more interested than others in dissemination over and above traditional publications.

Resources

It is important that the resources required to carry out the study are realistically appraised. Resources, whether human, material or financial need to be specified.

Personnel

The person(s) who will direct the project and the principal investigator(s), should be clearly identified together with the amount of time intended to be devoted to the project. It may be that this is a proposal for a full-time commitment or for only a few hours a week. Spell out the time implicated. Academic and clinical collaborators should be identified, and relationships with them and their responsibility and commitment to the project clarified. Where a complex study is involved the right mix of expertise may be an important element. It must be clear how they have contributed to the proposal.

It is especially important for inexperienced researchers to obtain the support of established research workers. In this respect it can be useful to show that active consultation has taken place in the development of a proposal. Indicate the kind of assistance offered by those experienced in research or with particular technical competence associated with data processing, analysis, costings and so on where formal supervision has been obtained, then provide credentials for the supervisor.

Other resources

Describing particular services or back-up facilities can strengthen a proposal. Good computer and library facilities fall into this category as do sufficient space and secretarial support. Where established networks are integral to a project or cooperation has been obtained from particular agencies or institutions, some indication of this, like a letter of agreement, may be included as a helpful appendix.

Budget

Preparing a research budget requires as much skill as preparing other parts of the proposal. It is amazing, when a maximum amount is specified in calls for proposals, how many are costed at just that amount! Part of the skill in budgeting lies in locating other people who know the prices of commodities – staff salaries as well as equipment and other consumables. However knowing the details of the data collection and processing makes costing much easier – how many hours it takes to collect data, how much travel time and mileage, how much data punching will be required. Preparing a budget means translating the time scale and plan of work into financial terms.

Novice writers have a tendency to want to skimp the budget, earnestly believing that if a project costs less, then it improves the chance of being funded. Undercutting the budget simply reflects inexperience. Sharp-eyed critics will quickly notice where there has been undue trimming and what is feasible in the costs quoted. Equally where excesses are included, like a new computer for a short project, or large travel budgets, they will be cut. Sometimes budgets can be a matter of negotiation if they are thought to be too high by virtue of over-elaborate sampling or extended time scales. However, to be caught short of cash and time can be disastrous and funding bodies do not take kindly to requests for extensions of time or increased budgets. In preparing a budget, use a checklist to include main headings like:

- Research staff salaries
- Secretarial staff salaries
- Data collection costs, including purchase of equipment and other materials, printing, travelling expenses, stationery and postage
- Data processing costs
- Book purchases
- Conference attendance
- Product development
- Dissemination
- Overhead costs.

It is sometimes useful to separate costs into capital costs, to include the purchase of equipment, and recurrent costs. It may be possible to obtain funds for books as well as travel to conferences. Put them in, there is no harm in trying! Some organizations, especially universities, ask for overhead costs. Check out whether this is so and the current rate. Parent organizations also wish to check a budget statement before it is submitted, and salaries and other costings usually have to be counter-signed by someone with specific expertise in this matter. An appropriate budget is always a matter of careful specification rather than just pulling some notional figure out of the air.

Curriculum vitae

Attach an appropriate curriculum vitae for all principal investigators. This is not always essential but is usually asked for and it does no harm to include one. Its contents should be appropriate and include details of:

- Name
- Age
- Qualifications
- Education
- Work experience
- Research experience
- Recent relevant publications.

One or two pages is usually sufficient to show whether the applicants have the appropriate experience and performance record to conduct the study.

Final review

It is likely that a research proposal will go through several drafts. Indeed there would be a major cause for concern if it did not! There are a number of things to be achieved by reviewing research proposals. Not least is to consider its physical presentation. Nicely spaced typescript with a major effort on legibility, lucidity and clarity of presentation are all important. While readers of a proposal will not be consciously evaluating it on how it is presented, nevertheless the relatively small amount of time it takes to ensure a pleasant layout which is easily followed will be time well spent. Devices like a bold typeface, underlining, spacing and use of diagrams, flow charts and tables are useful to attract the reader's eye. The latter are often more useful in presenting details than reams of text. Avoid small type in the text.

It is also useful to ask someone with experience of successfully submitting proposals to check over your efforts. Most people are pleased to assist, so long as there is evidence that you have made proper attempts to produce a good piece of work.

Some general comments

This chapter has discussed developing the research proposal primarily from the point of view of having it approved for funding. It should have demonstrated also the need to write down a clear statement of proposed research to assist researchers themselves. Matters of making explicit a proposed time schedule and proper project management techniques can be fundamental to the successful execution of a project. However, it is even more helpful to enlist the help of experienced researchers who have themselves submitted successful proposals, so that they may offer advice in the development phase of a study proposal. Others' experience in such matters is invaluable.

Some funding bodies offer the opportunity to submit an outline proposal for approval before a full proposal is submitted. This permits a degree of negotiation about the focus, content, methods and so on. Recent data showed that while 30% of applications to a funding body were funded, 38% of those which had been submitted for informal advice and comment were successful compared with 19% which had been submitted without prior notice (Watts, 1990).

Different bodies considering a proposal will be looking at quite different things, and it is important to identify their primary concerns and give special consideration to them. Check whether the funding body has any special requests in terms of the subject matter they are likely to fund, whether there is any specific geographical area or limits to funding. Some bodies may prefer a particular kind of proposal, for example they look more kindly on proposals asking for capital equipment rather than those asking for staff costs. In Chapter 3 some sources of research funding were identified. Check if they have any particular requirements in the manner in which a proposal is presented. This may involve no more than a telephone call to the appropriate secretary. Some organizations have a check list or a particular form on which proposals must be made. Notes of guidance may be available and it is wise to adhere to them strictly. Other organizations regard the form of the proposal as a measure of the worth of the researcher and offer no guidance on preparing a proposal.

It is also helpful to know how proposals are viewed. Sometimes they are sent to external referees with particular expertise for comment, whilst others are dealt with completely 'in house'. As well as scientific referees, the National Health Service, national nurse education bodies and government health departments may also have 'customer' referees who are looking for the utility of the research in practice or policy terms, rather than the quality of the science. Knowledge of the membership of a review committee can be useful in anticipating areas to which special attention or orientation should be given. When a committee of mixed expertise reviews proposals, then all members should be able to understand the nature of the study. At times there could be a problem of orientation – when biological or physical scientists are asked to review a proposal with a social science orientation. In instances like this, it is important to avoid excessive jargon while maintaining appropriate specificity.

There is skill in achieving a balance between identifying every single possibility and spelling out every detail and providing sufficient detail to convince reviewers that the applicant has the ability to complete a worthwhile study. To some extent the degree of specificity is related to the state of knowledge in a particular field and to the extent to which the study is exploratory or explanatory. Writers of proposals have to rely on their judgement to some extent but, as a general principle, it is better to include more information than leave out something others may regard as important. However the reviewing panel will be abreast of standard methods and these do not have to be detailed.

The length of the proposal can be of some concern. Sometimes length and number of pages or words is specified. This is not usually meant to be taken rigidly, but to serve as a guideline to prevent over-excesses. If lengthy details of specific steps are required then these can be included as appendices so as to avoid crowding too much into the main text and so losing the crispness of the presentation. The purpose of appendices is to provide additional supportive information for reviewers who do not feel that the main text is sufficiently detailed but should not require to be read to obtain a clear impression of the study.

This book is intended primarily for people who are new to research and this chapter may be used to assist some who have never before developed a proposal, or developed a successful one. Some funding bodies are keen to support new research workers but are not likely to want to risk large sums of money or invest in potentially unmanageable studies. It is wise then to begin in a relatively small way or to ask only for funding for the first stage of the project. This safeguards both the funding body and the research worker should something go drastically wrong. Better still would be to have an experienced researcher as a co-applicant.

Finally, do not be dismayed if a first attempt is rejected. One can always learn from it. Unfortunately, not all grant awarding bodies provide information detailing why a proposal is rejected and this is singularly unhelpful to the recipient of the rejection slip. However, Increasingly, referees' comments (in an anonymous form) are given to applicants. In some cases grant bodies may refer the project, that is suggest that the researcher re-work it under guidance. In some cases it is almost as if referral is the rule and few proposals are accepted the first time round. It is always helpful to obtain copies of proposals which have been accepted by the body to which you are applying. This does not imply slavish adherence to that particular format but it does give some indication of the type of proposal more likely to be welcomed and hence succeed in being funded.

Other useful hints on writing research proposals can be found in many general research texts such as those by Burns & Grove (1987), Polit & Hungler (1991), as well as Parahoo (1989) and Hodgson (1989). Sandelowski *et al.* (1989) and Cohen *et al.* (1993) provide guidance for writing a grant proposal in qualitative research while Watts (1990) describes the submission of proposals for health services research in a government agency.

References

Ayer, S. (1994) Submitting a research proposal for ethical approval. *Professional Nurse*, 9(12), 805–6.

Brewin, C.R. & Bradley, C. (1989) Patient preferences and randomised clinical trials. *British Medical Journal*, **299**, 313–15.

Burns, N. & Grove, S.K. (1987) *The Practice of Nursing Research*. W.B. Sanders, Philadelphia.

Cohen, M.Z., Knafl, K. & Dzurec, L.C. (1993) Grant writing for qualitative research. *Image: Journal of Nursing Scholarship*, 25(2), 151.

Hayes, M.E. (1989) *Project Management: From Idea to Implementation*. Kogan Page, London.

Hodgson, C. (1989) Tips on writing successful grant proposals. *Nurse Practitioner*, 14(2), 44, 46, 49.

Microsoft Corporation (1994) *Microsoft Project. Business Project Planning System.*

Parahoo, K. (1989) Writing a research proposal. *Nursing Times*, 84(41), 49–52.

Polit, D.F. & Hungler, B.P. (1991) *Nursing Research, Principles and Methods*, 4th edn. Lippincott, Philadelphia.

Sandelowski, M., Davis, D.H. & Harris, B.G. (1989) Artful research. Writing the proposal for research in the naturalist paradigm. *Research in Nursing Health*, 12(2), 77–84.

Watts, G.C.M. (1990) Development of health services research applications. *Health Bulletin*, 48(1), 41–9.

Weiss, J.W. & Wysocki, R.K. (1992) *5-Phase Project Management: A Practical Planning and Implementation Guide*. Addison-Wesley Publishing, Massachusetts.

Chapter 10

Gaining Access to the Research Site

David C. Benton and Desmond F.S. Cormack

Having identified a research question, conducted a systematic review of the literature and decided upon a research design, a further critical step that novice researchers often find difficult is gaining access to the research site. If research is to be conducted which requires access to either human subjects or confidential individual based patient information, then careful negotiations will need to take place if delays in this important step are to be avoided.

The process of negotiating access to the research site is often complex and challenging and will inevitably bring you into contact with a wide range of individuals and groups. This experience can be rather daunting for the novice researcher but should be viewed as a learning experience since it is an integral part of conducting a research study. Even an apparently straightforward study often involves negotiating access with a wide range of individuals and groups.

Since the introduction of the National Health Services (NHS) reforms, the issue of research access has become even more complex (Department of Health 1991). The introduction of a market ethos has resulted in some researchers experiencing a degree of difficulty in negotiating access. Not only are the managers of NHS Trusts conscious of the need to protect the interests of often vulnerable research subjects, but they may also be concerned, if such a research produces adverse findings, that their market position might be compromised if data relating to quality of care is handled in an insensitive way. It is therefore essential that the researcher is clear on how to proceed in gaining access to the research site.

The research site

In this chapter the research site is the term used to describe a wide variety of settings within which research may take place. It may be a hospital, a community based service, a private or voluntary sector institution, an individual's home or, in the case of population based research, a street corner where individual members of the public may be approached. To a certain extent the research question may need to be modified in light of the discussions and negotiations that inevitably will take place in pursuing access with the various gatekeepers to the research sites. Within this discussion, the gatekeepers are those individuals who can either facilitate or block access of the researcher in conducting the study. It is therefore critical that the researcher initiate discussion to gain access at an early stage.

For novice researchers it is often worthwhile considering discussing with peers their experiences in gaining access. Such discussion can often provide opportunities to rehearse the approach that may be taken. Also the assistance of an experienced researcher in going over your proposal may highlight issues that the gatekeepers may have problems with, or from an external perspective, may require clarification. This, therefore, will ensure that you have had an opportunity to consider such issues in a safe environment so as to formulate an appropriately detailed response to any points likely to be raised.

It is important to note that in negotiating access it is acknowledged that the gatekeeper can only give the researcher permission to **ask** potential subjects to participate. Negotiated access does not guarantee that the research subjects will agree to participate in the study.

Research where negotiated access is not required

If data are already published then no permission or negotiation needs to take place to gain access to the material. For example, library based historical research is an example of a research design that does not require the researcher to gain formal access to the research site. This, of course, is only the case if the research materials are in the public domain.

Frequently, specialist collections of material may require the permission of the librarian, particularly if they are of key historical value and/or are original source material which may be damaged by excessive handling. If this is the case, the researcher may need to convince the owner/librarian that their skill in handling delicate original data sources is adequate and they will not cause any damage.

Some researchers believe that collecting non-invasive data from the general public does not require special permission. To a certain extent this is true, however a researcher who approaches members of the public may fall foul of the law since they may be reported as causing a nuisance. It is always advisable for researchers to alert the local constabulary of their intentions to conduct such data collection. This is particularly the case when collecting data on a busy street where the process may cause obstructions or delays in the flow of pedestrians.

Accessing the gatekeepers

There are a range of gatekeepers who can facilitate or inhibit the researcher's access to a research site (Crowe, 1994). Gatekeepers generally fall into one of two camps, either professional or organizational.

Organizational gatekeeper

Conducting research within any health care institution or setting requires that the management of the organization is aware of the activity taking place. This is essential so that the potential cumulative impact of different studies can be appropriately monitored. A key gatekeeper is therefore the Chief Executive or General Manager of the organization. The names of senior officials of NHS institutions can be obtained from an up-to-date version of the *Hospitals and Health Services Year Book* (Institute of Health Service Management, 1994). However, in light of the rapid changeover of staff, it is always advisable to telephone the organization to validate the information gleaned from such texts. It is normal practice that such individuals should be approached in writing in the first instance. The researcher should give brief details of the study to be conducted, the likely impact for the organization and a request to meet with either the Chief Executive or their nominated deputy. Contacting the Chief Executive is a critical step, particularly if the study to be conducted requires access to case records. In the United Kingdom, a case record is the property of the Secretary of State for Health. However, safe custody is delegated to the Chief Executive of either the District Health Authority if the hospital is a directly managed unit, or to the Chief Executive of the Trust if the hospital/service has acquired Trust status.

Professional gatekeepers

If the researcher is seeking access to a particular patient group, then there may well be a number of professional gatekeepers who will require convincing that the researcher is both capable and competent to undertake the study. As multi-disciplinary working becomes the norm rather than the exception, so the range of professional gatekeepers has expanded considerably. It is therefore always best for the researcher to attempt to identify who might be involved in the care and treatment of the subjects/patients they intend to recruit into the study. By doing this a list can be generated of those individuals who may have a view on any research that is proposed to be conducted with 'their' patient. In the past it was generally acceptable to approach the head of the particular professional group to seek approval for access. However, with the fragmentation of hierarchical lines of management this is no longer always appropriate. It is therefore essential that the researcher is clear about how the various professional groups work within a potential research site. Only then can an appropriate approach be made to perhaps the professional head of nursing, medicine or any other allied profession. Many research studies have run into difficulty because of failure to approach the right people at the right time.

Having identified the professional gatekeepers, again a written response should be made with the offer of following this up with a face to face meeting.

Whether approaching organizational or professional gatekeepers, it is essential that the researcher is well prepared for this encounter. The researcher should take to the meeting an adequate number of copies of the research proposal. The initial contact with the gatekeepers can have a profound effect on how easy or difficult access to the research site will be. It is therefore advisable that you be clear before the meeting as to the ground that will be covered. Ideally you will have prepared an opening explanation of the study. This will stress the significance of the work, the commitment that will be required from the organization providing research access and, perhaps most significantly, what will be in it for them. At the very least, be prepared to offer a copy of the research results and come back and present the findings to the senior managers of the organization and/or those individuals that have been involved in the process. If the initial contact is managed well, then a commitment may be obtained from the senior officers to give support in gaining access lower down the organization. A letter of introduction may significantly influence the cooperation of others within the organization. It is, however, important that such a letter should not be used as a mechanism to coerce people into agreement, but it certainly can assist in providing additional authority to the researcher since hopefully it will make reference to the importance of the work and the commitment of senior management.

It is also important at this early stage to establish how ethics committee approval can be sought. The Department of health published a new guide to the establishment of research ethics committees and, on the whole, these are now functioning well up and down the country (Department of Health, 1991). A more recent publication on standards relating to the functioning of these committees has been produced (National Health Service Training Directorate, 1994). Access to both the guidance on the operation of committees and the standards of functioning can be a useful additional aid to the novice researcher seeking to negotiate access.

Access and power relationships

In the previous section, we have alluded to the fact that a letter of support from the Chief Executive or professional head can influence the participation and agreement of others in provision of access to research subjects. The problem of coercion becomes more acute if there is either a line relationship between the researcher and the subjects, or there is a care dependency relationship. For example, the authors are aware that nurse educationalists often use student nurses as the subjects for research study. If the research is conducted with their own students, then often students may feel that they have no option but to cooperate in the study. Similarly, nurse teachers may feel unable to refuse a head of department access to the teacher's own students since there is a clear hierarchical power relationship present.

The primary concern for all nurses should be the well being of their patient or those they care for. This tenet is enshrined within the UKCC document on exercising accountability (United Kingdom Central Council for Nursing, Midwifery and Health Visiting, 1989). A researcher who is a nurse and also wishes to conduct research within her own hospital or institution must be careful that both the research subject granting permission and the manager/professional head approving access must be clear of their role and not be swayed by personal knowledge of the researcher. It is therefore essential that adequate external advice is available to the researcher in ensuring that the decisions that are being taken regarding access within an institution where the researcher is known are comparable to those that would be taken if the researcher was proposing to do the study in an institution elsewhere.

Ethics committee approval

All research conducted within the auspices of the National Health Service and involving human subjects or personal information relating to them requires the approval of the local ethics committee. The responsibility for establishing an ethics committee lies with the Health Authority not the hospital or institution. Clear guidance has been developed by the Department of Health (1991) on how these committees should be constituted and run. This guidance was initiated since many researchers found that in the past ethics committees, if they existed, met on an infrequent basis and the decision making process was often unclear.

In more recent times, an additional set of documents on the standards by which ethics committees should be assessed has been developed. Ethics committees are encouraged to comply with these standards and to audit themselves against them. Access to both the guidelines for the establishment of ethics committees, and the standards of their functioning, can be a useful and informative source for novice researchers wishing to navigate their way through the process of successfully gaining ethics committee approval.

It is important to make contact with the ethics committee at an early stage to ascertain whether or not there is a specific protocol that requires to be followed in making an ethics committee application. For example, it is not uncommon for the format of the protocol to be specified in detail. The researcher will sometimes be presented with a computer disk with a draft format which needs to be completed. In addition to a proforma, extensive guidance explaining the type of response required for each section is often provided. Clearly, early access to such material is essential if delays are to be avoided.

Historically, research ethics committees tended to be most familiar with randomized control trials, for example assessing the effectiveness of new therapeutic agents. Thankfully, most ethics committees now have considerable experience with the full range of research designs. However, it is often in the researcher's best interest to identify who amongst the membership of the ethics committee has a particular interest or understanding of the approach being proposed. Initial contact with this individual may assist in ensuring that all necessary information is presented to the committee.

For those health districts with a large number of teaching establishments, a model of devolved responsibility is often in operation. This is where individual members of the committee will be given the responsibility of screening protocols and contacting the researcher at an early stage, conducting a detailed ethical review and presenting the work at the committee for debate. Obviously, it is in the researcher's interest to ascertain if such a model is in place since the member with devolved responsibility for their particular study may provide useful guidance at an early stage.

Litigation and insurance

The recent increases in the number of cases of litigation against researchers and the host organizations within which they operate has led to ethics committees being particularly conscientious in ensuring that the researcher and the organization have adequate insurance (Mander, 1992). Drug companies will provide insurance cover, sufficient to deal with any claims, for harm caused by the particular drug that is being tested. However, this does not usually cover errors in administration. If, for example, the researcher were to administer the wrong dose of drug, then it would be likely that the researcher rather than the company would be liable. This is a particularly complex field and it is down to the ethics committee to ensure that all research is adequately insured. It is therefore essential that the researcher discuss with the chairman of the ethics committee the type of insurance that their particular study will require, and the proof necessary to be presented as part of the application process.

Informed consent

Another area that often causes novice researchers some particular difficulties is that of informed consent. For research subjects to be able to make an informed choice they need adequate information, in a language that is readily understandable to them, giving details of what will happen to them and any associated risks. In the past many researchers were reluctant to provide such information since they would argue that to do so might influence the outcome of the research. Such an argument is no longer defensible and any researcher seeking to hide information from a subject will not be given research approval by the ethics committee.

Confidentiality and anonymity

Assurances regarding subject confidentiality and anonymity will also require to be addressed. It is often possible to offer people anonymity provided that the subjects are drawn from a large enough pool and that the reporting of results is done in a way that does not localize the information to a particular hospital department or ward. Researchers must therefore be careful when writing up their studies not to breach confidentiality or anonymity.

Numbers of subjects and their selection

Another area which the research ethics committees are particularly concerned with is the number of subjects to be approached and how they are selected. The researcher will need considerable clarity over this point if her study is to gain ethics committee approval. Clearly dependent on the research design, the number of subjects and the method of sampling may vary considerably. The researcher should, therefore, be prepared to defend both the size of the sample and the method of sampling against challenges from the committee. Clarity over the advantages and disadvantages of the various approaches that could be used to select the sample for the particular study being proposed is a worthwhile preparatory step.

Since the publication of guidance on the establishment of local research ethics committees, all committees must report on an annual basis the research that has been approved by the committee (Department of Health, 1991). This list can obviously provide the researcher with much useful information since it can identify work already going on in the field that may interact with the researcher's own planned study. Furthermore, it can also provide a ready-made network of individuals with an interest in the researcher's field. This information is in the public domain and therefore it is legitimate for a novice researcher to approach researchers already conducting work in the field. Early contact with such individuals can often provide valuable insights into how access to the research site can best be facilitated.

Approaching subjects

Having successfully navigated the gatekeepers, both professional and organizational, and gained the approval of the local ethics committee, research subjects still need to be approached. The method of selection will have been detailed as part of the research protocol as will the information that will be provided to ensure informed consent. However, the manner by which they are approached can have a significant influence on whether individuals agree or refuse to participate. A quiet, polite, unhurried and assertive approach is often the most successful. Sufficient time must be set aside so as to ensure that the potential subjects have adequate opportunity to ask any questions. Impatience or tactlessness not only result in research subjects declining to participate but may also result in the professional or organizational gatekeepers withdrawing access as reports of such behaviour are fed back. Generally speaking, subjects are usually more than willing to participate provided the researcher takes the time to explain what the study is about and gives the individual the respect they deserve. After all, without the good will of research subjects, researchers would be very limited in the type of study they could conduct.

Conclusion

Gaining access to a research site can be time-consuming. However, if the researcher identifies the necessary gatekeepers at an early stage, approaches them in a systematic way, and seeks the support of peers in the process, access to the research site is a relatively straightforward step.

Like many things in life, having successfully negotiated access to a research site for the first time, the second and subsequent occasions become far easier. This is not simply because the researcher is aware of who needs to be contacted, but also a track-record has been established. Accordingly, researchers need to pay particular attention to any promises made in relation to the feedback of research results, to ensure that access on a subsequent occasion is not denied.

References

Crowe, S. (1994) Who pays when trials go wrong? *Health Care Management*, 13–14, 16.

Department of Health (1991) *Local Research Ethics Committees*. Her Majesty's Stationery Office, London.

Institute of Health Service Management (1994) *The Hospital and Health Services Year Book*. Institute of Health Service Management, London.

Mander, R. (1992) Seeking approval for research access: the gatekeeper's role in facilitating a study of the care of the relinquishing mother. *Journal of Advanced Nursing*, **17**(11), 1460–4.

National Health Service Training Directorate (1994) *Using Standards for Local Research Ethics Committees*. National Health Services Training Directorate, Bristol.

United Kingdom Central Council for Nursing, Midwifery and Health Visiting (1989) *Exercising Accountability: Advisory Document*. United Kingdom Central Council for Nursing, Midwifery and Health Visiting, London.

B: Research Design

The research design represents the major methodological thrust of the study, being the distinctive and specific research approach which is best suited to answering the research question/s. As will be seen in Chapters 11 to 19 the major research designs – which are not always entirely mutually exclusive – each have individual advantages which make them appropriate in particular circumstances.

Selection of the research design is influenced both by the research question and the aim and objectives of the research. Selection of a research design is always preceded by clearly identifying the purpose of the research. In selecting an appropriate design, it is useful to have a general knowledge of a variety of designs and thereby be able to consider a range of possibilities, eliminate those which are not appropriate and select the one best suited to your particular study. As with many aspects of the research process, it is rarely possible to achieve perfection. In selecting a research design, bear in mind that whichever one is chosen, it will be imperfect and have some limitations with regard to your particular needs. However, careful consideration of research designs will enable selection of the one which has the 'best fit' for your particular study.

The chapters in this section are intended to give readers of research reports an insight into a few selected research designs. They are also intended to give researchers, working under supervision, an introduction to the major research methodologies, and to provide the basis for selecting a specific design which can then be studied in detail by making use of the references provided at the end of each chapter.

Chapter 11

Qualitative Research

Sam Porter

The first questions to be asked in relation to qualitative research are: what is it and what makes it different from other forms of research? The short answer to these questions is that the uniqueness of qualitative research lies in the fact that it does not focus primarily upon the identification and explanation of facts, but upon the illumination of people's interpretations of those facts. As a consequence, qualitative research is an appropriate mode of enquiry when researchers wish to study the understandings and motivations of their research subjects. These rather sweeping statements require clarification. The conventional way of providing this is to contrast qualitative with quantitative approaches.

Contrasting qualitative and quantitative methods

The first differences that can be noted between the two approaches is the focus of their analysis. While the focus of quantitative research is primarily upon *numbers*, often aggregated into statistics, qualitative research concentrates on *words*, in the form of speech or writing.

In addition to their focus of analysis, each approach is associated with a number of assumptions. Quantitative methods are often associated with the aim of identifying and explaining causal relationships between events. Thus, by noting that apples always fell to the ground when loosened from a tree, Newton was identifying a causal relationship. By propounding his law of gravity, he explained the relationship.

Qualitative researchers often argue that this sort of explanation is inappropriate when the subject matter of research is the actions of human beings. Apples have no choice but to fall to the ground; humans often do have a choice about the sort of behaviour they display. As a consequence, it is argued that research into human behaviour should focus on the motivations that people have for doing the sorts of things that they do. In short, qualitative research is often associated with the search for *reasons* rather than *causes*. This in turn means that, in contrast to quantitative methods, whose aim is often to *explain* why something happens, qualitative approaches seek to *understand* the interpretations and motivations of people.

While quantitative researchers often aspire to *objectivity*, the assumption that facts can and should be presented in a manner untainted by the feelings, opinions or bias of the researcher or researched, qualitative researchers emphasize the importance of *subjectivity*, the assumption that the sole foundation of factual knowledge is personal experience.

Belief in the significance of subjective factors in qualitative research is not limited to the subjectivities of research subjects. Qualitative analysts often assert the need for researchers to reveal the values, interests and influences associated with their own subjective experiences. This proess is termed *reflexivity* (Hammersley & Atkinson, 1983). Good qualitative research involves reflexivity at several levels. First, researchers identify the theoretical framework that they are operating within, along with the values and commitments that they adhere to. Second, they reflect upon how personal factors specific to their own experiences may affect the research. Finally, researchers describe and reflect upon the importance of the methods used in their research and the context within which it is conducted.

To signal their reflexivity, qualitative researchers often use the first person active to describe themselves, rather than the traditional third person passive ('I noted ...' instead of 'It was noted by the researcher ...'). In line with this qualitative tradition, I shall use the first person to refer to myself in both this chapter and Chapter 29.

Artificial divisions

Having set up a number of divisions between qualitative and quantitative methods, readers should be aware that neither style of research fits neatly into these categories. The purpose of this contrast is to give a flavour of the ideas underlying different approaches to research, rather than to make definitive statements about them. Indeed, I am acutely aware that, in contradiction to what I said above about reasons and causes, my own research (Porter, 1993a) provides an example of the use of qualitative methods to elucidate causal relations. One of the most encouraging aspects of recent advances in research has been the willingness of researchers to overcome divisions through the incorporation of that which is best from both traditions into their research designs.

The theoretical foundations of qualitative research

As with any system of investigation, qualitative research is founded upon a number of wider assumptions, which can be classified according to four levels of understanding (Bilton *et al.*, 1981). These levels are ontology, epistemology, methodology and methods. What is meant by these rather daunting philosophical terms, and how they relate to qualitative research, will be explained below. However, before examining the four levels, two points need to be underlined. First, it needs to be emphasized that the following is only one (albeit common) version of the assumptions underlying the use of qualitative methods; alternative groundings can be constructed. Second, these are assumptions and are therefore open to debate and disagreement. Despite being presented here in the form of a catechism, they should not be taken as gospel.

Level one: ontology

Ontology concerns questions about what exists.

Question: What is the subject matter of qualitative research?
Answer: Social reality.
Question: What is the nature of social reality?
Answer: Social reality only exists as meaningful social interaction between individuals.

Qualitative research has been much influenced by a branch of philosophy known as *phenomenology*. The basic premise of phenomenology is that the nature of the outside world can never be fully known. All that can be known are people's perceptions and interpretations of that world. After all, how do we know about anything, except through the use of our senses and mental faculties? In its strongest form, phenomenology asserts that reality is to be found in people's minds, rather than in external objects. One of the consequences of this position is that reality is not a fixed entity. It changes and develops according to people's experiences, and the social context within which they find themselves.

The significance of social context is crucial because it is through our social interactions with others – parents, teachers, friends and health care professionals, to name but a few – that our understandings and preconceptions about the nature of reality are formed. This is not just a one-way process, in that through our inter-actions with each other, we help to create the social reality around us. It is for this reason that it was stated above that social reality only exists as meaningful social interaction between individuals.

As a qualification it should be noted that, for some qualitative researchers, acceptance of the importance of social context implies that phenomenological understanding is not enough. They argue that social reality is more than indivi-duals' understandings; it also consists of the social structures that enable and constrain the actions and interpretations of individuals (Porter, 1993a). Never-theless, it remains true to say that phenomenology is the bedrock of most qualitative research.

Application of phenomenology to nursing leads qualitative researchers to con-centrate on people's experience of being ill. As Benner & Wrubel, (1989) put it, 'Illness as a human experience of loss or dysfunction has a reality all its own'. This line of reasoning entails a rejection of the traditional medical model of the ontology of illness, which equates the reality of illness with the physical manifestations of disease or disablement. The focus of the medical model is seen as unacceptably narrow, in that the reality of sickness cannot be reduced to the biochemical pro-cesses of the disease that a person is suffering from. Proper understanding must include the person's subjective experience and understanding of the illness, and the social context within which that experience and understanding occur.

The significance of this revision of the ontology of illness should not be underestimated. Jerrett (1994), in her phenomenological study of the experiences of parents with chronically ill children, makes the point well when she argues that 'their subjective experience is fundamentally important not just because it involves a personal reassessment of objective reality, but because lived experience is reality'.

Level two: epistemology

Epistemology concerns questions about what we can know about what exists.

Question: What counts as knowledge of social reality?
Answer: Our knowledge of social reality equates with our understanding of the meanings and motives which guide the social actions and interactions of individuals.

The connection here between epistemology and ontology is clear. If social reality consists of the experiences and understandings of people, then knowledge of reality will be knowledge of those experiences and understandings. An example of the application of this sort of epistemological assumption to nursing research can be seen in Melia's (1982) study of student nursing. For Melia, the reality of student nursing lay in the students' own constructions of their nursing world. Therefore, the interest of the research

'lay in obtaining the student nurses' view of nursing, in other words to allow the students to "tell it as it is" '.

For Melia, 'telling it as it is' involved gaining knowledge of the experiences, understandings and motives of the subjects that she was researching.

Gaining such knowledge is not as simple as it may at first seem. A thorny question that has long troubled phenomenological researchers is whether or not it is actually possible to get inside people's minds in order to fully understand their experiences. One problem here is that in a completed research report, the understandings of the subjects have been filtered through the understandings of the researcher, and it is very difficult to tell the degree of distortion that has occurred in this process. As Melia (1982) observes, the part played by the qualitative researcher in the production of data is crucial.

The epistemological claims of qualitative research are cautious; for many qualitative researchers absolute knowledge of reality is simply not possible – knowledge of social reality will always be coloured by the interpretations of the researcher (Porter, 1993b).

Level three: methododology

Methodology concerns questions about the manner in which knowledge about what exists can be gained.

Question: How can we know about the nature of social reality?
Answer: Social reality can be discovered by looking at it through the perspective of the individuals living in it.

Question: How can such a perspective be gained?

Answer: This perspective can be gained by using methods which illuminate the meanings and motives of subjects.

Qualitative researchers are required to interpret as accurately as possible the experiences, meanings and motives of subjects, from the perspectives of those subjects. Accuracy in the reproduction of subjects' perspectives largely depends upon the researcher's knowledge and familiarity of the social setting being studied. Gaining this familiarity takes a considerable period of time, spent either as a participant observer or an interviewer. The qualitative researcher needs to immerse herself as fully as possible in the lives or work of the people she is studying.

However, irrespective of the degree of involvement, the influence of the researcher's own perspective will remain, and it is necessary to construct a methodology which takes account of this. Here lies the importance of reflexivity. By openly examining and reporting on how their own experiences and understandings have impinged upon the nature of the research, researchers open up their influence upon the research to the scrutiny of readers, who can then make their own judgements about the authenticity and persuasiveness of the findings.

Thus Melia (1982), in a reflexive account of her research, outlined for the reader the degree of knowledge that she had of the social world of the student nurses in her study. She pointed out that, having trained and practised as a nurse, she had a degree of familiarity within the setting, with the jargon used and with hospital ways in general. However, she was also careful to point out gaps in her knowledge of the specific social world that she was examining. She noted that her experience of training was not the conventional three-year programme that her subjects were studying in, and that she had trained in a different institution to that in which they were training.

It can be seen how Melia's reflexive account gives her readers the opportunity to judge the degree of knowledge that she had about the world of her research subjects, and thus about the accuracy of her reproduction of their perspectives. In the absence of statistical tests for validity and reliability, this sort of reflexivity is crucial to qualitative research if it is to be persuasive.

Level four: methods

Methods are techniques used to collect evidence about what exists.

Question: What are the best ways to gather information about the meanings and motives of social actors?

Answer: Those methods which:
  (1) Enable researchers to become involved in the social world of the subjects they are studying. This involvement can give researchers direct experience of the meanings and motives of subjects.
  (2) Give subjects the opportunity to describe and explain, in their own words, the meanings and motives which provide the basis for their actions and interactions.

A number of methods have been devised by qualitative researchers to gather data, either by involving themselves in the subjects' social world or by allowing subjects to describe their understandings on their own terms. These methods include in-depth interviewing, oral history, participant observation and conversation analysis.

In-depth interviews

The most common qualitative method used in nursing research is in-depth interviewing. Other terms for this form of interviewing are 'unstructured' (if there is no prior format for the interview), 'semi-structured' (if there is some format, but the interview is allowed to expand beyond the bounds of that format), 'informal' or 'ethnographic'. The rationale for in-depth interviews is to give subjects the opportunity to describe their experiences in their own words.

In-depth interviewing can either be used as a free-standing method of enquiry or in conjunction with participant observation. When combined with participant observation, the information supplied by interviewees can explain and put into context what the researcher has seen during observation.

In in-depth interviews, the researcher starts out with only a general plan about the direction which the conversation will take. Qualitative researchers tend to avoid questionnaires or heavily structured interview formats for two reasons. First, it is argued that informal interviews provide a more natural setting. If people are allowed to chat freely about their lives in a non-threatening environment, they will tend to be more forthcoming. Second, it is contended that the way questions are constructed in structured interviews and questionnaires tends to reinforce the questioner's assumptions. This leads to two dangers. First, interviewees may feel pressurized into agreeing with what they perceive as the researcher's preconceptions about the 'right' answer. Second, there is a danger that the researcher will be entirely off the mark, asking the wrong questions about the problem they are investigating. If there is no opportunity for interviewees to have an input outside the confines of a pre-determined structure, then such errors may go unnoticed by the researcher. It is argued that in-depth interviews can overcome these problems because they involve less influence on the part of the interviewer and more influence on the part of the interviewee.

Many examples of this method could be chosen. One is Wuest & Stern's (1991) study of families of children with persistent middle ear problems. Wuest & Stern interviewed ten such families in order to learn about the factors that influenced family interaction. They discovered that one of the main concerns of family members was how to manage the day-to-day practicalities of family life. The interviews revealed that families felt they were not getting adequate support from health professionals to help them cope with their situation. Wuest and Stern concluded that nurses have the potential to become a major resource for families with chronically ill children by providing this service.

Oral histories

A variant of the in-depth interview is known as oral history. This is used if the social setting that the researcher wants to find out about existed in the past, thus making it impossible for the researcher to become directly involved in it. As in in-depth interviews, subjects in oral histories are given the opportunity to describe and explain their past experiences in their own words.

A good example of the use of this method in nursing research is Keddy *et al.*'s (1986) examination of the relationship between nurses and doctors that pertained in Canada in the 1920s and 1930s. To gain information about what it was like to be nursing in this era, Keddy *et al.* taped 34 semi-structured interviews with older nurses, asking them to recall past events and experiences from their work histories. One of the main themes that emerged from these interviews was the significance of nurses' relationships with doctors in this era, a relationship in which doctors enjoyed almost absolute authority.

Participant observation

Participant observation is the classic qualitative method. As its name implies, it involves researchers participating in the daily lives of their research subjects, while at the same time observing the actions and interpretations of subjects going about their day-to-day business. The aim of this qualitative method is to attain an 'insider's' view of the group under study. This is gained both by the researcher's direct experience of the social setting she is studying, and by the information given to the researcher during conversations with members of the group under study.

The recording of data gained from participant observation may be done through audio or video taping. However, the most common method of data recording is the use of fieldnotes. As the name suggests, these are observations written manually into a notebook by the researcher. They involve detailed descriptions of social situations and interactions that occur in the 'field' of research, field being the term used for the location where data are gathered.

Participant observation has a long history. However, it was not until the early twentieth century that it was developed as a method of scientific enquiry by European anthropologists such as Malinowski (1922), who used it to study non-Western cultures, and by the 'Chicago School' of sociology, who used it to examine sub-cultures closer to home.

Despite being a well established method of social research, participant observation does not enjoy great popularity in nursing research. There are good practical reasons for this, in that it is very difficult for a healthy researcher to participate in the social world of patients or clients. Given that the primary focus of qualitative nursing research is upon this group, the possibilities of participant observation, in contrast to those of in-depth interviewing, are extremely limited. However, qualitative nursing researchers can participate in the social world of clinical nurses. One example of this approach is my own work into the influence of gender upon nurses' professional relationships with medical colleagues (Porter, 1992). The data for that study were gathered during three months of participant observation conducted in an intensive care unit. By working in the unit as a staff nurse, I was able to immerse myself in the occupational lives of my research subjects.

First, I looked to see if there were any differences in the quality of interaction depending upon the sex of those involved. I found that while the gender of a nurse had little effect upon the quality of interaction between nurse and doctor, the gender of a doctor did, with female doctors often being more egalitarian in their dealings with nurses than their male counterparts. Examination of nurses' attitudes to gender issues showed that they resented doctors' expectations for them to act as handmaidens, and regarded it as perfectly valid to respond to medical pomposity in an assertive manner. However, while nurses were prepared to criticise doctors who were openly chauvinistic, they did not extend their critique to medicine as a whole, seeing sexism as an individual phenomenon rather than an institutional ethos.

It can be seen from this example that participant observation can be used both to discover the nature of interaction in a social setting, and to illuminate the understandings and motives of those involved in the interactions.

Conversation analysis

A more formal method of observation of social interaction is used in the technique of conversation analysis. The aim here is to study how people talk to each other in everyday settings. Emphasis lies in how conversations are technically constructed so as to accomplish ordered conversational interaction. Because even the smallest nuances in conversations are important in this type of research, the use of a tape recorder is essential. Even better is a video recorder, which also records gestures and facial expressions, thus giving a fuller picture of the processes of communication.

In this form of research, the researcher usually takes on a passive role, allowing research subjects to carry on normal day-to-day conversational activities, and recording them while they do so. The recordings of conversations are then transcribed using a specialist annotation, in which, for example, the lengths of pauses are timed to a tenth of a second, and interruptions and overlaps are marked. What is said is recorded phonetically, rather than being translated into standard English. While this sort of detailed analysis of mundane encounters may appear trivial, conversation analysts assert its importance on the basis that talk is the building block of all social interaction and that, conversely, broader social processes permeate down to conversational interaction.

A pertinent example of the use of conversation analysis can be found in Brewer *et al.*'s (1991) study of the conversations of children with severe learning difficulties. By studying the group dynamics of conversations, Brewer *et al.* discovered that, contrary to popular images that regard mentally handicapped children as communicatively incompetent, these children possessed considerable conversational skills. One child was seen to be highly adept at orchestrating encounters with others, skilfully organizing, structuring and controlling conversations. However, the other children were far from incompetent as co-conversationalists, and were capable of appropriate responses and turn taking. By methodically breaking down the talk of children with severe learning difficulties into the basic component parts of verbal interaction, Brewer *et al.* demonstrated the organized nature of their conversations, thus providing a useful challenge to preconceptions that we may have about the mentally handicapped.

The functions of qualitative research in nursing

As has been seen, the purpose of much qualitative research is to describe the meanings and motives of an identified group of people as faithfully as possible. The focus can be on patients, as in Johnson's (1994) study of how overweight people restructure their perspectives during the process of dieting; on relatives, as in Jerrett's (1994) study of parents with chronically ill children, or it can be on nurses themselves, as in Melia's (1982) study of the lives of student nurses.

However, research is not always descriptive. It can also be used to test theories. An example of this approach can be found in May's (1992) examination of the degree to which Foucault's (1973) notion of the 'clinical gaze', which characterizes the relationship between doctors and patients as entailing medical surveillance, can be applied to the nurse–patient relationship.

Qualitative research can also be useful in policy evaluation. An example of this approach can be found in Mason's (1994) study of community maternal and child health policies in Jamaica and Northern Ireland.

Conclusion: the increasing importance of qualitative research

The increasing significance of qualitative research in nursing is indicated by the fact that in the first edition of this book it did not merit a chapter of its own. It now merits several. There is good reason to believe that its importance will continue to grow. The change in nursing philosophy away from a mechanistic approach to patients, towards a more holistic perspective on care, leads to more emphasis being put upon the wants, needs and fears of patients. This change in emphasis inevitably entails the adoption of research methodologies which allow for the elucidation of those wants, needs and fears.

The shift towards qualitative research has been accelerated by the increasing influence upon nursing academics of feminist research concerns, which also place personal experience at the centre of the research agendum. Hagell (1989) makes this point very clearly:

> Nursing, as a discipline, has a distinct knowledge base which is not grounded in empirico-analytical science and its methodology but which stems from the lived experience of nurses as women and as nurses involved in caring relationships with their clients.

Given the convergence of nursing concerns and qualitative ideas about the importance of people's experience, there are good reasons to believe that qualitative methods will enjoy an increasingly prominent place in nursing research. Indeed, it could even be that the use of qualitative research will come to distinguish nursing knowledge from the sort of knowledge that other, more mechanistically orientated, health professionals aspire to.

References

Benner, P. & Wrubel, J. (1989) *The Primacy of Caring.* Addison-Wesley, Menlo Park, California.

Bilton, T., Bonnett, K., Jones, P., Stanworth, M., Sheard, K. & Webster, A. (1981) *Introductory Sociology.* Macmillan, London.

Brewer, J.D., McBride, G. & Yearley, S. (1991) Orchestrating and encounter: a note on the talk of mentally handicapped children. *Sociology of Health and Illness*, 13, 58–67.

Foucault, M. (1973) *The Birth of the Clinic.* Tavistock, London.

Hagell, E. (1989) Nursing knowledge: women's knowledge. A sociological perspective. *Journal of Advanced Nursing*, 14, 226–33.

Hammersley, M. & Atkinson, P. (1983) *Ethnography: Principles in Practice.* Tavistock, London.

Jerrett, M. (1994) Parents' experience of coming to know the care of a chronically ill child. *Journal of Advanced Nursing*, 19, 1050–6.

Johnson, R. (1994) Restructuring: an emerging theory on the process of losing weight. In *Models, Theories and Concepts*, (ed. J.P. Smith), pp. 31–46. Blackwell Scientific Publications, Oxford.

Keddy, B., Jones Gillis, M., Jacobs, P., Burton, H. & Rogers, M. (1986) The doctor–nurse relationship: an historical perspective. *Journal of Advanced Nursing*, 11, 745–53.

Malinowski, E. (1922) *Argonauts of the Western Pacific.* Dutton, New York.

Mason, C. (1994) Maternal and child health needs in Northern Ireland and Jamaica: official and lay perspectives. *Qualitative Health Research*, 4, 74–93.

May, C. (1992) Individual care? Power and subjectivity in therapeutic relationships. *Sociology*, 26, 589–602.

Melia, K. (1982) 'Tell it as it is' – qualitative methodology and nursing research: understanding the student nurse's world. *Journal of Advanced Nursing*, 7, 327–35.

Porter, S. (1992) Women in a women's job: the gendered experience of nurses. *Sociology of Health and Illness*, 14, 510–27.

Porter, S. (1993a) Critical realist ethnography: the case of racism and professionalism in a medical setting. *Sociology*, 27, 591–609.

Porter, S. (1993b) Nursing research conventions: objectivity of obfuscation? *Journal of Advanced Nursing*, 18, 137–43.

Wuest, J. & Stern, P. (1991) Empowerment in primary health care: the challenge for nurses. *Qualitative Health Research*, 1, 80–99.

Chapter 12

Grounded Theory

David C. Benton

A casual review of any scholarly journal that publishes nursing research will reveal a wide range of methods used by nurse researchers encompassing both quantitative and qualitative approaches. However, a similar review of the same journal ten years ago would yield a quite different picture. In the past ten years, it has been observed that there has been a noticeable increase in the number of published studies which use qualitative techniques (Chapman, 1989). Omery (1987) suggests that this increase can be attributed to the fact that nurses now feel confident enough as researchers to select the most appropriate methods to meet the needs of the topic under study. Aamodt (1982) has argued that any method which facilitates the discovery of variables associated with the provision of care can contribute to the development of nursing knowledge and the associated theory base. Furthermore, Aamodt (1982) suggests that inductive approaches to the development of theory can be readily employed by nurses who wish to undertake research and to practise related topics.

One means of inductive theory generation which has been consistently utilized by nurses since its development by Glaser and Strauss (1967), is that of the *grounded theory* method. This method has been used by nurse researchers to develop inductive theories on topics as diverse as couple communication patterns, quality of care from the patients' perspective and competence validation and cognitive flexibility (Hilton, 1993; Wilde *et al*, 1993; Loving, 1993). Field & Morse (1985) have identified that there is a need for nurses to develop their own theories of health care, theories which have been developed directly from the everyday practice of members of the profession. Since grounded theory entails the development of theory from data which have been methodically obtained from the real life setting, it is ideally suited to the needs of nurses who wish to investigate topics about which little is known.

Many aspects of nursing are qualitative in nature and as yet under researched (Chapman, 1989). This fact, along with the need to develop a nursing knowledge base, has resulted in the utilization of the grounded theory method. It is the intention of this chapter to clearly identify the processes involved in undertaking a grounded theory study and provide guidance which will assist you, should you wish to conduct research using this method.

Grounded theory method

The grounded theory method is ideally suited to the investigation of those topics about which there is little prior knowledge. The method developed by Glaser & Strauss (1967) requires that you approach data collection without a preconceived framework. Without an open-minded approach, there is a danger that significant material will be ignored since data that are seen as not fitting the existing model may be disregarded. The use of the grounded theory approach will enable you to develop theories based on the reality of the topic under study. This process will encourage you to explore data so as to discover the basic social and psychological processes operating within the area of enquiry.

Unlike quantitative methods, the grounded theory approach does not proceed in a linear fashion. Grounded theory is typified by the concurrent activities of data collection, organization and analysis. This process continues until a theory is developed which is of sufficient detail and at a sufficient level of abstraction to explain the variation in the data observed. The process by which the grounded theory is generated is known as the constant comparative method, a method by which every element of data is compared with every other element.

Data sources and methods of collection

Data are commonly generated through field observation or by examination of documentary evidence. Field observation is a process where data are generated by observation, interview or video or audio taping. This entails close inter-personal contact with the subjects of the study. To help you understand the role you play in this process, it is advisable to keep a daily journal or diary. Thoughts, impressions, or emotional reactions experienced, can all be recorded and may assist in under-standing the material gathered.

Data collection initially starts with an attempt to examine the wider issues sur-rounding the topic under study. Only when you have established the wider context should more focused investigation begin. Luker & Chalmers (1989), for example, describe the process of client referral as it emerged from an in-depth study of health visiting practice.

Interview and observation are two techniques frequently used to generate data for a study utilizing the grounded theory method. These techniques are not unique to grounded theory and are described in detail in Chapters 21 and 23 respectively. Nevertheless, Strauss (1987) has suggested that data obtained from these sources can be confusing at first. However, since organization and analysis of the data begin at an early stage, this should enable you to identify areas which can be clarified in subsequent interviews or observations.

Theoretical sampling

Theoretical sampling is the term used to describe the manner in which data sources are identified and selected for inclusion in a study and is integrally linked with the constant comparative method of data analysis. Initial decisions about samplings are based upon general understanding of the area under investigation. This initial decision is the only decision that you can pre-plan, since the selection of all other data sources is controlled by the emerging theory. Unlike other forms of research, such as the experimental or survey design, you are unable to identify the size and characteristics of the sample at the outset of the study. In a grounded theory design, you are only able to identify the sample, retrospectively, once the theory has been generated.

Individuals, groups, or situations, are selected to provide comparison data. Theoretical sampling can either attempt to minimize or maximize the differences between the comparisons being made. By minimizing differences, you can collect data which can assist you in identifying the basic properties of categories and the specific conditions under which they exist. Furthermore, minimizing differences can also assist you in identifying those fundamental ways in which categories vary. Maximizing differences between data sources increases the chance of identifying different properties of the categories and finding those properties which are most stable.

Reliability and validity of data

Goodwin & Goodwin (1984) have reported that there is a tendency to ignore the issues of reliability and validity or to consider them irrelevant, when undertaking research based in the qualitative paradigm.

If research is to be of value, then it must address the issues of reliability and validity. Glaser & Strauss (1967) and Stern (1985) have argued that reliability is established by taking findings back to those respondents who provided the original data from which you generated the theory. Respondents can then confirm or refute the theory developed. Stern (1985) points out that if the process is used on an ongoing basis, then it is similar to the test/retest approach to establish the reliability that is used in quantitative research.

Validity of the theory can be established on the same basis as that advocated for reliability. By taking developing theory back to the original informants, you can receive feedback which can be used to establish validity.

Grounded theory does address the issues of reliability and validity. More general issues concerning reliability and validity as applied to qualitative research are addressed in Chapter 11. However, Heinz *et al.* (1990) identify a specific approach for examining a complete piece of work for both reliability and validity. By using independent experts, it is possible to examine various aspects of the process of developing grounded theory for reliability and validity. It is suggested that not only can the method provide data on the reliability and validity of a study, but it is also capable of identifying investigative bias and conceptual clarity.

Data recording

The grounded theory approach is dependent upon the accuracy of the source data; thus, data recording is a vital step in the entire process. Data are most frequently recorded by use of audio tape or/and written notes. Alternatively, you may choose to use video tape which, in addition to a verbal record, can also provide data on non-verbal behaviour. If audio tape is used then it is necessary to add non-verbal data at the stage of transcription. Transcription is the process where the audio record is typed ready for coding and analysis.

The choice of audio, video or written data recording will be dependent upon a number of issues. The recording and transcription of audio or video tape requires access to equipment and possibly secretarial resources. Written methods of recording are less expensive, but the data may not be as accurate or complete unless you are able to use shorthand. Consequently, since completeness and accuracy are important, and if adequate resources are available, tape should be used. However, dependent on the location and preferences of the respondents, it may not be possible or appropriate to use recording devices. Informants may refuse to participate if tape is used, or they may be working in areas where background noise could result in a poor quality recording, incapable of transcription.

If you are unable to use any form of data recording technique during the interview or observation, then it is important that a permanent record is made as soon after the event as possible. Go somewhere quiet and either write or dictate notes, identifying and recording as much detail as possible.

Whichever approach is used, it is important that certain information always appears on the data record. First, the name of the interviewer/observer and the date, time and place where the interview/observation occurred. Second, the individual, group or subject being interviewed/observed. For clarity, all pages should be typed double spaced and with ample margins. Ideally, the interviewer data should appear on one side of the page and the interviewee data on the other. All pages should also be numbered and referenced so as to ensure that data do not go missing or appear out of context. Figure 12.1 illustrates as an example of how a transcribed interview should appear. Please note that the name and source of data would not normally appear on published material: in this case, all identifying characteristics are fictitious.

Explaining terminology

There are a number of terms that have particular meaning when applied to the grounded theory approach. These include substantive codes, categories, properties, theoretical constructs, core categories and saturation. An understanding of the meaning of these terms and the relationship between them is vital if you are to undertake a study using a grounded theory design.

Substantive codes

When data are collected, you should examine the various incidents so as to label those items or words which you feel contribute to the comprehension of the underlying processes. Coding of the actual substance of the data is referred to as

Interview:	John Brown, Director of Quality
Date and Time	10/08/1994 10:30AM
Location	Rural Health Authority
Researcher	Mary Smith Page 3 of 28

Interviewer
What were your hopes for the post?

Interviewee
While there might have been more lofty aims to do with intergrating research into practice and all that sort of thing, it was much more about safeguarding nursing. It was about getting influence, I felt that nursing had lost influence when general management came in. Because of the kind of research that was put forward I got the feeling that general managers didn't value what was being done. To get any sort of credibility there was a need to take the initiative by getting it right. Playing the game by their rules.

Fig. 12.1   Excerpt from interview illustrating a suitable layout.

substantive coding. At this early stage of coding, individual words or short phrases are highlighted in the text and codes written in the margin. To ensure detailed theoretical coverage, each sentence and incident should be coded into as many substantive codes as possible – a process known as open coding. This may result in some data being coded into more than one substantive code. This process can be supported by the use of computer technology and software but this will be discussed elsewhere (Chapter 30).

Categories and properties

Glaser & Strauss (1967) suggest that categories can be thought of as analogous to variables in quantitative research. Categories are produced when a number of substantive codes are condensed into a higher level of abstraction. Categories are commonly used to describe a class of individuals, events, situations or phenomena that have certain characteristics in common. To have meaning, a category must be capable of being uniquely defined. For example, when examining data about the help seeking behaviour of alcohol abusers, the category 'support person behaviour' emerged, which referred to 'nurses', 'doctors', 'psychologists', 'social workers', 'family', and 'friends' who exhibited certain characteristics.

In grounded theory, the characteristics of a category are referred to as the 'properties' of the category. By studying the properties exhibited in different occurrences of the category throughout the text, similarities and differences can be identified, thus refining the definition of a specific category or, conversely, leading to the generation of new ones. Furthermore, such examination will allow you to identify the situations or conditions under which the categories occur.

Theoretical constructs

Having identified the substantive codes and then derived categories, there is a need to interweave the component parts into a coherent entity which has meaning both to you as a researcher and to those who contributed to the data. Theoretical constructs are the means by which the various categories are linked. However, it is important not to attempt to develop theoretical constructs at too early a stage as there is a danger that vital codes, categories and properties will not yet have been discovered (Corbin, 1986).

Corbin (1986) suggests that one means of identifying theoretical constructs is by asking questions of the categories so as to attempt to move categories from lower to higher levels of abstraction. Specifically, 'what is the category conveying?'. Alternatively, you can hypothesize about the relationships that may exist and test them back in the field.

Glaser (1978) suggests that by posing a series of six questions, it is easier to identify relationships amongst categories. The six questions should address cause, context, contingency, consequence, covariance and conditions. Figure 12.2 illustrates how these questions can be posed in general terms, and, in addition, a supplementary question is identified that can assist in theoretical construct formation.

(1) 'What is/are the cause(s) of behaviour manifest in a particular category?'
(2) 'Under what context does the category manifest itself?'
(3) 'Is the category contingent upon any circumstances?'
(4) 'What are the consequences of the existence of this category?'
(5) 'Does a change in this category result in a change in another category – do two or more categories covary one with another?'
(6) 'What are the conditions for the existence of this category?'
(7) 'How do cause, context, contingency, consequence, covariance and conditions interrelate?'

Fig. 12.2 Questions to assist the development of theoretical constructs (modified from Glaser, 1978).

Core categories

By linking categories together, one, and occasionally more, core categories will evolve. When you generate a theory, the core category should be at its centre and should be capable of explaining much of the variation in behaviour discovered in the data. Most other categories and their properties should relate to the core category, integrating in such a way as to produce theory that is capable of explaining the maximum amount of variation in behaviour.

Strauss (1987) identified a number of criteria that can be used to assist in the identification of the core category in study data. Figure 12.3 summarizes criteria for a core category.

(1) It is central to the theory.
(2) It is capable of accounting for a large percentage of variation in the pattern of behaviour.
(3) It must appear frequently in the data.
(4) It is clearly related to the majority of other categories.
(5) It takes longer to define the precise nature of the core category and its properties than other less central ones.
(6) A core category has clear implications for more general theory.
(7) As the core category is developed and its properties discovered, theory formation as a whole will move forward.

Fig. 12.3   Criteria for a core category.

Saturation

A category is said to be 'saturated' when examination of the data reveals no further properties and the categories are completely developed. In other words, examination of data yields only re-occurrences of material that has already been discovered, coded and integrated. When attempts to identify new data from diverse sources find nothing new, at this stage a category can be termed saturated. This implicitly implies that a category developed by studying only one data source cannot be considered saturated. Glaser & Strauss (1967) suggest that single sources can at best yield only a few categories and some of their properties. If you therefore intend to undertake a piece of research which uses the grounded theory method, you will require access to diverse data sources if you are to achieve saturation of categories.

Constant comparative method

The constant comparative method lies at the heart of the grounded theory approach and is the principal method of data analysis used in theory generation. This method of analysis entails the comparison of incidents with incidents, allowing the generation of categories. Incidents are then compared with categories, a strategy which allows you to identify the properties of the categories (see Fig. 12.4). In the early stages of category development, the comparison of incidents with categories will generate anomalies, and it is at this point that you should stop coding and record a memorandum on your thoughts on the matter (such memos are discussed in detail later in this chapter). This process then progresses to the comparison of category with category, category with construct, and construct with construct. Comparison of similar incidents will assist you in defining the basic properties of categories; it will also help you to identify the context under which the category exists or

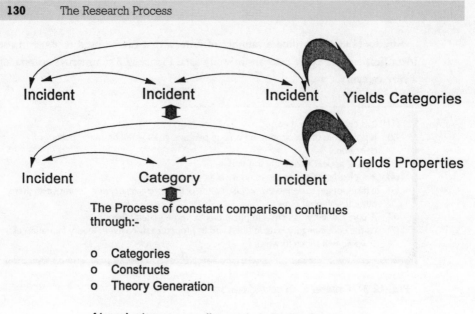

The Process of constant comparison continues through:-

o   Categories
o   Constructs
o   Theory Generation

At each stage anomalies and similarities are used to clarify boundaries and relationships

Fig. 12.4   Schematic illustration of constant comparative method.

operates. Specific differences between incidents aids the clarification of boundaries and the relationship or links that exist between categories.

As the process proceeds, you will eventually discover that you are no longer identifying new properties of categories and that the relationships between categories begin to crystallize – saturation has been reached. No longer are you discovering major anomalies in your categories, and modifications are more in terms of clarifying the relationship which link the categories and constructs together. When you have reached this stage, it is likely that you will be able to write a theory that is dense and capable of describing the basic social processes involved in the area under study. However, it is important to compare the various categories for underlying similarities which will allow you to reduce any duplication of properties or categories before you write the theory.

Memos and memo writing

Memos and memo writing, in the course of grounded theory research, are a means by which you facilitate and record the analytical process. Memo writing is at the very centre of the grounded theory method. By recording thoughts, questions and hypotheses in a permanent form, you will find it easier to track the development of categories, properties, theoretical constructs, the core category and ultimately the theory. However, memo writing is much more than simple note taking.

Memo writing should start soon after the first data have been gathered and you have started to code and analyse the content. At first, memos may be rather superficial in nature, but they will become more abstract as increasing amounts of codes, categories and properties are discovered. The memos should be thought of as a tool to assist you in exploring the developing categories and the relationship between them. Memos are written by you and are intended for you. Unfortunately, this process can be time consuming and monotonous, but it is essential to the development of theory.

For clarity, memos should be recorded on separate cards and not on the data source. Index cards are ideal, facilitate cross-referencing, are inexpensive and easy to store. Furthermore, when recording memos it is important that, in addition to the memo, certain other information is noted so as to allow you to identify what prompted your thoughts, views, questions or hypotheses. For example, the memo should be dated, titled by the categories to which it refers and references to the point that initiated your thinking. Figure 12.5 illustrates these points and gives an example of a memo written at an early stage of analysis based on the data contained in Fig. 12.1.

12.05.94   Professional Empowerment
Source   John Brown Interview 10.5.94 Page 3

A number of words and phrases seem to link together. These include getting influence, credibility, taking the initiative. I wonder how other professions see nursing research. Is nursing research seen as a way of winning back power lost as a result of organizational change?

Fig. 12.5 Index card illustrating memo writing.

Figure 12.5 illustrates that memos need not be long. However, it is important that they are recorded immediately, when thoughts are still clear. Hence always keep some index cards near at hand and record memos as and when thoughts occur. You often find that this can be at unexpected times and not just when you are working with data.

Sorting

Having accumulated a large number of memos, it is then necessary to sort them to facilitate the development of your theory. Initial memos, which focus on substantive codes, can be sorted so as to enable you to identify categories and their properties within the data. When adequate numbers of memos relating to categories have been written and are sorted, it is likely that a core category and basic social processes can be identified. Hence, sorting is seen as a means of achieving higher levels of abstraction.

When sorting, it is advisable to start by ordering memo cards by category. All memos relating to one category can then be compared for the existence of consistency. When reading through the sorted memos, frequent cross-referencing to other categories may indicate that it is possible to reduce these into one category at a higher level of abstraction. Any anomalies discovered may suggest the need to develop another category or at least gather further data so as to explain the differences.

Using literature

When conducting research which attempts to test existing theory, literature is used to place the research in context, describe its significance, identify variables and address issues of method, instrumentation, subjects and setting. Literature is consulted prior to the study so as to identify the hypothesis under examination. Although previous published research may be used to compare or contrast findings in the 'discussion' section, the literature is predominantly accessed, reviewed and critiqued prior to commencement of the study. However, a research study that uses a grounded theory design uses literature in a significantly different way. First, an initial literature search can provide evidence that little is known about the subject under study, thus supporting the need for research and, more specifically, the appropriateness of a grounded theory approach. Second, an in-depth critique of literature prior to data collection and analysis should not be undertaken since this may provide you with a framework which includes categories that are inappropriate or incomplete. Third, literature should be treated simply as another data source. That is, it should be examined, coded, analysed and have memos written about it. Finally, access to literature should be on-going. Concepts reported in published material can be examined at various stages throughout the duration of the study compared with those developed in your theory. Such an approach is particularly useful when addressing issues of reliability, validity and generalization. The existing literature can thus be used to support the developing theory.

Theory writing

Theory writing is an integral part of the grounded theory method and can be thought of as a natural extension of the memo writing process. As categories are discovered then saturated, theoretical constructs are proposed and evaluated, memos will concurrently become more abstract. By examining these abstract memos, a developing theory can be identified. Hence, writing the theory is not a deliberate and separate act, but an on-going process. Nevertheless, when writing the theory, a number of points must be considered.

First, the theory should describe the underlying basic social psychological process which accounts for the majority of variation in the data gathered.

Second, you will have been working with the data for a considerable period of time. What seems perfectly clear to you may not be as easily comprehended by colleagues. To a certain extent, this is guarded against by constantly taking your developing theory back to those who are providing data. However, peer review is a useful way of checking that the theory is understandable and not open to mis-interpretation.

Third, is the theory dense? It is essential that you examine your theory and assure yourself that all categories are saturated and that they are all connected via constructs in a meaningful way. Furthermore, it is necessary that conditions under which categories exist or operate are well defined, described, supported by suffi-cient evidence from the data.

Fourth, the theory presented must be linked to existing knowledge. If you have used existing literature and documentary sources during the process of theory development, this should not present a problem. However, if discrepancies between the existing literature and the newly developed theory remain, they must be explored and explained.

Finally, a well written grounded theory must be testable. That is, hypotheses (sometimes referred to as propositions) should be clearly stated. By stating hypotheses, you will provide direction for subsequent investigation. However, more importantly to those who provided the data, hypotheses should offer new insight into the practice, situation or event under study.

Conclusions

The grounded theory approach is a means of identifying the basic social psycho-logical processes involved in the situation under study and as a result can be considered as a powerful means of developing nursing's knowledge base. By using this method, a theory evolves from nursing practice, consequently it is likely that it is directly relevant to the clinician, thus offering greater understanding of everyday care. In conclusion, if you believe, as does the author, that understanding is necessary for the provision of high quality care, then research using the grounded theory approach has much to offer the nursing profession.

References

Aamodt, A.M. (1982) Examining ethnography for nurse researchers. *Western Journal of Nursing Research* 4(2), 209–21.

Chapman, C. (1989) Research for actions: the way forward. *Senior Nurse* 9(6), 16–18.

Corbin J. (1986) Qualitative data analysis for grounded theory. In *From Practice to Grounded Theory – Qualitative Research in Nursing*, (eds W.C. Chenitz & J.M. Swanson). Addison Wesley, Menlo Park, California.

Field, P.A. & Morse J.M. (1985) *Nursing Research – the Application of Qualitative Approaches.* Chapman and Hall, London.

Glaser, B.J. (1978) *Theoretical Sensitivity.* Sociology Press, Mill Valley, California.

Glaser B.J. & Strauss, A.L. (1967) *The Discovery of Grounded Theory.* Aldine Publishing, New York.

Goodwin, L.D. & Goodwin, W.L. (1984) Qualitative versus quantitative research or qua-litative and quantitative researcher. *Nursing Research* 33(6), 378–80.

Heinz, P.S., Scandrett-Hibden, S. & McAulay, L.S. (1990) Further assessment of a method to estimate reliability and validity of qualitative research findings. *Journal of Advanced Nursing* 15(4), 430–5.

Hilton, B.A. (1993) A study of couple communication patterns when coping with early stage breast cancer. *Canadian Oncology Nursing Journal* 3(4), 159–66.

Loving, G.L. (1993) Competence validation and cognitive flexibility: a theoretical model grounded in nursing education. *Journal of Nursing Education* 32(9), 415–21.

Luker, K.A. & Chalmers, K.I. (1989) The referral process in health visiting. *International Journal of Nursing Studies* 26(2), 173–85.

Omery, A. (1987) Qualitative research designs in the critical care setting: review in application. *Heart and Lung* 16(4), 432–6.

Stern, P.N. (1985) Using grounded theory method in nursing research. In *Qualitative Research Methods in Nursing*, (ed. M.M. Leininger). Grune and Stratton, Orlando.

Strauss, A.L. (1987) *Qualitative Analysis for Social Scientists*. Cambridge University Press, Cambridge.

Wilde, B., Starrin, B., Larsson, G. & Larsson, M. (1993) Quality of care from a patient's perspective: a grounded theory study. *Scandinavian Journal of Caring Sciences* 7(2), 113–20.

Chapter 13

Quantitative Research

Diana E. Carter

Introduction

Quantitative research has been defined as 'a formal, objective, systematic process in which numerical data are utilized to obtain information about the world' (Burns & Grove, 1987). Objective and value free collection of data in controlled settings following a predetermined research design is the underlying aim of this type of research and may go some way towards providing an explanation of cause and effect. Sometimes referred to as the traditional research process, it is regarded as being the acceptable method for developing a science.

The quantitative approach emerged from the branch of philosophy known as logical positivism, which was founded on the belief that the world could be viewed as a machine, and that the task of science was to discover the laws by which the machine operated. Having discovered these laws and learned about them, the achievement of perfect predictability was seen as a natural follow-on. The means of understanding the world can be seen in the emphasis that was placed on the measurement and quantification of observable data.

At one time, a bipolar approach to research methods prevailed. On the one hand, there were the proponents of quantitative research who argued that such an approach provided a more objective knowledge base to guide practice. Then there were other researchers who emphasized the advantages of the qualitative approach in the understanding of life experiences and their meanings. However, there is now a general recognition that each approach can make a valuable contribution to the investigation of phenomena significant to nursing.

The research approach adopted will depend on several factors including the nature of the phenomena to be investigated, the aim of the research and the state of existing knowledge. Some studies may be exclusively quantitative or qualitative, while others may effectively combine these approaches.

If the collection of more numerical and measurable information is a priority, a quantitative approach is called for. Such an approach can be seen in the study of nurses' perceptions of the needs of the suddenly bereaved in the accident and emergency department carried out by Tye (1993). That study used a structured, self-administered questionnaire and incorporated a five-point Likert-type rating scale which allowed responses to be standardized and statistically analysed.

However, as Corner (1991) suggests, using different approaches in a single study can provide a much richer and deeper understanding of what is being investigated than would otherwise be the case. Corner used a triangulation research approach to investigate the attitudes and educational preparation of newly qualified registered nurses to care for patients with cancer and to evaluate an educational intervention on cancer care for nurses, arguing that such a combination facilitated a greater understanding of the complexity of nursing practice.

Reality and its measurement

From a quantitative point of view the world is seen as stable and predictable, and the researcher believes that 'truth' is absolute and there is one single reality that can be defined by careful measurement. As Leddy & Pepper (1989) explain, numbers (for example, amount, position, time, location) are used to describe both humans and the universe in such a way as to quantify their properties. Achieving such quantification calls for precise measurement tools that will generate numerical data which can then be subjected to statistical analysis (see Chapters 27 and 28) in order to reduce and organize them and determine significant relationships. As with logical positivism, 'truth', according to the quantitative researcher, is to be discovered in common laws, principles and norms, and having discovered these it will then be possible to achieve the goal of quantitative research, which is generalizability. Generalization involves the application of trends or general tendencies (identified by studying a sample) to the population from which the research sample was drawn.

Reductionism

The process for discovering reality in quantitative research is reductionistic, which involves systematically reducing or breaking down complex information or situations into their simpler component parts in an attempt to understand the whole (see Fig. 13.1). This is illustrated in a study by Braithwaite & McGown (1993) which aimed to examine the effects of distress on the capacity of informal caregivers of stroke patients to absorb information about stroke and caregiving. It involved use of a 10-question multiple choice test to measure carers' knowledge about stroke before and after a short seminar. A psychiatric screening instrument was used to measure carers' mental health, while the stress of caregiving was assessed by means of a 16-item scale. A measure of stroke patients' functional disability was obtained by asking carers how much assistance they provided. This was achieved by asking them to use a three-point scale to indicate how much assistance they provided in relation to 11 activities of living. Finally, carers were asked to indicate (using an eight-item behaviour check-list which tapped mood disturbance and difficulty relating to others) the extent to which the recipient of care was psychologically and socially disabled. Thus, the researchers broke the whole into parts that could be

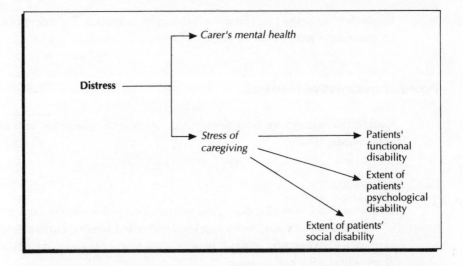

Fig. 13.1 Illustration of a reductionistic approach to distress experienced by caregivers.

examined, as could the relationships among the parts in order to gain knowledge of the whole. The underlying assumption is that the whole is the sum of the parts and the parts organize the whole.

Objectivity — *Avoiding bias*

Whereas qualitative methods facilitate study designs where the researcher and subject are part of a two-way process in which understanding develops in the development of theory (Corner, 1991), the quantitative researcher objectively distinguishes self from the subjects of the investigation, believing that boundaries must exist between them in order to ensure objectivity. Objectivity is achieved by the researcher remaining detached from the study and endeavouring to avoid influencing the study (including the subjects) with his own perceptions and values. Avoiding researcher involvement will help to guard against biasing the study towards these perceptions and values. It is acknowledged that the qualitative researcher also strives to achieve objectivity, but some of the methods of data collection used (for example, participant observation) can, by their very nature, sometimes allow subjectivity to enter into the research situation. In quantitative research the position is held that subjectivity (for example, values and feelings) cannot enter into the measurement of reality. Human behaviour is held to be objective, purposeful and, providing a valid and reliable tool is used, measurable.

I had preconceived ideas from my own practice

Quantitative measurement

A prominent feature of the data collected using the quantitative approach is that they can be measured and quantified by statistical analysis. It should however be noted that qualitative methods (such as unstructured interviews and participant observation) may also provide data which can be quantified. Further information on quantitative analysis can be found in Chapters 27 and 28.

Types of quantitative research

Quantitative research includes descriptive, correlational, quasi-experimental and experimental research.

Descriptive research

As discussed in Chapter 17, descriptive research aims to describe the characteristics of individuals and groups, such as nurses, patients and families, environments, for example the environment in which nursing is given, and situations and events such as specific nursing interventions.

For example, Sarna (1993) described the prevalence of types and dimensions of disruption in physical activities experienced by patients with non-small cell lung cancer. The subjects were all individuals who had been histologically confirmed as having non-small cell lung cancer. Using a variety of data collecting instruments, she was able to describe the extent to which the subjects were able to perform everyday activities such as bathing, dressing and climbing stairs.

Descriptive research is also a type of quantitative research which can be used to determine the frequency with which a particular variable occurs, as seen in Colbert's (1994) investigation of women consulting their GP following discovery of a breast lump. In that study it was found that of the sample selected, while 49% visited their GP within one week of finding a breast problem, 6% waited between seven and 12 months while a further 3% delayed for over a year.

Instruments used to obtain data in descriptive studies include questionnaires, interviews and observation.

Questionnaires

Questionnaires are designed to elicit information through the written responses of subjects. Although structured to the extent that each respondent will be faced with exactly the same questions in the same order, the degree of structure of individual items within the questionnaire can range from open-ended questions to closed-ended (fixed alternative) questions. The decision as to which type of question to ask will be determined to a large extent by the nature of the information required.

Narayanasamy (1993) used closed-ended questions to determine nurses' awareness and preparedness to meet patients' spiritual needs. For example, in response to the question 'To what degree do you feel your patients' spiritual needs are met?' respondents had to select one of five fixed responses:

(1)   Completely met
(2)   Well met

(3)   Adequately met
(4)   Poorly met
(5)   Not met at all.

Alternatively, the question could have been left open-ended: 'To what degree do you feel your patients' spiritual needs are met?' and respondents simply left to answer in their own words. However, an advantage of the former question is that it would be an easy matter for the researcher to tabulate the number of responses to each alternative in order to gain insight into the degree to which the respondents felt their patients' spiritual needs were met. With the open-ended question the researcher would need to develop categories and assign the open-ended responses to these so that tabulations could be made. The relative strengths and weaknesses of open and closed questions are discussed in more detail in Chapter 22.

Interviews

Interviews involve the researcher interacting with the respondent to elicit the required information verbally. As with questionnaires, interviews can vary in the degree to which they are structured. However, quantitative research generally uses structured interviews in which an interview schedule ensures that each respondent will be asked exactly the same questions in the same order, although once again, the degree of structure of individual items within the schedule can range from open-ended questions to closed-ended (fixed alternative) questions. The data collected are handled in the same way as questionnaire data, with the number of responses in each category being tabulated. Colbert (1994) used structured interviews in her study to determine why some women delay seeking help when they discover a breast problem, having established appropriate response categories following a small pilot study. (Further discussion on interviews as a method of data collection can be found in Chapter 21.)

Observation

Whilst observation is a commonly used method of data collection in qualitative research, quantitative research also uses observation techniques to produce numerical data. The observation techniques used employ previously developed mutually exclusive category systems so that the behaviour or events which are the focus of the observation can be organized and structured.

Observers may also make use of check-lists and rating scales. Check-lists are used to indicate whether or not a particular behaviour or event occurred and the number of times it was observed to occur, while rating scales allow the observer to rate the behaviour or event on a scale, thus providing more information than the dichotomous data from check-lists which simply indicate whether or not it occurred. (More information on observation is given in Chapter 23.)

Correlational research

In this type of quantitative research, the aim is to systematically investigate and explain the nature of the relationship between variables in the real world. The quantifiable data from descriptive studies are frequently analysed in this way. For example, analysis of the data obtained from parents and children through interviews, questionnaires and analogue scales by Gillies *et al.* (1994) in an investigation of post-operative pain in young children showed that although all the children studied were prescribed paracetamol, children under the age of three were more likely to be given the drug than those over three years of age.

Experimental research and quasi-experimental research

Experimental research is the most appropriate for testing cause-and-effect relationships, and is considered to be the most powerful quantitative method because of the rigorous control of variables. Quasi-experimental studies are not quite so powerful in that they lack the intensity of control which is an inherent feature of experiments. (Experimental research is further discussed in Chapter 14.)

Control

Whatever type of quantitative research and data collecting instruments you decide to use, if the findings are to accurately reflect the reality of the situation being studied your study requires to be designed in such a way as to maximize the amount of control over the research situation and variables. Through control, the influence of extraneous variables (variables which are not being studied but which could influence the results of the study by interfering with the actions of the ones being studied) is reduced.

Some of the mechanisms of control at the quantitative researcher's disposal are now discussed.

Sampling

When conducting research it is important to select a sample of subjects that is as representative as possible of the population being studied in terms of variables such as age, social class, educational level, etc. This is because the characteristics of the participants in a study have been suggested as the most common extraneous variables. If, for example, the study aimed to investigate the effect of a ward-based teaching programme on newly diagnosed diabetic patients' knowledge of their condition and its management, age and educational level could function as extraneous variables. Both variables might be related to the outcome of interest, which in this case is the patients' knowledge of their condition and its management, in that they affect how much knowledge patients gain quite independently of the teaching programme. Thus their effects are extraneous.

Random sampling techniques will help to ensure the representativeness of the sample in that each member of the population will have an equal chance of being included in the study. (Chapter 19 gives more details of sampling techniques.)

Randomization

Randomization helps the researcher to control possible extraneous variables. Using the previous example of an investigation of the effects of a ward-based teaching programme on diabetic patients' knowledge of their condition, having identified the population (patients with diabetes) the researcher would select a sample at random. This could be achieved by, for example, selecting every fourth patient from a computer-generated print-out of the population of diabetic patients. Thus, each member of the population has an equal chance of being selected and, if the sample is sufficiently large, it will be representative of the population in terms of age and sex.

It is often thought (erroneously so) that randomization is relevant only in respect of experimental research where subjects are randomly assigned to various treatment and control groups. However, it is also very relevant in relation to the data collecting instruments used in non-experimental research. For example, to investigate patients' attitudes towards information given to them during their hospital stay, it might be decided to use a series of written statements with which subjects are asked to agree or disagree. Ideally, the researcher should ensure that the order of these statements is randomized so that, for example, there is no pre-determined pattern in terms of positive and negative statements which could unwittingly interfere with subjects' responses.

The Hawthorne effect

If people are aware that they are participating in a study it is natural that they might alter their behaviour as a result, perhaps by modifying their responses to questionnaire items or by acting in a more friendly manner knowing that they are being observed, in an attempt to present themselves in a better light. This psychological response is known as the Hawthorne effect and the quantitative researcher who is trying to measure reality needs to make every effort to minimize this. There are various ways in which this can be achieved. For example, the researcher may decide to give the subjects a simple explanation of the study but omit to advise them of the actual relationship she is interested in. In an experimental study, provided subjects' rights are not infringed, you could choose not to inform subjects whether they have been assigned to the treatment or the control group.

Constancy of conditions

Ensuring that the study design is such that the conditions inherent in the research are the same for all participants is an important consideration for the researcher. Three aspects are briefly considered here: the research setting itself, control of input and time factors.

The research setting

In the interest of achieving constancy, consideration needs to be given to the degree of control exerted over the actual research setting. Mentioned earlier was the study by Braithwaite & McGown (1993) who were interested in the capacity of caregivers to learn about stroke relative to their measured degree of emotionality, and who measured caregivers' knowledge before and after a two hour seminar on the subject. To accommodate as many caregivers as possible they offered the seminars on several occasions. In that example, it would be important for the researchers to ensure not only that the same information was given to all the subjects using the same medium, but also that environmental conditions remained constant (for both the knowledge testing and teaching). Any discrepancy in terms of the research setting could be reflected when the subjects' knowledge is tested. If the environment in which the knowledge testing and teaching were given was not held constant then the outcome (that is, the caregivers' measured knowledge of stroke) may not be so much a reflection of the seminar (or their level of emotionality) but more a reflection of the effects of the environmental conditions in which the knowledge testing and teaching were carried out. In that particular example, it would not be too difficult for the researchers to partially control the research setting by ensuring that all knowledge testing and teaching were carried out using the same environmental conditions for all, such as an empty seminar room.

Clearly, the more the research setting can be controlled, the more effective the researcher will be in reducing the influence of extraneous environmental variables, and the more accurate will be the examination of the cause-and-effect relationships of the variables studied.

Control of input

A lot of nursing research is concerned with measuring the effects of specific nursing interventions and it is therefore important that control over these interventions is exercised. In studies such as the one cited above by Braithwaite & McGown (1993) it would be relatively easy to ensure that the same person provided the same information for the subjects. However, during the course of studies of nursing interventions, many members of the health care team are likely to come into contact with the subjects who form the sample, and their uncontrolled, unmeasured input is likely to be different for each subject.

In some instances, the role of the subjects' families and friends may influence the situation the researcher is trying to control. Additionally, if knowledge levels are a focus of interest in a study the intervention (say, a teaching programme) may stimulate the subjects to find out more about the topic themselves. Thus, if Braithwaite & McGown (1993) tested their subjects' post-seminar levels of knowledge at a later date it would be difficult to determine whether any measured increase in knowledge was an effect of the seminar or a reflection of additional information gleaned from other sources. This type of input is often very difficult to control. Information given to the subjects about the study is within the researcher's control, and one should ensure that each subject receives identical information about, for example, the purpose of the study and the use that will be made of the data.

Time factors

Depending on the time of day subjects may be more or less attentive to information being given. The time interval between an intervention and the measuring of the effects of this could also influence the findings. Similarly, subjects' responses to testing may also be influenced by whether this is carried out in the morning or the afternoon, and by the timing of data collection in relation to other events. For example, all the women interviewed by Colbert (1994) in her study to determine the reasons why women delay in consulting their GP when they discover a breast lump were interviewed immediately after their initial meeting with the oncologist. It was argued that at this time the women's anxiety would have been allayed and that there would be a greater willingness to express their thoughts and feelings. Irrespective of the rationale behind such a decision in this particular study, the important point to note is that the timing of the interview was held constant for all subjects.

Conclusion

The quantitative–qualitative debate has waned in recent years and it is now generally accepted that both approaches have the potential to make valuable contributions to the development of nursing knowledge. Indeed many studies combine both the qualitative and quantitative approaches to good effect, each approach serving to complement the other and each generating different kinds of knowledge that will be useful in practice.

References

Braithwaite, V. & McGown, A. (1993) Caregivers' emotional well-being and their capacity to learn about stroke. *Journal of Advanced Nursing*, **18**(2), 195–202.

Burns N. & Grove, S.K. (1987) *The Practice of Nursing Research: Conduct, Critique and Utilization.* W.B. Saunders, Philadelphia.

Colbert K. (1994) Why opt for an unnecessary delay? Delays in presentation of breast cancer. *Professional Nurse*, **9**(9), 643–5.

Corner, J. (1991) In search of more complete answers to research questions. Quantitative versus qualitative research methods: is there a way forward? *Journal of Advanced Nursing*, **16**(6), 718–27.

Gillies, M.L., Parry-Jones, W.L. & Smith, L.N. (1994) Postoperative pain in children under five years. *Health Bulletin*, **52**(3), 193–5.

Leddy, S. & Pepper, J.M. (1989) *Conceptual Bases of Professional Nursing.* Lippincott, Philadelphia.

Narayanasamy, A. (1993) Nurses' awareness and educational preparation in meeting their patients' spiritual needs. *Nurse Education Today*, 13(3), 196–201.

Sarna, L. (1993) Fluctuations in physical function: adults with non-small cell lung cancer. *Journal of Advanced Nursing*, 18(5), 714–24.

Tye, C. (1993) Qualified nurses' perceptions of the needs of suddenly bereaved family members in the accident and emergency department. *Journal of Advanced Nursing*, 18(6), 948–56.

Chapter 14

Experimental Research

Allan S. Presly

This chapter is not designed to enable you to carry out experimental research unaided, but is intended to familiarize you with the more common types of experimental design, so that accounts of research can be read more critically and with greater understanding. It is also intended to help you learn enough about experimental research to be able to make a provisional decision on which research design might be most suitable for your needs. You can then go on to find out more about this design, and to seek advice from an experienced researcher in the field.

As the name implies, experimental design refers to the overall plan of any experimental research project. It is important to note the term *design*, as it emphasizes that all good research should have been planned or worked out in advance. This is to ensure, as far as possible, that the researcher, at the end of an experimental research project, can make a statement of the kind: 'The introduction of, or change in variable *A* (the independent variable) caused the change in *B* (the dependent variable)'. This will only be possible if the experimental design has ruled out the possibility that a variety of things other than *A* could have caused the change in *B*. That is, if it is claimed that it has been proved that treatment *A* causes improvement in condition *B*, the research design has to be such that other possible variables such as better nursing care, bedrest, or better diet in hospital, have not caused the improvement.

There is no single all-purpose experimental design. Many different ones have been proposed to tackle different sorts of problems, but they all have in common the fact that they are intended to help eliminate explanations of research findings other than the one in which the researcher is interested.

Three main types of design will be discussed. In the first of these, a comparison is made of two or more *independent groups* of subjects treated under different conditions. In the second type of design, *repeated measures* are carried out on the same group of subjects, but under different conditions. In the third design, *a single subject* only is used, and the subject's response studied under different conditions.

Comparison of independent groups

Let us assume that the researcher is interested in what causes the birth weight of babies to vary. Obviously, human beings vary naturally among themselves in all sorts of ways even when they come from very similar backgrounds. Birth weight is no exception to this. That is to say, most characteristics of human beings show a range of variation which, within certain limits, is considered normal. This could be said not only of physical factors such as height and weight, but also for psychological and social factors such as intelligence or sociability.

Sample means

Suppose then that all the babies born in a large city in one year are examined and their birth weight recorded. The average (or more correctly the *mean*) birth weight of babies in that city might be calculated and found to be 3.2 kg. Checking all the babies' weights, or assessing all the members of any research population of interest, is often an impossible task. More often one would select a sample of the population and try to generalize on the basis of that. Thus, a random sample (see Chapter 2) of 50 babies born in the city in a given year could be selected and the mean birth weight calculated. A result very close to the result which would have been obtained from the whole population is likely to be obtained. If this exercise was to be repeated with a second random sample of 50, a mean weight close to (but probably not identical to) the true mean would be obtained. If this sampling of sets of 50 were repeated over and over again, the means would not be exactly the same. If, however, the samples are truly random, the sample means will tend to cluster, or be distributed, around the true mean, some lower and some higher. This variation will be accepted as normal variation in mean birth weights.

Figure 14.1 shows this normal variation in diagrammatic form. *O* represents the true mean birth weight of all the babies in the city. Each *X* represents the mean obtained from a random sample of 50 babies. It can be seen that in three samples the mean was the same as in the total population; in three samples it was slightly above and in three samples slightly below. This is taken as a normal acceptable variation in mean birth weights. Any one of the random samples will give a mean which will adequately represent the mean of the whole population.

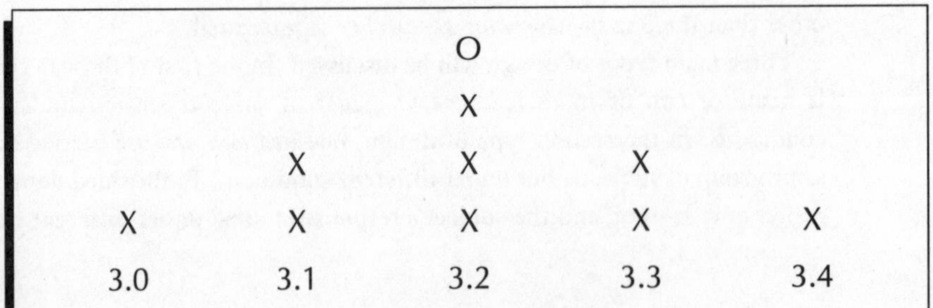

Fig. 14.1 Normal birth weight variation (example).

Forming an experimental hypothesis

If these findings were made public, it might be the case that one health visitor might indicate that she has kept records of birth weights of babies in her practice. The mean she gets is considerably lower (2.8 kg) than that found by the researcher and it looks as if it is outside the range of normal variation which has been established by the researcher's sampling procedure. What might be the explanation of this? A first step would be to compare the health visitor's sample with the one used by the researcher. Only if her sample could be considered a random sample from the total population can it be directly compared. It might then be discovered that this health visitor works in a rundown city area with poor housing conditions and amenities. If so, her sample must be regarded as a biased one and not properly representative of the whole population; thus, her mean cannot be directly compared with that in the original research. Something other than normal variation due to sampling must be found to explain the difference.

There are a number of factors which might account for such a situation in a poor area; less money, poorer attendance for ante-natal care, poorer nutrition, higher rates of smoking and alcohol use, and so on. Any of these variables might be the reason for the lower mean birth weight, but from this information alone there is no way of knowing which. It could be any one of them or a combination of several (see Dowding, 1982). One way to find out would be to design an experiment. If it is hypothesized that poor nutrition in the mothers is the most likely cause of low birth weight, how can this be tested separately from the effects of all the other possible factors? One suggestion is a comparison of two groups of babies who are similar in all respects except for the nutritional state of their mothers. That is, by comparing two groups in this way one can control for, or eliminate from consideration, all the variables except the ones of interest, birth weight, the dependent variable, and the nutritional state of the mothers, the independent variable. The research can then set out to discover what effect planned variation in the one (nutritional state) causes in the other (birth weight). More technically, the hypothesis is that if the nutritional state of pregnant mothers is improved, then the mean birth weight of their babies will increase.

A typical experimental design to test this hypothesis could be a comparison of independent groups.

(1)   A large group of pregnant women from a defined area would be selected. Ideally, it would be selected to be representative of all such women from that area, by means of random sampling, for example. In practice, however, it is more likely to be drawn from a population readily available, such as those attending one large hospital rather than from several hospitals scattered across the area. This is sometimes known as a 'convenience sample'. It would thus not be as representative as might be desirable. Members of the group would then be randomly allocated to two equal sub-groups, an experimental group and a control group.

(2)   The independent variable, the nutritional state of the women, must now be manipulated in one group and not in the other. That is, one new factor, and

only one, is introduced into one group (the experimental group) which is not present in the other (the control group). It could be argued that the nutritional state of pregnant women might be improved through dietary advice and supervision by health visitors, and a programme of such advice to be given to only one group of women could be arranged. The details of the dietary advice programme would then be worked out: where, how often and in what form, and by whom the advice would be given. This will ensure that the procedure of the experiment will be the same for all subjects and that the experiment can, if necessary, be replicated exactly by someone else.

(3)   Birth weights would be recorded in the same way for each group, preferably by someone who is not aware of which group the woman falls into. The birth weights provide the experimental data and from them the mean birth weight for each group can be calculated.

(4)   The question in this experiment is whether the mean birth weight of the experimental group is greater than the mean of the control group. However, suppose it is established that this is the case but only by a very small amount. It would be difficult to conclude with any certainty that the experiment has been a success since it is known (see Fig. 14.1) that mean birth weights of different samples vary slightly anyway. Therefore the real question then becomes: 'Is the difference between the average birth weight of the experimental and control groups greater than would be expected if any two random samples from the same population are compared?'. That is, is the difference apparently produced via the independent variable greater than would be expected by chance?

(5)   It could clearly be difficult to reach agreement on this simply by inspecting the mean weights, especially where differences were small. It is to help reach such agreement that some inferential statistical methods have been developed (see Chapter 28). These are specifically designed to assess what the normal variation in birth weight is likely to be and whether the experimental group mean is outside this range.

(6)   Suppose that the application of such statistics allows us to conclude that there is a significant difference between the experimental and control group means, with the mean weight of the experimental group being significantly higher. It can then reasonably be concluded that better nutrition in pregnant women will result in an increase in the mean birth weight of babies.

The foregoing example is only one of many possible types of experimental design although it is probably the simplest and most commonly used. It is widely used to evaluate new drugs and new treatment procedures, and numerous examples can be found in many research journals. See, for example, the report by O'Sullivan & Jacobsen (1992), which is an assessment of the effectiveness of a health care programme for teenage mothers. Miller *et al.* (1990) used a comparison of two independent groups to assess patients' compliance with a programme of diet and exercise following myocardial infarction. A third example is the report by Gift *et al.* (1992).

No-treatment and placebo control groups

In a typical treatment trial, the experimental group might receive the new treatment and the control group, none. This use of a no-treatment control, however, has been shown to be not entirely satisfactory. There is an ethical problem in withholding treatment, even temporarily, from those patients who might benefit from it, but there is also a scientific problem. The belief that one is being appropriately treated for a given condition even when one is not, has been shown in itself to produce some improvement. This alone might account for the difference between a group receiving genuine treatment and a group receiving none. This is commonly referred to as the 'placebo' effect. It has become the usual procedure in treatment research, therefore, to include a placebo control group rather than a no-treatment control group to compare with the experimental group. In nursing research, a placebo might be a lotion made up in exactly the same form as the treatment lotion but containing a substance known to have no effect on the condition concerned. This would then have the effect of making the procedure much more similar between treatment and control groups than a treatment/no-treatment comparison.

Referring back to the previous example, it could be argued that the difference produced in the birth weights might not have been due to the dietary advice. It could be, for example, that through more regular contact with the health visitors, mothers were more likely to attend clinics, and that this factor, rather than improved nutrition, made the difference. It would, therefore, have been a better designed experiment if, for example, the control group mothers received the same number of visits from health visitors but during these visits no dietary advice was given. This would then be a form of placebo rather than no-treatment control. It would be a better test of the value of dietary advice since it would eliminate another possible explanation of our result. An example of this type of design can be found in the study by Creason et al. (1989) on reducing levels of incontinence in aged female nursing-home residents. One group (experimental) received regular reminders about toileting; the second group (placebo) received the same amount of additional social contact, but no such reminder; the third group (no treatment) continued under the same conditions as before.

'Blind' assessment

In this and other types of research design, it has also proved to be the case that those assessing the effects of treatment can be influenced by knowing whether a patient was receiving the real treatment as opposed to the placebo. There will naturally be a greater inclination to see improvement in those in the experimental (treatment) group and so possibly to exaggerate the overall differences between the groups. It has thus become common practice that the assessors are not made aware of which group a patient belongs to, a procedure known as a 'blind'.

Theoretically, there is no limit to the number of groups which can be included in an experiment. One might perhaps have three randomly selected groups in a treatment evaluation experiment, one treated with the new treatment, one with a placebo and one with a treatment previously found to be helpful for the condition being studied. In this case, the new treatment must prove itself superior not only to the placebo, the 'expectation-of-treatment' effect, but also to the existing remedy. Again, there is no reason why two new procedures or treatments cannot be evaluated at once, for example, two new teaching methods versus an existing one, two different types of dietary advice or two or more doses of a new drug against a placebo. Provided that groups are selected at random and the only procedural difference among the groups is in the level of the independent variable, type or dose of drug, type of dietary advice or teaching method, any number of groups can be included in this research design. Agars & McMurray (1993) for example assessed the effectiveness of three different methods of teaching breast self-examination, each method being applied to a different group of subjects. A fourth group acted as a 'no-treatment' control group. In a study by Caruso *et al.* (1992) patients with fever were randomly allocated to four different groups in a trial of the effectiveness of four different cooling blanket temperatures.

Repeated measures

The comparison of independent, randomly selected groups does have one major disadvantage. It may require a larger number of possible subjects than are readily available in the time required. One alternative, therefore, is to use what is known as a 'repeated measures' design. In this design, both procedures or treatments are given to the same sample in succession rather than separately to two different samples. At first sight this design appears to have considerable advantages. There is an obvious saving in the number of subjects required since the same group is used twice, or more often if necessary. Also, random sampling of independent groups will result in some, usually slight, differences between the samples which might affect the outcome of the experiment. This is obviously ruled out in a repeated measures design, as the sample used for each treatment is identical. However, this design has one major disadvantage. The effect of the second treatment or procedure may be influenced by the fact that the subjects have already undergone the first. There may be a 'carry-over effect' in that by the time they received the second treatment, the sample of subjects is not exactly the same as the one which received the first. Reid *et al.* (1993) used a repeated measures design to examine the effects of different lengths of shifts on the quality of nursing care, and they note in their report some of the difficulties with this research design.

Cross-over design

Another design which was developed to try to cancel out the effects of any carry-over is known as a 'cross-over' design where half the subjects, group A, will receive treatment I followed by treatment II, and the other half, group B, treatment II followed by treatment I. This does not eliminate the carry-over effect, but it may be reduced. It can be argued that any difference that may then be found between group A and group B cannot be put down to the fact that treatment II always follows treatment I or vice versa. Although this design is still commonly used, it is now known that it does not reduce the effects of carry-over as much as was once thought. Considerable caution should thus be used in interpreting any results from such an experiment.

An example of a repeated-measures design with cross-over is to be found in the article by Campbell (1989) where a comparison was made of the effectiveness of two types of milk in treating infant colic. Figure 14.2 shows the design of this experiment.

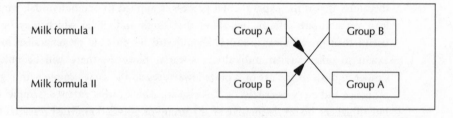

Fig. 14.2   Repeated-measures design with cross-over.

A group of babies with severe colic was selected. They were randomly allocated to two groups, A and B. Before the experiment began, an initial assessment of the degree of colic was made over a one-week period. This is called a baseline. It is an essential element in any experimental design as it represents accurately the situation existing before any change is introduced. Group A then received milk formula I for 1 week followed by milk formula II for a further week. Group B received formula II followed by formula I. The degree and frequency of colic was assessed by the mothers at regular intervals.

If all the babies had received formula I followed by formula II, and if formula I had apparently proved to be superior, that conclusion would have been open to the criticism that it was simply the fact that formula I was tried first which explained the outcome. By giving half the babies formula I first and the others formula II first, this criticism is apparently overcome. This supposed solution to the problem of order and carry-over effects is known as counterbalancing. Even with counter-balancing, however, the repeated measures design still has problems concerning the applicability of conventional statistical methods. Also, as noted earlier, the capacity of the cross-over variation to eliminate carry-over effects remains in some doubt.

This experiment by Campbell (1989) also provides an example of 'blind' assessment, referred to earlier. The milks were packaged in identical coded tins, and the code was not made known until the end of the experiment. Thus the mother's assessment could not have been influenced by knowing which formula her baby was receiving at any given time.

Another study which used a repeated-measures design, with counterbalancing was by Deiriggi (1990). She used this design to assess the effects of water-bed flotation on the energy levels of premature babies. A similar example can be found in the report by McCain (1992).

Single subject

The third type of experimental design is usually referred to as 'single-subject' or 'single-case' design. As the name implies, this design uses only one subject who is exposed to the different treatments or experimental conditions in sequence. One of the arguments put forward in favour of this design is that the traditional method of comparing average scores of independently selected groups may give little useful information about how any individual in those groups may respond or how any similar individual, as opposed to a similar group, will respond in the future. The mean results may not in fact fit any one subject very well. It is argued, therefore, that if the experimental process is applied to one individual, we will at least get accurate information about that single individual which may be more useful than group means, and it should still be possible to generalize to some extent to other similar individuals. Clearly, however, there will be objections similar to those of the use of repeated measures on the same sample with regard to sequence and carry-over effects. It is also arguable to what extent a 'sample' of one individual can be representative of any group or population. Most research theory follows the argument that the larger the sample which can be assessed, the more representative it is likely to be and therefore the more widely the results can be generalized.

Typically, in a single-subject design, the subject will be studied first under baseline conditions, the conditions which prevailed before any experimental change was made. During this period, all the relevant variables will be measured, and in some ways, this phase can be compared to a no-treatment condition in group research. Following the baseline period, one new factor is then introduced, the independent variable, and the effect on the selected dependent variable assessed. Provided the introduction of this factor is the only change, and that conditions are otherwise identical to the baseline, then it is argued that the change in the independent variable caused the change in the dependent variable.

The work of Turnbull (1993) is an example of the use of a single-subject design in nursing research. His experiment was designed to assess the effectiveness of two methods of reducing excessive consumption of water (polydipsia) by a patient with mild learning difficulties and a schizo-affective psychosis. The design and results of the experiment can be seen in Fig. 14.3.

In experimental phase A1 (baseline) the amount of water drunk over a 10 day period was recorded before any change was made. In phase B1 (first treatment phase) a system of rewards was introduced for reduced water consumption and, as can be seen, the level of water consumption decreased substantially. In phase A2 (return to baseline) the rewards are withdrawn and the conditions were thus the same as in phase A1. The water consumption duly returned to the previous levels. In phase B2 (second treatment phase) the rewards were re-introduced, resulting in a reduction in consumption level similar to phase B1. Finally, in phase C (third treatment phase), a specific reduced target (five drinks per day) was agreed with the patient, as well as continuing the reward system. The results clearly show a further substantial reduction in water consumption.

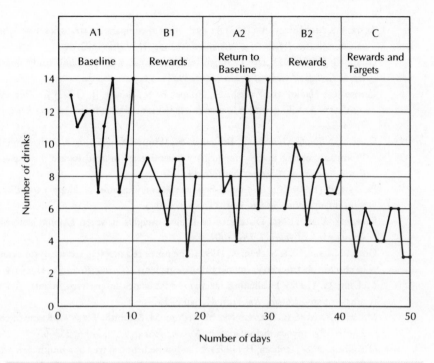

Fig. 14.3 Example of single-subject research design: reduction in excessive water consumption over a period of 50 days.

In this experiment, the dependent variable was the level of water consumption. There were two independent variables, the reward system and the target setting. The repetition of the AB sequence (A1B1 followed by A2B2) strengthens the overall conclusion that the introduction of rewards produced a reduction in consumption, and was further reduced in phase C. A causal connection was thus demonstrated between the independent and the dependent variables. It is not being claimed that this result applies to any other patient with similar problems. This patient was not selected as a 'sample' of such patients. However, it cannot be denied that this single-case experiment gives a clear indication as to what is more than likely to happen in other similar cases.

The three basic experimental designs, *comparison of independent groups*, *repeated measures* and *single-subject*, have been described. All have their advantages and disadvantages. Which type applies when any particular research question arises is not an easy matter and expert advice should always be sought before such a decision is made. Although the purpose of these basic experimental designs, and of many variations not mentioned here, is to allow clear-cut conclusions to be drawn, it must be said that the best-planned research will answer some questions, but will raise at least as many more that require further research. That is how science progresses.

References

Agars, J. & McMurray, A. (1993) An evaluation of comparative strategies for teaching breast self-examination. *Journal of Advanced Nursing*, **18**, 1595–1603.

Campbell, J. (1989) Dietary treatment of infant colic: a double-blind study. *Journal of the Royal College of General Practitioners*, **39**, 11–14.

Caruso, C., Hadley B., Rakesh, S., Frame, P. & Khoury, J. (1992) Cooling effects and comfort of 4 cooling blanket temperatures in humans with fever. *Nursing Research*, **41**, No 2, 68–72.

Creason, N.D., Grybowski, J., Burgener, S., Whippo, C., Yeo, S. & Richardson, B. (1989) Prompted voiding therapy for urinary incontinence in aged female nursing-home residents. *Journal of Advanced Nursing*, **14**, 120–6.

Deiriggi, P. (1990) Effects of water-bed flotation on indicators of energy expenditure in pre-term infants. *Nursing Research*, **39**, No 3, 140–5.

Dowding, V.M. (1982) Distributions of birth-weights in seven Dublin Maternity Units. *British Medical Journal*, **284**, 1901–4.

Gift, A., Moore, T. & Socken, K. (1992) The use of relaxation to reduce dyspnea and anxiety in chronic obstructive pulmonary disease patients. *Nursing Research*, **41**, No 4, 243–6.

McCain, G. (1992) Facilitating inactive/awake states in preterm infants. A study of 3 interventions. *Nursing Research*, **41**, No 3, 157–60.

Miller, P., Wikoff, R., Garrett, M., McMahon, M. & Smith, T. (1990) Regimen compliance 2 years after myocardial infarction. *Nursing Research*, **39**, No 6, 333–6.

O'Sullivan, A. & Jacobsen, B. (1992) A randomised control trial of a health care program for first-time adolescent mothers and their infants. *Nursing Research*, **41**, No 4, 210–15.

Reid, N., Robinson, G. & Todd, C. (1993) The quality of nursing care on wards working 8 and 12 hour shifts. *International Journal of Nursing Studies*, **30**, 403–14.

Turnbull, J. (1993) Treatment of polydipsia using a contingency management procedure incorporating a self-management approach: a single case study. *Behavioural and Cognitive Psychotherapy*, **21**, 275–9.

Action research is a relatively new approach in nursing but is rapidly attracting considerable interest because it is so highly suited to the kind of problem-solving and evaluation research which the profession needs. As well as being very similar in its methods to the stages of the nursing process, action research has parallels with other current trends within nursing. Nursing development units are being set up so that practitioners can implement and monitor research-based care and try to narrow the theory–practice gap. Action research also attempts to close the gap between the theory and practice of research, and to help participants to learn about doing research. The role of the researchers in action research is also to assist practitioners to take control of and change their own work. This parallels moves for nurses into patient/client advocate roles, empowering people to have more autonomy and control over their own health care.

This chapter will discuss these issues in greater detail, show what action research is, how the approach has come into being, and detail some action research projects in nursing.

What is action research?

Action research is a way of doing research and working on solving a problem at the same time. Researcher and participants work together to analyse the situation they wish to change: this may include doing some baseline measures using questionnaires, observation or other research methods. After this assessment they can then plan the desired change, set their objectives, and decide how to bring about the change. While they are putting their plans into action, they continue to monitor progress, changing their plans if this is judged appropriate. At the completion of the change process, they will make a final assessment and draw conclusions, perhaps writing a report on the project for themselves and/or others.

According to Smith (1986), 'action research, as the name implies, is a process containing both investigation and the use of its findings'. She used an action research approach in a hospital for the care of elderly people to facilitate changes which would improve the quality of life for patients. Action research was chosen for this project because it places emphasis on the developmental aspects of research and can cope with the resistance which is often encountered when changes are introduced. Results are fed back into the change process while the research is on-going, and the participating nurses are involved in the research alongside the research team. By being so closely involved in the study, the researchers are able to gain deep understanding of the setting and put forward realistic plans for changes (Smith, 1986).

Sandow (1979) used action research in an intervention study in which she acted as a resource person to groups of parents of handicapped children and evaluated the outcomes. Sandow is not a nurse, but both her subject matter and methods were similar to that of Smith. Sandow sees action research as offering 'a bridge between pure and applied research'. There are at least two participants – the practitioner/evaluator and the recipient of the service, who is both *subject* and *client*.

In summary, action research provides a method for improving working methods based on research organized by professionals. It takes a critical view of existing practices, and it provides a theoretical basis for professional decisions. In describing the role of the teacher–researcher in action research, Carr & Kemmis (1986) accurately portray the role of the nurse–researcher too.

Action research in facilitating change

What these definitions have in common is an emphasis on action research as a method of facilitating change through involving and motivating participants in a given project. Involvement is crucial for the researcher too, for it allows her to gain a much deeper understanding of the setting and the change processes than she would otherwise have. In other words, both sides in the research encounter stand to benefit. Participants are helped to implement the changes they desire and at the same time learn about how to do research, while the researcher also extends her knowledge and experience of the process of research and learns about the particular area being studied.

Contained within these definitions are clues about why the action research approach has been developed and what its origins are. These points will be dealt with in more detail in the following section because they lead on to a discussion of the particular methods used in action research projects, and to what makes action research distinct from previously established approaches.

Why action research?

Action research can capitalize on the advantages and compensate for the limitations of the traditional quantitative and qualitative approaches. These are discussed in detail in Chapters 11 and 13 respectively, but it is necessary to outline some of their features here in order to explain how the critical approach of action research has come about.

Quantitative research

Quantitative research was the original approach adopted by natural scientists studying psychics, chemistry, astronomy, biology, and so on. This approach relied on the observation of phenomena and their behaviour, whether these were stars, chemicals, animals, or subsystems of these, such as the renal or cardiovascular systems. The fundamental aim was to control natural events by being able to predict what would happen and then to intervene to change things (Allen, 1985). For example, if a law can be established which shows that bacterium X requires certain conditions to live and reproduce, then intervening to alter these conditions will result in the death of the strain and the treatment or prevention of infection.

Quantitative researchers claim that their research methods are objective. The researcher studies a particular subject without having any preconceptions or preferences about the outcome of the study, and without interfering in the natural course of the events. In this sense, natural science claims to be value-free in that the personal values of the scientist are irrelevant to the scientific study.

It is equally possible to show that beliefs and values enter into all stages of the research process, from decisions about which methods to use (for example whether experiments on animals will be used), right through to what level of statistical significance to choose as accepting or rejecting the research hypothesis.

Furthermore, quantitative scientists are increasingly realizing that their research does have an intrusive effect on the subject matter they are studying. It seems obvious, for example, that experimental psychologists studying rats will influence the rats' behaviour by the way they handle them. Rough handling will induce stress and alter biochemical measures of anxiety which may well have an effect on the findings.

Qualitative research

In response to these and other criticisms of quantitative science, qualitative workers have developed different methods which they claim are more suited to the different methods which social scientists study, namely human beings. This second approach has also been called *interpretive* science because its goal is understanding rather than control. Qualitative social scientists aim to understand or interpret people's behaviour by learning how they themselves make sense of the world in which they live. Communication is the means whereby interpretive scientists come to share the same understandings as their subjects and arrive at a consensus interpretation of the meaning of events.

The *ideal* form of interpretive study is anthropology, where anthropologists spend an extended period of time living among a group of people in order to understand their way of life. Classically, anthropologists knew they had truly understood the society under study when they could live like a *native* in that society quite naturally and spontaneously without having to think about how to behave. Today it is perhaps more common for this type of method to be used to study a group in one's own society but the methods are basically the same, as is the end point and aim, of being able to understand by empathy and consensus how and why the people beings studied behave as they do.

Like quantitative approaches, qualitative approaches have their limitations. In both approaches, the researcher is the *expert* who chooses what and how to study, who has the knowledge and expertise, and who does research *on* the subjects – whether these are rats, bacteria or humans. In other words, the research relationship is a hierarchical power relationship, and research subjects give up their time and energy to take part in the research but receive little or nothing in return. Both types of research can therefore be described as exploiting their subjects.

Inequality between the researcher and those studied in both quantitative and qualitative approaches is also evident in the degree of *exposure* each receives. Research subjects make themselves vulnerable by disclosing their activities and meanings, and sometimes their deepest and most personal secrets to researchers. Researchers' personal lives, beliefs and feelings, however, are left out of the research. This can add to the false *objectivity* of research because readers who do not know about the researchers' personal views cannot judge the extent to which these have influenced their interpretations of the data.

Related to these inequalities are the different rewards which researchers and researched obtain from participating in the study. Research subjects often gain nothing, other than perhaps the gratification of having a researcher show an interest in them and take what they are saying seriously. Once the researcher has collected that data, however, nothing changes for the subjects – they are left with their problems and concerns, and life goes on much the same as before. The researcher, on the other hand, stands to gain a great deal in terms of career advancement, financial rewards and an enhanced reputation from publishing the research report.

A further limitation of interpretive research is that it gives a false impression about reality, but in a different way from that of quantitative research. Whilst not claiming objectivity, it does give the impression that the basis of all human relationships is communication. Therefore if something goes wrong in social life, we can put it right by improving communications. While there may be something in this, it is very often the case that features that lie beyond communications are at the heart of the problem and it is misleading to imply that people can change their own situations fairly easily by improving communications. For example, the nurse–doctor relationship is based on differences in power which can lead to doctors telling nurses to mislead or lie to patients about their diagnosis. Nurses are often afraid to 'disobey' doctors in this respect, and no amount of attempts to improve nurse–doctor communications may be able to persuade some doctors not to behave in this way. Nurses are not able to make fundamental changes in this aspect of their practice by improving communications because the underlying power structures which have been in place for centuries remain.

Critical science

In response to these and other criticisms and limitations of both quantitative and qualitative approaches (Allen, 1985; Webb, 1989), a third approach called critical science has emerged. Allen states that,

> 'the fundamental goal of critical science is to establish the conditions for open, unconstrained communication. This entails exposing hidden power imbalances'.

He likens the critical research approach to informed consent, in which all participants can act with autonomy and responsibility because obstacles which block or distort communication have been removed.

Critical science as an approach has therefore been developed to overcome problems and limitations with earlier quantitative approaches. Action research is one method of carrying out critical science, just as experiments are a quantitative method, and participant observation and unstructured interviews are qualitative methods. Having examined the origins of critical science and action research, it is now possible to look in more detail at how research is carried out.

Performing action research

Several writers have put forward schemes to illustrate the stages involved in carrying out action research, and it is easy to see how these mirror the problem-solving strategies which are also reflected in the nursing process. Towell & Harries (1979) describe a 'general model of the change process in project work', whose five major stages are illustrated in Fig. 15.1.

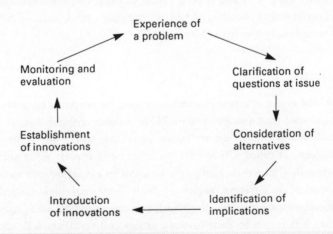

Fig. 15.1 The stages of action research.

However, there are additional activities which run alongside and concurrently with these stages: these include seeking assistance, establishing a project committee, investigation to illuminate issues, choices by staff and working through their implications, and review of the changes introduced.

Whereas previous approaches to research have used a one-directional approach, moving from one stage to the next and so on to completion of the study, on-going monitoring, feedback to participants and modifications to the innovation being introduced are a crucial feature of action research.

Lauri (1982) emphasizes this constant reviewing and modification in her four-point list of the stages of action research:

(1) Preliminary diagnosis and the collection of baseline data.
(2) Processing the results with participants.
(3) Re-planning and re-implementation of the activity to be changed.
(4) Assessment of the changes and utilization of the results.

In summary, she writes that

> 'constant monitoring and evaluating of the activity is one of the leading principles of the action research'.

Hunt (1987) similarly drew attention to the cyclical nature of the action/evaluation process, feedback to participants as the study progresses, collaboration in setting and monitoring achievement of objectives and use of group dynamics in carrying out the research.

Implicit in these descriptions of the action research process is that participants will be willing volunteers. They must want to examine their own practices and change them if deficiencies or better methods are identified. Otherwise, the action research will fail because collaboration will not be achieved between researcher and participants (Webb, 1989). The starting point for action research is thus the recognition by workers of problems in their present working practices and a wish to change their activities (Lauri, 1982). Consent and collaboration may have to be renegotiated as the action research progresses, particularly if staff turnover in the research setting is high (Meyer, 1993).

Triangulation

A vital aspect of action research is its use of a variety of methods which give more valid data than a single method. This is called triangulation, as discussed earlier, and this is a term derived from surveying, where surveyors use a measuring instrument called a theodolite mounted on a tripod. What surveyors are doing when they take their readings is to measure a building or a road junction from a number of different angles in both horizontal and vertical planes. These measurements then give them such a complete and detailed picture of the site that they can return to their drawing offices and construct scale diagrams and even models of it.

This complete and full picture is what social researchers also aim for in using a triangulated approach. They might use several different methods to cross-check on data, for example, backing questionnaire data up with observations as already discussed. Or they might study more than one group of research subjects in different settings to compare their behaviour. Yet again, several different researchers might participate in the project, each bringing their own perspectives and skills to collecting and interpreting the data.

Methodical eclecticism

Methodological eclecticism is a technical term linked with triangulation by its rejection of the straitjacket of either quantitative or qualitative methods. Being eclectic means choosing freely from what is available according to one's preference. So a person with eclectic tastes in music might like Chopin, jazz and 1960s music rather than sticking to one particular style. In action research, this free choice of different methods allows the advantages of some methods to offset the limitations of others, and enables one to 'have one's cake and eat it'!

Reflexivity

Reflexivity is another important concept within critical science and therefore also within action research. This term refers to the need for researchers to put themselves 'on the line' in their research reports in the same way that participants are made vulnerable by revealing their innermost thoughts and emotions. As well as making the research encounter a more equal one, and removing the exploitation which can be part of traditional approaches, researchers need to 'come clean' about themselves for other reasons. Readers of research reports can only make judgements about the quality of the research and the researcher's interpretations if they have access to all the data that went into the report. The beliefs and attitudes of researchers are part of this data and should be made available in the report.

Because action research is concerned with developing research methods as well as with introducing and evaluating changes in practice, researchers also need to write about the process of carrying out the project from their own points of view. If research methods are to develop and people are to learn from others' successes and failures, researchers have a scientific obligation to 'tell it like it is'. They should be honest about how they did the research so that others may benefit and not feel inadequate if they have to deviate from their own research recipe for some reason.

If one were to search for one word to describe how action research is done, perhaps 'openness' would be the best one. Action research should be marked by an open attitude to the participants and the changes they wish to make in their work, to the research methods used, to making changes along the way, to investing the researcher's 'self' in the project and to writing up the study in an honest and revealing manner.

Action research in practice

A look at two examples of nursing action research will illustrate how these underlying ideas are put into practice.

Putting research findings into practice

Hunt (1987) used action research in a project designed to assist a group of nurse–teachers to translate research findings into practice. Teachers and librarians from nine schools of nursing were invited to participate in the project, and in the first phase the librarians helped the teachers to carry out a literature search to identify research-based nursing practice literature. In phase two, evaluation and synthesis of the literature was carried out, using guidelines to standardize the critiques and develop the teachers' skills in this area. Subgroups of teachers worked on different topics and, in phase three, groups (focusing on mouth care and on pre-operative fasting) attempted to translate their findings into practice.

The mouth care group prepared written summaries of their work and discussed these in workshop and study days with colleagues from both education and service areas. The procedure committee was also given a copy of the summary and teachers announced that this would form the basis of their teaching of learners after a certain date. Changing mouth care practice also involved liaising with the central sterile supplies department as well as the supplies department to curtail supplies of mouth care packs and substitute small toothbrushes.

The whole process took several years to run through, and even after this period of time some ward sisters did not use the guidelines although they had been involved in the workshops which discussed the changes. Hunt (1987) concluded that:

> 'this indicated the extent of the autonomy exercised by ward sisters in ignoring policy decisions and the lack of an effective management system to ensure that agreed practice changes were implemented and maintained'.

With regard to pre-operative fasting, the same process was gone through, albeit with slight variations. A similar lack of response on the part of some staff was felt by Hunt to reflect 'the traditional patient–professional relationship of passivity and control, in spite of the developing rhetoric' about patients' active participation in their own care.

Certain features of action research emerge clearly from Hunt's report, including the participation of teachers as research subjects in solving the practical problem of translating research findings into action. Evaluation was also continuous, in that reports on the three stages of the project are given. There is also a reflexive and critical discussion in the latter part of the article about methods used, and the degree of success or failure they achieved. What seems to be missing is an account of the part played by the action researcher – presumably Hunt herself. It would have been fascinating and highly illuminating for later researchers to gain insight into the experiences of the researcher throughout the protracted process of trying to introduce change. What was the precise nature of her input to the project? How did she cope personally with the stress of her involvement over many years in a project that met with limited success? How did she attempt to overcome resistance?

Relationships in an action research project

Webb's report on her personal experiences of carrying out an action research project, on the other hand, does focus on these issues (Webb, 1989). She spent three months working as a participant observer on her study ward, collecting baseline data using stress and ward learning environment questionnaires, measuring workload, and attempting some further measures. The aim in this initial period was to get to know the ward and its staff, to understand its methods and problems as an insider and to build up credibility with staff in preparation for the subsequent action phase.

The conflicts of being closely involved in a ward where there were deep interpersonal conflicts are discussed. The strategies used – whether successful or not – to cope with ethical and practical dilemmas are described, and the writer's personal learning through the project are presented. Webb tells how difficult it can be not to take sides in a situation of conflict, and how this is made worse when, as a participant, a researcher becomes part of the conflict. Because she intended to act as a facilitator for the subsequent action phase of the project, Webb did not think it appropriate to take sides in a dispute because this could alienate participants. At the same time, she witnessed, and was on the receiving end of, difficult situations in which it was hard not to convey her feelings, and impossible not to be personally affected by the events.

To take one example, a discussion arose during ward report about a doctor having given confidential information to a patient's divorced wife when she had come to visit her ex-husband. The information concerned a diagnosis of cancer, which had not been given to the patient himself. Most nursing staff were angry about the doctor's action, felt that it was a breach of confidentiality and that the doctor should not have behaved in this way. The ward sister, however, felt that it was up to the doctor to make his own decisions on the basis of his medical training, which she explained was longer and deeper than nursing training. Consequently she felt that it was not appropriate for nurses to challenge such a decision. Like most of the nurses present, Webb disagreed strongly with the ward sister's view, but felt that in the context of the project she (as a researcher) should be restrained in the way she expressed herself. It was more difficult when staff openly talked to the researcher about interpersonal problems on the ward. Webb tried to deal with these situations by using active listening techniques, and trying to get the nurses to explore how they could have acted differently to resolve the difficulties constructively.

Webb (1989) concludes that, despite the precarious nature of her negotiations through this phase of the project, action research is a powerful method for studying and implementing change in nursing research.

Action research: the answer to all our problems?

Action research is 'the method of choice' for nursing research, according to Greenwood (1984). However, there is a danger in assuming that there is a ready answer to every problem. Those who have used action research in nursing have drawn attention to two important limitations in the approach, and these concern power and resources.

Power

In Meyer's attempt to increase lay participation in care, doctors' authoritarian practices had this effect. By paying lip service to changes but not actually modifying the way they worked, doctors acted as a brake on developments (Meyer, 1993).

In a project to develop the roles of ward sisters, Alexander & Orton (1988) found that in practice nurses in general, and ward sisters in particular, lacked power to influence important aspects of their work. On the other hand, Hunt (1987) reports that sisters were able to resist changes in practice precisely because they did have a great deal of power. The differences between these two suggestions may be explained by organizational factors in the hospital. Within a ward, a sister may have a great deal of power to influence practices. But when 'outside' factors are considered, others may have greater power. This is particularly likely to be the case with resources.

Resources

Almost all nursing action researchers report that lack of resources can be a strong barrier to implementing change. Some writers talk of staffing issues, while others mention workload. However, these are the same thing in the end because if there are too few staff then the workload for those small numbers of personnel becomes too great.

Booth & Davies (1991) used a Nursing Development Unit approach to introducing and monitoring change and did this themselves, without the help of an *outside* researcher. They found that when the workload was high they had to hold up further changes until a quieter time. Smith's attempt to improve practice in an elderly care setting was also impeded due to insufficient numbers of nursing staff and fluctuations in staffing and workload (Smith, 1986). In Johns & Kingston's (1990) project on a children's ward, management policies inhibited change because they opposed the use of a *bank* scheme to solve staffing problems.

Staff changes during the course of the action research caused difficulties for both Armitage *et al.* (1991) in a mental health setting and Meyer (1993) in a general nursing context.

Workload fluctuations were also given by Edwards *et al.* (1991) as a reason why their attempts to improve discharge planning did not progress smoothly. Similar problems faced Alexander & Orton (1988) in their ward sister development work.

Whilst action research has great potential to help promote change within nursing, then, it is a mistake to think that it can solve all our problems. Where nurses lack power and are unable to control staffing resources, it is likely that their attempts to develop practice will run up against barriers.

Conclusions

In summary, this chapter has attempted to show how action research is an approach which draws on the best of other approaches, and uses research to respond to the needs of those who are being studied as well as those of the researcher. This process brings out into the open many of the taken-for-granted assumptions of previous approaches. Issues of power, autonomy, ownership and research purposes are placed on the agenda. However, action research cannot provide a ready answer to these dilemmas; as Light & Kleiber (1978) state,

> 'where each researcher draws her/his ethical and practical lines must be her/his own decision'.

Nevertheless, they believe that action research leads to 'more human, more moral, and more perceptive field research'.

References

Alexander, M. & Orton, H. (1988) Research in action. *Nursing Times*, 84, 38–41.

Allen, D.G. (1985) Nursing research and social control: alternative models of science that emphasize understanding and emancipation. *Image: The Journal of Nursing Scholarship*, XVII(2), 58–64.

Armitage, P., Champney-Smith, J. & Andrews, K. (1991) Primary nursing and the role of the nurse. *Journal of Advanced Nursing*, 16, 413–22.

Booth, J. & Davies, C. (1991) The management of change on a nursing development unit. *Nursing Practice*, 4(2), 12–15.

Carr, W. & Kemmis, S. (1986) *Becoming Critical*. Falmer Press, London.

Edwards, J., Riley, P., Morris, A.M. & Doody, J. (1991) An analysis of the quality and effectiveness of the discharge planning process. *Journal of Nursing Care Quality*, 5(4), 17–27.

Greenwood, J. (1984) Nursing research: a position paper. *Journal of Advanced Nursing*, 9, 77–82.

Hunt, M. (1987) The process of translating research findings into nursing practice. *Journal of Advanced Nursing*, 12, 101–10.

Johns, C. & Kingston, S. (1990) Implementing a philosophy of care on a children's ward using action research. *Nursing Practice*, 4(1), 2–9.

Lauri, S. (1982) Development of the nursing process through action research. *Journal of Advanced Nursing*, 7, 301–7.

Light, L. & Kleiber, N. (1978) Interactive research in a health care setting. *Social Science and Medicine*, 12, 193–8.

Meyer, J. (1993) New paradigm research in practice: the trials and tribulations of action research. *Journal of Advanced Nursing*, 18, 1066–72.

Sandow, S. (1979) Action research and evaluation: can research and practice be successfully combined? *Child: Care, Health and Development*, 5, 211–23.

Smith, G. (1986) Resistance to change in geriatric care. *International Journal of Nursing Studies*, 23(1), 61–70.

Towell, D. & Harries, C. (1979) *Innovations in Patient Care. An Action Research Study of Change in a Psychiatric Hospital*. Croom Helm, London.

Webb, C. (1989) Action research: philosophy, methods and personal experiences. *Journal of Advanced Nursing*, 14, 403–10.

Chapter 16

Historical Research

Anne Marie Rafferty

The study of nursing history appears to be enjoying something of a renaissance. Its star has risen and fallen with the fashions of curricular change and oscillations in the political temperature. Once regarded as a central part of the liberal education of a nurse, history declined in status to that of disposable luxury in the technology orientated 1980s. The status attached to history by society appears to reflect the esteem in which liberal values in education are held at any given time. In so far as nursing reflects in microcosm the wider changes in society, history can be regarded as a metaphor for the fluctuating fortunes of liberal educational values more generally.

Shifting sands

Compared to the history of medicine or science, little has been written about the purpose of history and the function of the historian in nursing. Yet nursing is not without its historiographical commentators. Prominent among these have been Lynaugh & Reverby (1986) in the USA and Davies (1980) and Maggs (1978) in the UK. Such commentaries have marked a watershed in the writing of nursing history on both sides of the Atlantic. What they have advocated and practised was a move from the hero-centred view of history, to a more critical form of research which located nursing within a wider social and political context. The movement within American nursing history culminated in the early 1980s in the edited collection of Lagemann (1982), which brought together a series of essays that asked new kinds of questions about nursing politics and nursing work.

Pre-eminent among these questions are those pertaining to race, class and gender in nursing. Innovative work emerging from Australia, South Africa and the USA considers ways in which these questions intersect with and react upon eachother (Marks, 1994; Strachan, 1995). Such research complements that of earlier American nurse historians, who were amongst the first to include questions of race and ethnicity within their research repertoire (Carnegie, 1991).

Throughout the 1980s sporadic methodological commentaries emerged from nurse historians keen to reflect upon their craft. Apart from Dzuback's (1982) annotated bibliographical guide to the American literature, MacPherson & Stuart's (1994) review essay probably represents the most compact and wide-ranging commentary on the state of the historical art in nursing in the 1990s. Together, these works have helped to create a new intellectual community within nursing and an audience for the consumption and appreciation of nursing history.

Why study history?

People study history for a variety of reasons; for pleasure, as a form of intellectual training, for the light it sheds on contemporary problems and as a contextual guide to decision-making. Marwick (1970) argues that the study of the past contributes greatly to our understanding of contemporary problems, human behaviour and the forces driving social change. In Britain, the use of historical evidence in justifying the case for change in the United Kingdom Central Council for Nursing, Midwifery and Health Visiting (UKCC)'s Project 2000 document owed much to the inspiration of Celia Davies as project officer and her research experience in historical sociology (UKCC, 1986).

As individuals we tend to be attracted to different subject areas, kinds of work and social environments for various reasons; some people love laboratory work, others libraries; some thrive on social and collaborative contact, others on solving problems solo; some rejoice in computer graphics, ruminating over data sets and statistical tests, while others prefer the *in situ* analytic art of participant observation. But the key ingredient that unites many researchers is passion, emotional and often political commitment to their chosen subject of study. This can apply as much to scientists as historians and the history of science provides ample evidence of cases where faith and political beliefs can be as important an impetus to innovation as reason (Pickering, 1992).

Context and chronology

Research is concerned with asking questions, gathering evidence, describing and explaining the nature and strength of the relationship between variables. Historical research is also concerned with such questions and although it may be difficult to calculate the precise nature of the relationships between historical variables, it is also worth recalling how difficult it is to pin down causation in health care too. What differentiates the historical enterprise from the scientific, however, is the former's focus upon context and chronology as explanatory power. As the historian E.P. Thompson reminds us

'The discipline of history is above all, the discipline of context; each fact can be given meaning only within an ensemble of other meanings' (Thompson cited by Lynaugh & Reverby, 1986, p. 4).

Intricacies of interpretation

Unlike the scientist, the historian is not concerned with exercising control over variables in the same way a scientist might, reducing the number of variables for analysis nor holding these constant over time. Rather the historian has to work with 'natural' experiments; those which posterity, the preservation policies of organizations, gatekeepers and legal regulators of access to records allow. That does not mean to say that every historian will use the same piece of evidence in the same way or arrive at the same conclusions using a similar set of sources. Interpretation lies at the heart of the historiographical endeavour. Historians will attach greater or lesser significance to the influence of particular variables upon events and outcomes.

It is, for example, a commonplace assumption that nursing history responds mainly to changes in medical theory and practice; that both are sensitive to and shaped by similar pressures. Medical history had traditionally provided much in the way of context and point of orientation for nurse historians, but this symmetry and synchronization is now being questioned as taken for granted and axiomatic. Indeed, when it comes to the percolation of medical innovation through to clinical nursing, the relationship is likely to be more complex and interactive than merely reactive. Furthermore there is surprisingly little research evidence to support an inevitable convergence of the boundaries of clinical medical with nursing practice. Much of this has to do with the virtual neglect of clinical nursing practice as a subject for historical research, a neglect that is only now beginning to be redressed.

To take one example, the bacteriological revolution of nineteenth century medicine is generally acknowledged as a major transformative event in scientific medical history, yet we know almost nothing about its impact upon the theory and practice of nursing. Ironically, almost as elusive is the effect of Pasteur and Koch's 'germ theory' and Lister's antisepsis practice upon the daily routine of rank and file medical theory and practice! The deeper we dig beneath the apparently smooth surface of medical innovation, the more fissured and complex the pattern of dissemination and adoption becomes. Florence Nightingale was not the only opponent of the 'germ theory' of disease; many medical practitioners and leaders of medicine rejected Lister's theories and interventions (Granshaw, 1992). Similarly what might be construed as the breakthrough events in nursing's political calendar, such as the Nurses Registration Act of 1919, may barely feature as a footnote in the medico-political discourse of the day.

Carr (1970) has defined history as

'the continuous interaction between the historian and his facts, an unending dialogue between the present and the past'.

Although it may seem on the surface that historians are at the mercy of their sources, all researchers are in fact dependent upon their evidence and subject to economic and ethical constraints. Historical research is particularly sensitive to chronology of the question(s) being asked.

In attempting to identify the 'causes' of wound healing, for example, a historical survey of past treatments may cast light on the mechanisms underlying changes in the theory and practice of wound care. The Hippocratic and Galenic medical theory of the fifth century BC to the second century AD, for example, maintained that suppuration and the production of so-called 'laudable pus' was an essential part of wound healing (Cartwright, 1977). This reasoning contrasts vividly with current theory of wound care, the object of which is to prevent infection.

What the historian attempts to understand is how such theory was shaped and the factors that brought about change at any given point in time. Studying the history of nursing research helps us to understand that knowledge is provisional and apt to alter with the generation of fresh findings. While more sophisticated analyses of the theory/practice gap and implementation process in nursing research are beginning to emerge (see Chapter 33), historical studies of specified nursing 'inventions' can enhance our understanding of the politics of innovation and research utilization.

Calculating change

Unlike research involving calculations and statistical inference and interpretation, history does not lend itself easily to estimating the precise effect of confounding variables, those which produce an interactive effect and therefore require correction to ascertain the effect of each individually. History is not, however, devoid of, nor divorced from the world of statistics. The advent of information technology has penetrated every sphere of life, including history, so much so that quantitative methods in the history of medicine were the subject of a book by Porter & Wear (1988). The Society for the Social History of Medicine recently sponsored a conference on history and computing, a growing area of interest for researchers skilled in the management of large data sets, working at the interface between demography and history.

Yet some historians have gone as far as talking about the strength of their evidence in terms of causation. Stone (1972) in his discussion of the causes of the English Civil War, divides the casual factors into three chronological groups: long-term preconditions, medium-term precipitants, and short-term triggers. 'Causes' here may be more readily conceived of in terms of necessary and sufficient conditions rather than ranked precisely into a hierarchy of contributory factors.

To take a recent example in this country, if studying the origins of Project 2000 and the 'causes' of its success, one of the major questions the historian would ask is why has Project 2000 apparently succeeded as a reform strategy where others seem to have failed (UKCC, 1986)? What have been the factors which have promoted its implementation? The merits of the case; demographic pressures; the social, political, and economic environment; the fit with government policy, administration of the health, educational and social services; or all of these, and if so, were all equal in importance? Immediately, we are confronted with the problems of historical evaluation. What in historical terms counts as success or failure? How can we measure historical change? Which outcome variables should we consider? Whose view(s) should we take into account, practising nurses, nurse leaders, the project team, government officials? Which sources should we use and how should we prioritize these? How should we order our enquiry?

Value of and value in history

Perhaps the value of historical research in nursing can best be illustrated by an example which has provided a corrective to the historical record. This *revisionist* approach is admirably illustrated by Baly's study of Florence Nightingale and the politics of the Nightingale Fund (Baly, 1986). Much of Baly's research is devoted to the exposure of a number of myths concerning the Nightingale School and its training methods.

Contrary to popular wisdom, St Thomas's was not originally considered by Miss Nightingale as an ideal institution for the Nightingale School on account of its insalubrious location and its matron, Mrs Wardroper, whose competence to supervise nurse training was doubted by Miss Nightingale. Furthermore, far from providing a codified scheme of instruction and a model of training ready for export, the training provided was haphazard, the wastage rate high, and only modest numbers of well educated women came forward to be inculcated with the *new* spirit of reformed nursing. Diaries, for example, which were kept by the probationers for inspection by Miss Nightingale, indicated that most of the probationers' time on the wards was unsupervised and that the intellectual content of lectures was pitched deliberately low and required supplementary interpretation and coaching from the Home Sister (Baly, 1986, p. 174).

Continuity and change

History helps us to understand the process of change, be it in methods used to treat pressure sores or the introduction of new ways of organizing care. One of the first evaluation studies of team nursing, for example, was published in the late 1950s by a Canadian nurse (Jenkinson, 1953). Where did the idea and method originate? Was it significant that this innovation was promoted by a nurse from North America? What was it about the organizational climate at the hospital in question (St George's, London) which favoured the introduction of new ideas? Was the then matron, Muriel Powell, a crucial influence in supporting the change? In relation to nursing research, historical research can help us to understand more fully the factors which transform a 'good idea' into standard practice and help explain why some research findings are implemented and not others.

Historical research provides one way of investigating the dynamics and direction of change. The historian's own views, opinions and preconceptions as well as research funding policy may be crucial determinants of the questions selected for study and the mode of investigation adopted. Individuals may be attracted to different disciplines, topics and techniques in research for a variety of reasons, some of which may be very personal. In qualitative research, the researcher's belief system may be taken for granted as intrinsic to the research process and even formally integrated into the fabric of the account and analysis (Walker, 1994). In scientific research, the accent is on eliminating the influence of the investigator, although studies in the history and sociology of science confirm that researchers' values, personal histories, belief systems and ambitions can be important motivators of research (Pickering, 1992).

Sources and sampling

It may at this point be worthwhile considering the range of resources upon which the historian of nursing might draw in order to construct an account. First I shall discuss access and availability. While both historians and scientists may have to negotiate access to the research site through gatekeepers such as ethical committees, health service managers and keepers of manuscripts, the historian may have her work predetermined by virtue of the preservation or destruction of records. The potential to generate data anew rests with the scientist. The historian traversing unknown territory may have little idea of what, if anything, sources, once located, will reveal.

Historical sources are subject to a particular set of regulations concerning access and closure which may be crucial in determining the research that can be undertaken. The '30 year rule' in the UK closes access to public records for 30 years after the date of the last item in the file. 'Public' may be defined as those records deriving from organizations which are accountable to public bodies such as Parliament. All records of National Health Service authorities fall into this category, and administrative records are only open 30 years after the date of the last item contained in the file. Medical records of patients in that country are only open to the public after 100 years. In exceptional cases, organizations may decide to waive the rules normally governing access to material under their jurisdiction and open files earlier than the statutory period to *bona fide* researchers, provided precautions to safeguard anonymity and the conditions of the Data Protection Act in publications are adhered to.

Public records may be stored at the Public Record Office (PRO), the Scottish equivalent, Scottish Record Office (SRO), or a local repository such as the Greater London Record Office (GLRO) or regional records offices such as County Records Offices or local repositories such as (in Scotland) the Lothian Health Board Medical Archives Centre at Edinburgh University Library. Some hospitals store their own records, but the stage of preservation varies enormously. Private organizations may also maintain their own records.

The Royal College of Nursing (RCN) employs a full-time archivist for this purpose, who is based at the Scottish Headquarters in Edinburgh. The Wellcome Institute's Contemporary Medical Archive contains a number of different sources that are relevant to nursing, including the records of the Health Visitors Association.

Supplying sources

The scholarly and innovative merit of an historical work may hinge upon the extent to which it is based upon primary sources or reinterprets secondary sources in a novel way. Primary sources are the raw unedited data (the minutes, papers and correspondence of organizations such as the now defunct General Nursing Council for England and Wales), upon which historical interpretation is based. Secondary sources refer to the digested, interpreted or reported data of primary historical material. Generally, the secondary literature is mastered before the primary data are mined to provide the necessary contextual material for the account, but this order may not be strictly adhered to as new lines of inquiry emerge. Arguments will usually be suggested by the data, and are subject to change as different types of sources emerge and are explored and re-read at different stages in the research. Interpretation is a dynamic and interactive process.

In keeping with developments in other areas of historical research, notably that in the history of medicine, the scope of nursing has broadened recently to encompass a wide range of sources. There is no standard method for the organization or compiling of sources or evidence. These might include not only official and semi-official printed or written documents and private papers, but also literary accounts, biography, autobiography and fiction. More recently, oral testimony has yielded useful data on the experiences of working nurses. Little account as yet has been taken of patients' views but film, television, video, architecture, art and photographic material have recently been incorporated within the inventory of sources and methods (Hudson-Jones, 1988). It remains to be seen what the impact of the telephone and the information superhighway are likely to be in supplying the sources of the future.

One of the major advantages of using a range of tools and sources as data is the potential for verification of evidence and interpretation. Thus, official documents may be used in combination, if possible, with private diaries and oral testimony to check and confirm a line of inquiry. Different perceptions of the same situation or event are likely to emerge from different individuals with different agendas and interests. The uncovering of 'multiple realities' may be the very point of the investigative exercise and is especially important in tracking the pathways of decision-making in policy analysis. In many ways, historical research may be considered akin to qualitative research in its acknowledgement of multiple realities and triangulation of methods.

Voyage of discovery or journey without maps?

On a practical level, historical research can be both frustrating and rewarding. Hours spent searching for a particular source of evidence may yield little. Equally, it is possible to stumble on a goldmine of information: a personal diary, an album of photographs, a clutch of newspaper cuttings. The records of the past were not written with the needs of the historian in mind, although public bodies do have preservation policies implemented by officials trained to evaluate the historical importance of documents. These policies may be regulated by resources and other factors not necessarily within the control of historians themselves. As nurses and historians, we should take an active role in trying to influence preservation policies to maximize their utility for future generations of historians, nurses and researchers.

Although it is probably advisable to build a research project around a solid set of records, this assumes the archives have been used by, or are known to, the researcher. This presupposes that the researcher has already undertaken sufficient work to have refined the research question in order to identify specific sources. Few may be able to afford the luxury of such in-depth preparatory or pilot work before submitting proposals for funding to vetting agencies. Nonetheless, it is possibly inadvisable to depend upon only one source of data no matter how potentially rich.

The direction and outcome of the research will be dependent upon the use that can be made of the sources and, consequently, the question asked may change dramatically in the course of investigation. The order of inquiry is negotiated and loose; there is no orderly progression of steps or stages to follow and one is likely to come and go between primary and secondary material in response to the data.

Practicalities such as the employment of an archivist may be crucial in determining the use of sources. The listing of holdings and cataloguing of material greatly enhances the efficiency of information retrieval. Much may also depend upon the experience and efficiency of the researcher. While nurses with a first degree in history will have an advantage in undertaking historical research, much of what trained historians perhaps take for granted has to be learned along the way for nurses who do not.

Generally speaking, however, the problem of historical research is not one of finding sufficient material, but of containing the huge volumes of paper generated by organizations. Documents, journals and personal papers should be systematically screened for relevant material and this can mean hours of laborious scrutiny and scanning. All research has its routine tasks, but this is labour which may be crucial to how the account will be organized and presented. In determining the division of labour, it may be advisable to tackle the records of one organization at a time. If events are particularly current, it is desirable to interview the participants themselves.

Oral history requires specific methodological and ethical considerations and has acquired the status of a sub-discipline within history itself (Thompson, 1978). It may serve a variety of purposes: to fill gaps in the documentation, uncover details of decisions, generate evidence missing from the records or allow the clarification of factual points. In some cases it may be the only evidence available. There are many pitfalls, as well as great potential in the use of oral testimony, some of which have to do with the power relations and social characteristics of the interviewer and interviewee. Oral history may be invaluable as an insight into an individual's thought processes, the discovery of new and important information and, more generally, in enriching the quality of data.

As a testament to its commitment to nursing history and leadership, the Royal College of Nursing (RCN) sponsored a project concerned with collecting the career histories of a cohort of retired nurse leaders. This *top-down* history is being supplemented more recently, by a *bottom-up* approach to the oral history of nurses who were trained in and practised in the 1930s.

Social and socializing history

So what have been the characteristic features of historical research in nursing? Much of nursing history has been used to serve a number of professional even 'professionalizing' ends (Rafferty, 1991). Early writing in nursing history was more concerned with synthesizing existing knowledge rather than producing new knowledge through fresh investigation. The use of previously unexploited primary evidence and the development of novel interpretations is the *raison d'etre* of research. Both characteristics have been exemplified in studies of British nursing since the early 1960s. Davies' (1980) innovative edited collection of social scientific aspects of historical nursing research provided a focus for feminist and labour history interpretations of nursing history. Maggs (1978) was one of the first nurses to treat nursing history as a case study in social history.

Pilgrims of progress

It may be tempting to view the changes of the past as somehow inevitable and as the fulfilment of progress, and much history has been written from this point of view. This assumes that the past is governed by law-like mechanisms and ignores the conflict and complexities of rival forces competing for power. Much of the recent research in the history of nursing rejects this view as failing to account for the tensions between historical agencies and the intricacies of power differentials which favour one set of conditions rather than another. The past as representing *progress*, while psychologically gratifying, prejudges the past, and forces it into a mould which empirical research may contradict. For example, although increases in nurses' pay in the UK have occurred since the introduction of the National Health Service, the fluctuating pattern of relativities suggests that the story of nurses' pay has not been one of onward and upward (Gray, 1989).

Mining metaphors

In many ways, historical research may be compared to mining; extensive exploratory work may be necessary to refine an area for further investigation. Diligent excavation may reveal a wealth of resources. For this reason, and the fact that only in exceptional cases will records be susceptible to computer analysis, the process of extracting and analysing the data and formulating interpretations is time-consuming and labour intensive. One cannot readily feed the data into a computer and run a battery of tests or a statistical package to identify trends or characteristics. Much of the analysis has to be conducted without such aids to efficiency. Historical research can be expensive in time and resources, and there are no immediate practical spin-offs in terms of a product to justify research investment. It also tends to be an individualistic enterprise and less frequently undertaken as part of a multi-disciplinary project. One does not see much of the group research activity of science in history, although the history of the International Council of Nurses has been written as a team effort and collaborative project (Brush & Stuart, 1994). Historical research has helped to shed important light upon the multiple metaphorical meanings of nursing and has provided a vehicle for setting a challenging political agenda for nurses.

Repertoire of resources

Access to historical research in nursing is mediated through normal academic channels, but inquiries are welcomed by the History of Nursing Society based at the Royal College of Nursing in London, which also holds conferences and meetings and publishes a journal, the *International History of Nursing Journal*. In theory, one can study nursing history wherever there are resources to do so; the Public Records Office in London and the Greater London Records Office both produce broadsheets outlining their holdings on nursing history. The Wellcome Institute has a large collection of relevant archival material in their Contemporary Medical Archive.

The task of research, whether it involves registering for a higher degree or not, is eased considerably where there is intellectual and practical support. Help and advice can be offered by members of the RCN Society and also through the Wellcome Units for the History of Medicine based in Glasgow, Manchester, Oxford, Cambridge, the Wellcome Institute in London and the Department of Nursing and Midwifery Studies at the University of Nottingham.

In the USA, a Center for the Study of the History of Nursing and Archival repository is affiliated to the University of Pennsylvania School of Nursing and a new journal, *Nursing History Review*, is in its third volume. The centre has its own archivist. A second centre has recently been established in the University of Virginia. The Mary Adelaide Nutting Collection at Teachers College, Columbia University, New York, contains important educational and clinical material and texts. Historical options are offered in masters and doctoral programmes at the University of California at San Francisco jointly between the School of Nursing and the Department of History of Health Sciences. Fairman (1987) has produced a useful inventory of the repository holdings of nursing history archives in the USA.

Conclusion

The above discussion represents only the briefest outline of some signposts to historical research in nursing. Until the early 1960s, the writing of nursing history was dominated by nurses and nurse leaders who used history as a vehicle to justify professionalization. The arrival of researchers whose primary academic training was not in nursing, for example sociologists, historians of medicine, feminist, labour and social historians, exerted an important impact upon the direction of the discipline. The pre-eminence of the professionalization agenda, which characterized the early writing in nursing history, was not necessarily broken by social scientists but was theorized and researched in a different way.

Interest in nursing by social and feminist historians and historians of medicine has led to a new set of questions being asked about nursing as women's work, the effect of race, class and gender, and other socio-political and economic factors upon the working experience of nurses, their place within the health care division of labour and relationships with patients. The latter has paradoxically proved to be the most intractable form of analysis.

History has implications for nursing research. Above all it can provide a powerful tool for helping us to understand the theory/practice gap in nursing research. Historical research has much to contribute to reflective practice, the management of change and our understanding of the process and politics of innovation. It could facilitate the framing of a research policy for nursing and help us unravel and celebrate the genius of nursing's inventiveness, past, present and hopefully to come.

Acknowledgements

I should like to thank Margo Szabunia and Barbara Brush for providing constructive comments on a previous draft of this chapter.

References

Baly, M. (1986) *Florence Nightingale and the Nursing Legacy.* Croom Helm, London.

Brush, B. & Stuart, M. (1994) Unity amidst difference: the ICN project and writing international nursing history. *Nursing History Review,* **2**, 191–204.

Carnegie, M.E. (1991) *The Path We Tread: Blacks in Nursing 1854–1990,* 2nd edn. National League for Nursing, New York.

Carr, E.H. (1970) *What is History?* p. 24. Macmillan, London.

Cartwright, F.F. (1977) *A Social History of Medicine.* Longmans, London.

Davis, C. (1980) The contemporary challenge in nursing history. In *Rewriting Nursing History*, (ed. C. Davies, pp. 1–17). Croom Helm, London.

Dzuback, M.A. (1982) Nursing historiography, 1960–1980: an annotated bibliography. In *Nursing History: New Perspectives, New Possibilities* (ed. E.C. Lagemann), pp. 181–210. Teachers College Press, New York.

Fairman, J. (1987) Sources and references for research in nursing history. *Nursing Research,* **36**(1), 56–9.

Granshaw, L. (1992) 'Upon this principle I have based a practice': the development and reception of antisepsis in Britain, 1867–90. In *Medical Innovations in Historical Perspective*, (ed. J. Pickstone). St Martin's Press, New York.

Gray, A.M. (1989) The NHS and the history of nurses' pay. *Bulletin of the History of Nursing Group at the Royal College of Nursing,* **2**(8), 15–29.

Hudson-Jones, A. (ed.) (1988) *Images of Nurses: Perspectives from History, Art and Literature.* University of Pennsylvania Press, Philadelphia.

Jenkinson, V. (1953) Case assignment method of nursing. *Nursing Mirror,* **116**, i–iv.

Lagemann, E.C. (ed.) (1982) *Nursing History: New Perspectives, New Possibilities.* Teachers College Press, New York.

Lynaugh, J. & Reverby, S. (1986) Thoughts on the nature of history. *Nursing Research*, **36**, 1(4), 68–9.

MacPherson, K. & Stuart, M. (1994) Writing nursing history in Canada: issues and approaches. *Canadian Bulletin of Medical History*, **11**(1), 3–22.

Maggs, C.J. (1978) Towards a social history of nursing, parts 1 and 2. *Nursing Times*, **74** (occasional papers), 53–8.

Marks, S. (1994) *Divided Sisterhood: Race Class and Gender in the South African Nursing Profession*. MacMillan, London.

Marwick, A. (1970) *The Nature of History*, p. 17. Macmillan, London.

Pickering, A. (1992) *Science As Practice and Culture*. University of Chicago Press, Chicago.

Porter, R. & Wear, A. (eds) (1988) *Problems and Methods in the History of Medicine*. Croom Helm, London.

Rafferty, A.M. (1991) Historical knowledge. In *Knowledge for Practice* (eds K.M. Robinson & B. Vaughan). Heinemann, London.

Stone, L. (1972) *The Causes of the English Revolution*, pp. 47–144. Routledge, Kegan Paul, London.

Strachan, G. (1995) 'A good nurse cannot be bought with money': the development of the professional and industrial roles of the nursing organisation in Queensland, Australia, 1904–1950. *Nursing History Review*, **3**, 235–56.

Thompson, P. (1978) *The Voice of the Past*. Oxford University Press, Oxford.

United Kingdom Central Council for Nursing Midwifery and Health Visiting (1986) *Project 2000: A New Preparation for Practice*. UKCC, London.

Walker, K. (1994) Confronting 'reality': nursing science and the micropolitics of representation. *Nursing Inquiry*, **1**(1), 46–56.

Appendix 16.1: Useful addresses

UK

Royal College of Nursing
Scottish Board
42, South Oswald Rd
Edinburgh, EH9 2HH

Wellcome Institute for the History of Medicine
183, Euston Rd
London NW1 2BE

Department of Nursing and Midwifery Studies
Queen's Medical Centre
University of Nottingham
Nottingham, NG7 2UH

USA

Center for the Study of the History of Nursing
School of Nursing
University of Pennsylvania
420, Guardian Drive
Philadelphia, PA 19104-6096

Center for Nursing Historical Inquiry
School of Nursing
University of Virginia
Health Sciences Center
Mcleod Hall
Charlottesville
Virginia, 22903-3395

University of California at San Francisco
c/o The Library
School of Nursing Collection
Special Collection
San Francisco, CA 94143-0840

Mary Adelaide Nutting Collection
Columbia University
Teachers College
Milbank Memorial Library
Special Collections
New York, NY 10027

Chapter 17

Descriptive Research

Diana E. Carter

Introduction

As the term implies, research which is 'descriptive' is concerned with description which can include description of types, classes, qualities or characteristics of a focus of interest. Daily (either verbally or in writing), as we communicate with others, we inevitably include descriptions within our accounts. However, whilst personal experience suggests that such accounts may not always be accurate, complete or unbiased, the process of describing is familiar to all of us.

The aim of descriptive research is to discover new facts about a situation, people, activities or events, or the frequency with which certain events occur. This is achieved through the systematic collection of information about the phenomenon of interest and forms an essential phase in the development of nursing knowledge, in that it provides the basis for future research, generating questions and hypotheses for experimental study. As with other types of research, descriptive research begins with the identification of a problem or problematic situation. The description and analysis of that situation may reveal relevant factors or relationships hitherto undetected which in turn could form the basis for further research.

Many areas of nursing have been investigated in descriptive studies, including the equipment used in the provision of that care and the specific nursing practices involved, as for example the study of the use of syringe drivers by David (1992). Other areas of investigation have included the environment in which nursing care is given as well as the characteristics of nurses and patients themselves, as in the comparative study of patients' and nurses' opinions of the role of nurses in informing breast cancer patients (Suominen *et al.* 1994).

The nature of descriptive research

The focus of descriptive studies is on the situation as it is and no attempt is made to manipulate variables. This focus might include conditions that exist, practices that prevail, beliefs and attitudes that are held, on-going processes and developing trends. The data which are obtained can then be used to justify and assess current conditions and practice, or to make plans for improving them.

Descriptive studies vary enormously in their scope and complexity. For example, a large sample of subjects drawn from a defined population may be studied. This is referred to as *survey research*. At the other extreme, a case study design involves the extensive study of a single unit (an individual, family or group). In this instance, while the number of subjects is small, the number of variables examined tends to be large because there is a need to investigate all the variables that may have an effect on the situation being studied. Similarly, the information obtained in descriptive studies may be quite diverse, ranging from data on easily defined objective facts such as age, gender, income and education level, to subtle and personal realms of human experience such as feelings or attitudes. The methodology of descriptive studies can also show wide variation, the methods of data collection including the use of questionnaires and interviews which sometimes incorporate rating scales (for example, Likert scales) and visual analogue scales, and observation techniques.

Descriptive research frequently precedes experimental studies in that it often serves to generate hunches about the relationship among the various phenomena studied which can then be tested in an experimental study which may confirm or reject the hunches. Descriptive studies are generally guided by research questions and/or research objectives rather than a research hypothesis as such. As mentioned above, there is no attempt to introduce anything new or to modify or control the situation being studied, and because there is no manipulation of the variables under study, and as no attempt is being made to establish causality, descriptive researchers do not use the terms 'dependent' and 'independent' when referring to variables. Whilst relationships between variables are identified in order to obtain an overall picture of the phenomena being examined, examination of the types and degrees of relationship is not the primary purpose of a descriptive study.

However, in common with all types of research, the descriptive researcher is trying to achieve a clear picture of the situation, and protection against bias is an important consideration. Measures taken to achieve this protection include definition of variables, sample selection and the use of valid and reliable instruments and methods of data collection.

Definition of variables

Conceptual and operational definitions are the two types of definition to which researchers refer. A conceptual definition conveys the general meaning, in much the same way as does a dictionary definition (LoBiondo-Wood & Haber, 1986). However, this type of definition does not help in relation to the measurement of a particular variable. The researcher has to go further than this and describe what is to be measured and how this will be carried out. This is known as an operational definition (or operationalization), and involves specifying the tools or instruments required to make the observations or measurements (see Chapter 6). Having operationalized a variable it then makes possible the replication of the study by others, and it also renders the findings of the study more reliable.

Sample selection

Samples vary considerably in the extent to which they represent the population, but the researcher who pays particular attention to the representativeness of the sample increases the possibility of generalizing the findings to a larger group.

Many descriptive studies include a large number of subjects obtained through random sampling, which it is hoped will increase the generalizability of the findings to a wider population. However, some studies use non-random sampling techniques, and while they may produce important relevant findings, such findings cannot automatically be extrapolated to similar situations. More details of sampling techniques can be found in Chapter 19.

Valid and reliable instruments

Instruments to be used for the collection of data must first of all be tested for reliability and validity. Reliability refers to the degree of constancy or accuracy with which the instrument measures an attribute, while validity is the degree to which it measures what it is supposed to be measuring. There are many methods of assessing aspects of an instrument's reliability, and also a variety of approaches in relation to validity which are referred to elsewhere in this text.

Perhaps an important point to note here is that even though an instrument has been previously tested in another study, it is advisable to re-test it as it has been shown that neither reliability nor validity is constant and both can change over time.

Methods of data collection

As mentioned above, data collection in descriptive studies may involve the use of interviews, questionnaires and observation techniques.

Interviews and questionnaires

Interviews and questionnaires both involve direct questioning of subjects. Qualitative descriptive research frequently employs unstructured interviews, while quantitative descriptive studies, which call for instruments that will facilitate the collection of numerical (quantifiable) data, often use questionnaires and structured interviews. Both interviews and questionnaires are useful for obtaining data about the subjects of a study. The data may pertain to:

(1) *Personal background information:* this includes demographic information such as age, marital status, educational level and professional qualifications.
(2) *Behavioural information:* this may describe what the subjects did in the past, as in the study by Colbert (1994) which investigated the length of time women delayed consulting their GP following detection of a breast lump; what people do at present, as for example how often the subjects in Richmond's (1993) study tested their own blood glucose levels; or subjects' intended/expected

future behaviour as in Hewlett's (1994) investigation of the functional ability of patients with rheumatoid arthritis and their perceived future disability.

(3) *Level of knowledge or information on a particular topic:* as in the study by While & Rees (1993) which investigated and described the knowledge base for prescribing in district nurses and health visitors.

(4) *Opinions, attitudes and values, or how the subjects feel, or what they believe:* as exemplified in Richmond's (1993) study where subjects were asked if they worried about the complications of diabetes and those who ran their blood glucose levels higher than normal were asked if they did this for fear of a hypoglycaemic attack occurring.

Questionnaires may also incorporate the use of Likert-type rating scales where, in relation to each item, subjects are asked to indicate the point on the scale which most effectively represents their opinion. In his study of nurses' perceptions of the needs of suddenly bereaved families in the accident and emergency department, Tye (1993) asked nurses to rate whether each of nine nursing actions was 'not helpful; slightly helpful; moderately helpful; very helpful or one of the most helpful'.

Visual analogue scales can also be employed and have been found particularly useful in obtaining descriptions of the severity of pain experienced by patients. Figure 17.1 shows an example of a scale on which respondents could be asked to indicate their pain severity, with 0 representing no pain and 10 the most severe unbearable pain.

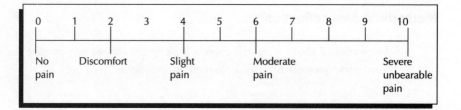

Fig. 17.1 Visual analogue scale for pain.

The use of this type of scale is not confined to investigation of pain. For example, in a study of nurses' views of infection control Gould & Ream (1994) used a visual analogue scale to elicit nurses' perceptions of hepatitis as a serious disease, as did Crouch & Dale (1994) in their study of feelings engendered in nurses during triage assessment in the accident and emergency department.

Observation

Observation techniques are also frequently used in descriptive nursing research studies. The focus of observation may be the behaviours and characteristics of individuals, as for example in Seed's (1994) study of student nurse socialization, and may include physical appearance, verbal and non-verbal communication behaviours, and actions. Environmental characteristics may also be observed as an individual's surroundings can have a considerable effect on behaviour.

Where a particular situation is being observed, the researcher's participation in that situation can range from one of non-participation, where the emphasis is solely on the observation and recording of events, to one of participation, where the researcher is actually a part of the situation as well as an observer and recorder of events.

If using interviews, questionnaires or observation as means of collecting data, some consideration needs to be given to the validity of each of these methods. For example, subjects' verbal or written responses to interview questions or questionnaire items about how they actually carry out a particular task may bear little or no resemblance to how they actually perform it. Similarly, there is no guarantee that the behaviour observed is a true reflection of how subjects behave when there is no observer present. Interviews, questionnaires and observation are dealt with in more detail in Chapters 21, 22 and 23. The remainder of this chapter will look at the different types of designs that can be used when conducting descriptive research.

Descriptive designs

Exploratory descriptive design

Opinions differ as to which non-experimental research approaches should be classified as *descriptive*, and some research texts do not include exploratory research in this category. One reason for this is that in descriptive studies the research question presupposes a prior knowledge of the problem and the researcher must be able to define what and who are to be measured and the techniques of doing so. However, description is integral to the process of exploration.

As the name suggests, this type of design is appropriate for areas about which nursing has little theoretical or factual knowledge. The researcher is exploring a particular area to discover what is there, the meanings attached to the discoveries and how these can be organized. This type of study calls for intuition and insight on the part of the researcher. It also calls for a degree of flexibility so that any new leads can be followed up, so moving the study into new areas as the researcher proceeds and as her knowledge of what is being studied increases.

The approach in such studies is frequently, but not exclusively, qualitative (see Chapter 11), integrating a variety of data collecting methods such as participant observation and unstructured interviews. This type of approach does not rely on pre-coded instruments and the possibilities of discovery and understanding unknown phenomena are enhanced.

Because of the exploratory nature of the study, few if any of the variables are under the researcher's control and are simply discovered and observed as the researcher comes across them.

Simple descriptive design

In this type of design, the variables of interest have been previously studied, either independently (as in an exploratory study) or with other variables. The variables are partly controlled by the situation (as in exploratory designs) but they are also partly controlled by the researcher, who chooses the sample for the study. This design is used when the researcher wishes to examine the characteristics of a single sample, as shown in Fig. 17.2.

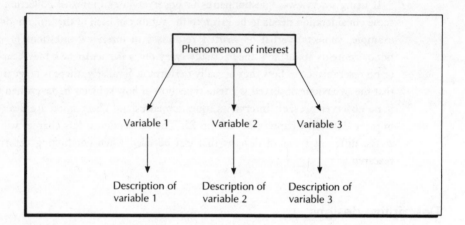

Fig. 17.2   Simple descriptive design.

After determining the phenomenon of interest, the researcher identifies and defines the variables within this and then proceeds to use the appropriate data collecting technique in order to obtain data which describe the variables. The number of variables to be examined and described will be determined in part by the study. For example, a survey of the use of syringe drivers by David (1992) collected data from patients' records on the following variables: the frequency and duration of syringe driver use, drugs and drug combinations used, how often patients had more than one syringe driver at a time, the frequency of and reasons for needle re-siting and critical incidents occurring during syringe driver use. The resultant data provided a useful general picture of syringe driver use and identified a need for further research in this area.

Comparative descriptive design

The comparative descriptive design is appropriate if the researcher wishes to examine and describe the variables in two or more groups. Figure 17.3 shows an example of the comparative descriptive design.

This type of design can be seen in the study carried out by Suominen *et al.* (1994), which compared patients' and nurses' opinions regarding the role of nurses in giving information to breast cancer patients. The study involved administering near-identical questionnaires to patients who had undergone surgery for breast

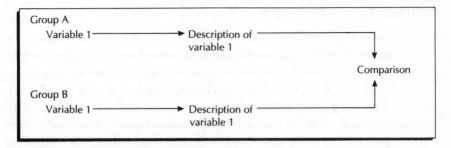

Fig. 17.3   A comparative descriptive design.

cancer and nurses who cared for breast cancer patients. The researchers were then able to compare patients' and nurses' opinions on variables such as patients' perceived knowledge levels about their illness situation and information received by patients before and during hospitalization and to carry out statistical analysis based on a multivariate technique.

Case-control study designs

A case-control study is one in which a group of *cases* (for example, patients with a post-operative wound infection) is identified. A second group of *controls* is then selected. This latter group will comprise post-operative patients who are similar in many respects (for example, in terms of the surgical operation they have had) except that their wounds are not infected. The two groups can then be compared with respect to the variable (for example, skin preparation) which is thought to have precipitated the development of wound infection post-operatively.

From the data presented in Fig. 17.4 it can be seen that the majority of cases (that is, those patients who had developed post-operative wound infections) had received skin preparation D pre-operatively, whereas relatively few controls (patients whose wounds had not become infected) had had their skin prepared this way.

	Nature of skin preparation			
Group of patients	A	B	C	D
Cases	7	3	18	72
Controls	67	19	6	8

Fig. 17.4   Case-control study of pre-operative skin preparation; results are expressed as percentages of patients.

The majority of case-control studies (like the above example) are retrospective in that they look back into the history of the subjects and investigate and describe what happened to them in the past before they were selected for study.

Retrospective study designs

Because retrospective studies attempt to link the present situation with what happened in the past, they are sometimes referred to as *ex post facto*. In other words, both the proposed cause and the proposed effect have already happened, and the researcher attempts to identify the factor(s) which resulted in the effect. However, it has to be recognized that the researcher's knowledge of the proposed cause and proposed effect can sometimes bias the investigation. Additionally, there is the problem that if the researcher is interested in something which happened a long time ago and which has resulted in the effect, then the subject's ability to accurately recall the information may be somewhat suspect.

Longitudinal designs

Longitudinal designs facilitate the collection of data over a period of time, and are useful if, for example, the researcher wanted to examine changes in a group of subjects over time (Fig. 17.5).

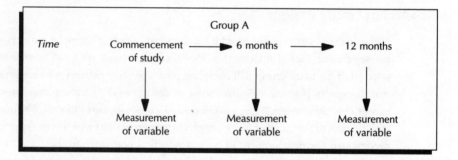

Fig. 17.5 Longitudinal design.

Such a design was employed by Seed (1994) in her study of student nurse socialization, in which the emergent views of a cohort of student nurses were explored over a three year period using a combination of data collecting methods, namely participant observation and interview. Data were collected during a four hour visit to each student by the researcher every 12 weeks for three years. As a result, the researcher was able to describe students' changing perceptions about the people they were nursing.

As can be readily appreciated, the use of a longitudinal design tends to be expensive and also calls for long term researcher and subject commitment in many instances. On the other hand, it is generally recognized that research problems which involve trends, changes or development over time are best addressed through longitudinal designs.

Cross-sectional designs

This type of design involves the collection of data at one point in time. It is a design that would be appropriate for examining groups of subjects in various stages of development simultaneously (Fig. 17.6).

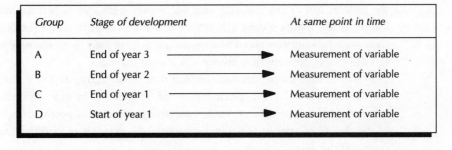

Group	Stage of development		At same point in time
A	End of year 3	⟶	Measurement of variable
B	End of year 2	⟶	Measurement of variable
C	End of year 1	⟶	Measurement of variable
D	Start of year 1	⟶	Measurement of variable

Fig. 17.6 Cross-sectional design.

If, for example, the researcher wished to study the development of manual dexterity in student nurses, by employing a cross-sectional design, she would be able to describe groups of subjects at different stages of their training programme at one time. Hence the collection of data can be 'telescoped' into one period, the duration of which is determined only by the length of time it takes to collect the data.

While this type of design may be more economical in terms of time and money than the longitudinal design, it does make the assumption that the stages of development are part of a process which will progress across time. A comparison of longitudinal and cross-sectional designs is shown in Fig. 17.7.

Longitudinal	Cross-sectional
Costly in terms of time, effort and money	Less time-consuming, less expensive, more manageable
Confounding variables could affect the interpretation of the results	Confounding variables of maturation resulting from elapsing time not present
Early trends in the data can be investigated	
Subjects may respond in a socially desirable way that they believe is congruent with the researcher's expectations.	

Fig. 17.7 Comparison of longitudinal and cross-sectional designs.

Prospective study designs

Prospective studies are very like longitudinal studies in that they start in the present and end in the future. Looking to the future, the researcher is interested in describing the effect(s) of a cause (or causes) which may already have occurred. Such a design was employed by Hewlett (1994) within her study of changing disability in patients with rheumatoid arthritis. Initially, the patients' functional ability was measured with the Stanford Health Assessment Questionnaire (Kirwan & Reeback, 1986) in which the patients had to rate the ease with which they were able to perform different categories of activities of daily living. Six months later, using the same questionnaire, these same patients were asked whether each activity of daily living was now more or less difficult to perform than six months ago, or the same.

However, such studies are less common than retrospective studies in that it can take a long time for the phenomenon of interest to become evident. It is acknowledged that prospective studies are stronger than retrospective ones because of the degree of control that can be imposed on extraneous variables that may confound the data.

Conclusion

Many variables in nursing are not amenable to experimental manipulation, and this is one reason why descriptive studies can be of great value. The descriptive researcher, in search of meaning, is concerned with observing, describing and documenting aspects of events, phenomena or situations as they occur naturally, and the information obtained can often form the foundation for the development of nursing theories.

This chapter has introduced some of the aspects related to descriptive research and has briefly considered a number of types of descriptive designs which are frequently employed by researchers conducting this type of research.

References

Colbert, K. (1994) Why opt for an unnecessary delay? Delays in presentation of breast cancer. *Professional Nurse*, **9**(9), 643–5.

Crouch, R. & Dale, J. (1994) Identifying feelings engendered during triage assessment in the accident and emergency department: the use of visual analogue scales. *Journal of Clinical Nursing*, **3**(5), 289–97.

David, J. (1992) A survey of the use of syringe drivers in Marie Curie Centres. *European Journal of Cancer Care*, **1**(4), 23–8.

Gould, D. & Ream, E. (1994) Nurses' views of infection control: an interview study. *Journal of Advanced Nursing*, **19**, 1121–31.

Hewlett, S. (1994) Patients' views of changing disability. *Nursing Standard*, **8**(31), 25–9.

Kirwan, J.R. & Reeback, J.S. (1986) Stanford Health Assessment Questionnaire Modified to Assess Disability in British Patients with Rheumatoid Arthritis. *British Journal of Rheumatology*, **25**, 206–9.

LoBiondo-Wood, G. & Haber, J. (1986) *Nursing Research – Critical Appraisal and Utilization*. Mosby, St Louis.

Richmond, J. (1993) An investigation into the effects of hypoglycaemia in young people aged 16–30 years. *Journal of Advanced Nursing*, **18**(11), 1681–7.

Seed, A. (1994) Patients to people. *Journal of Advanced Nursing*, **19**(4), 738–48.

Suominen, T. Leino-Kilpi, H. & Laippala, P. (1994) Nurses' role in informing breast cancer patients: a comparison between patients' and nurses' opinions. *Journal of Advanced Nursing*, **19**(1), 6–11.

Tye, C. (1993) Qualified nurses perceptions of the needs of suddenly bereaved family members in the accident and emergency department. *Journal of Advanced Nursing*, **18**(6), 948–56.

While, A.E. & Rees, K.L. (1993) The knowledge base of health visitors and district nurses regarding products in the proposed formulary for nurse prescription. *Journal of Advanced Nursing*, **18**(10), 1573–7.

Chapter 18

Evaluation Research

Senga Bond

What sets evaluation research apart from other forms of research is its prime intention of contributing to policy making – be it at the level of an individual work unit like a school of nursing or a hospital ward or, at the other end of the continuum, at the highest level of government. Evaluation is conducted with the purpose of informing decision-makers to enable them to make better decisions. Given that evaluations are done in the real world of providing services, education or whatever, rather than as 'academic' projects, it encounters all of the features that make organizations tick. If all research is political, evaluation research is more so.

Well conceived, well designed and conducted and thoughtfully analysed evaluations have the potential to provide insights into how services or projects are operating, the extent to which they are meeting intended goals or the needs of recipients, their strengths and weaknesses and their cost effectiveness. By doing so they provide fruitful directions for the future. Evaluations should provide relevant information for decision-makers and so contribute to setting priorities, guiding the allocation of resources and guiding the modification and refinement of structures and processes. With such a broad range of possible functions it is not surprising that evaluation conforms to a number of different models, differentially appropriate to a range of circumstances and interests and having particular strengths and weaknesses in different contexts.

The purpose of evaluation

Table 18.1 points to some different evaluation models and the particular characteristics they emphasize. This list should immediately alert the potential evaluator to the wide range of activities and meanings involved in the idea of 'an evaluation' and the range of investigative activities that could be used. Usually, however, there are three main categories of purpose which guide the request for, or the decision to undertake, an evaluation. These are needs assessment, formative evaluation and summative evaluation.

Needs assessment

The first is not evaluation of an existing project at all but a means of seeking an

Table 18.1 Some models of evaluation (based on Herman *et al.*, 1987).

Model	Emphasis
Goal-orientated evaluation	Evaluation should assess the extent to which the specified goals of an innovation are achieved, i.e. the effectiveness of an innovation.
Decision-orientated evaluation	Evaluation should facilitate intelligent judgements by decision-makers.
Responsive evaluation	Evaluation should describe the processes involved in a scheme or innovation and relate this to the value perspectives of key people.
Evaluation research	Evaluations should focus on explaining the effects of innovations and generating generalizations about their effectiveness.
Goal-free evaluation	Evaluation should assess the effects of innovations over and above their own specified goals and focus on the extent to which client needs are met as well as unintended consequences.
Advocacy–adversary evaluation	Evaluation should derive from the argumentation of contrasting points of view.
Utilization-orientated evaluation	Evaluation should be structured to maximize the utilization of its findings by specific stakeholders and users.

assessment of needs, problems or conditions which should be taken into account and addressed in future planning. In this kind of situation there is generally a need for information, or a feeling that things are not as they should be and there is a need to clarify goals, assess the extent to which they are shared, identify whether clients perceive problems and decide whether there needs to be new forms of action. Examples of this kind of enquiry would be 'What is the overall magnitude of the population requiring a service?', 'What is the nature or range of facilities likely to be required?', 'How will a new service be monitored?', 'What might users feel about services being proposed?'.

Formative evaluation

This kind of evaluation has its main thrust in providing information which will improve the running or development of an on-going service in relation to its value. It will involve monitoring the implementation of an innovation, the functioning of an existing service and the processes of achieving goals. The thrust is to understand how well a service or project is moving towards its objectives so that remedial action may be taken when things seem to be going amiss and modifications are required, or to recognize when things are going well. Parlett & Hamilton's (1977) influential paper deals with conducting formative evaluations.

This time-consuming activity involves detailed assessments of the many processes involved in an innovation and feeds back activities to the participants so that they can act on the insights gained. In some respects formative evaluation embodies components of action research (see Chapter 15) since its thrust is to make changes for improvements. These changes may involve personnel, their activities, the organization of services or technologies in use. An example of formative evaluation is work undertaken to study management practices in a new residential unit, staffed by nurses, for the care of long-term psychiatric patients (Garety & Morris, 1984). This study relies on already developed scales to assess staff orientation and attitudes as well as direct observation of the ways that staff interact with patients in order to decide whether care practices are related to styles of interaction with patients, and so to improve them. At a different level a current study is comparing locality purchasing of health services by three Health Commissioners in a formative and comparative mode using case study methods developed by George & McKeown (1985) and data collected in a focused way, dealing selectively with those aspects of the case believed to be relevant to the study (Pettigrew *et al.*, 1992). Meetings are arranged at regular intervals to feed back findings to stakeholders at different levels to assist in improving processes identified as necessary or important aspects of enabling locality purchasing.

Summative evaluation

The main goal of summative evaluation is to present information about the effectiveness and value of an innovation. It may relate to the decision to continue or discontinue an innovation and whether or how to expand or reduce it.

Carrying out this kind of evaluation may involve only one example or case, or comparison, either between different innovations within a programme or with a control group which is not receiving any intervention. An example of one of the largest summative evaluations of a new health service is the work carried out on National Health Service Nursing Homes set up in three experimental sites and compared with hospital accommodation (Bond *et al.*, 1990a, b, c). Most evaluations are carried out on a much smaller scale, although the study by Smith & Cantley (1985) is an excellent demonstration of the depth of work necessary to understand the processes within even a single small organization providing, in this instance, day care.

Comparing evaluation and research

It should now be clear that there are many reasons for doing evaluations and many different ways of going about it. Thus different people involved in evaluations will not only see different purposes in it, but will hold conflicting expectations of it. Some would regard as acceptable evaluation by participants sitting around a table sharing their opinions and arriving at a conclusion. At the other extreme are large scale, well designed research studies. Most evaluation falls somewhere in between.

Evaluation applies the methods of social research, so that the principles and methods which apply to the other kinds of research described throughout this text apply here too. What distinguishes evaluation research is not method or even subject matter, but intent – the purpose for which it is done.

Table 18.2 describes some characteristics which apply to evaluation and to research. The focus in evaluations relates to the underlying purposes and, while evaluations are intended to inform decisions, and hence action, there is nothing inherently action-orientated about research per se (with the exception of action research). While nursing research tends to have an applied focus, it need not have, since the prime purpose is to seek new understandings and add to our knowledge base. There is increasing recognition that, for research to influence practice, greater attention has to be given to involving the potential users at an early stage. This is a prime characteristic of well conducted evaluations. Thus evaluation research straddles the twin ideals of knowledge generation for local use and informing decisions, and has to adapt to fulfilling both purposes.

Most evaluations are local, although they may have more general implications depending on the settings and methods used. Research has as a main characteristic the generalizability of its findings. Thus evaluation research must be set at this wider level and make clear the parameters which limit the extent of its general-

Table 18.2 Characteristics of research and evaluation.

Characteristic	Evaluation	Research
(1) Focus	Decisions – evaluation seeks understanding to facilitate decisions	Conclusions – research seeks understanding as its primary goal
(2) Generalizability	Low – results are often applicable only to the setting studied	High – results should be applicable to comparable settings
(3) Valuing in inquiry	Worthwhileness	Truth
(4) Measurement principles	Important	Important
(5) Scientific principles	Important	Essential
(6) Sampling techniques	Desirable	Crucial
(7) Random selection of subjects	May be feasible	Important if possible
(8) Descriptive and inferential statistics	Utilized	Utilized
(9) Audience	Identified and important	May or may not be identified
(10) Politics	Recognized and accommodated	Usually considered improper
(11) Replicability	Usually not possible	Very important
(12) Setting	Very significant	Minimally important
(13) Reporting	Internal and political	External, public and open
(14) Theory building	Not usually	Central and important

izability. If we take the study of National Health Service Nursing Homes as an example, there are some findings which may have relevance for the private nursing home sector, especially related to the staffing, organizational styles of the home managers and care practices. However, the study was wholly based in the National Health Service, and we know that the clients in the National Health Service nursing homes were more psychologically dependent than were those in private establishments (Bond *et al.*, 1989). While the findings have general relevance there would be danger in extrapolating some findings for this reason apart from any others.

Those who seek evaluations are interested in the worth of findings in terms of their value for decision-making. This tends to be the major criterion in considering whether the evaluator has done a good job. For research, the essence lies in the validity of the findings – what confidence can be placed in them – irrespective of any other value it may hold. Evaluation research has to conform to the cannons of science and measurement principles to arrive at information which is valid. While evaluators also use methods which conform to measurement principles, adhering to good science is usually less important than empiricism. Often evaluations are the art of the possible – and often it is not possible to adhere to good science, because the practical context in which evaluations are done just does not permit this. For instance, it is not always possible to set up different ways of providing a service or introducing a new policy directive or to sample adequately those who are exposed to new developments, for practical or political reasons. The evaluation exercise is then carried out in such a way that the findings are restricted and interpretation not straightforward. Thus while the statistical and measurement aspects of evaluations may be similar to those carried out in research, the underlying design and/or sample selection are often, of necessity, less rigorous, although opportunities may arise to select cases which are theoretically sensitive and after good comparisons. Thus, the findings in evaluations are even more constrained than are those of research.

Evaluations tend to be sought, or are carried out, in-house while a consultant may be employed. The customer and audience for the evaluation therefore is well identified in advance and should have had a major say in how the evaluation has proceeded. The relevance of the findings, however, may prove to be of value to a wider audience, but this is not necessarily the case. In basic research, the audience is not targeted in advance, unlike research with clear practical relevance in commerce, industry or public service. Indeed, research, especially fundamental research, should in many respects be impartial to particular applications, and focus exclusively on a search for knowledge. Marie Curie had no application in mind in her life work to isolate new chemical elements. The search was to increase knowledge. In research per se then, the closer it is to pure research the more the political context is played down, while in evaluations and evaluation in research, the political context is both recognized and taken into account while the researcher, rather than the focus of the study, attempts to remain impartial. Thus, in doing evaluation research there has to be a balance between disinterest and the political context in which the results are to be produced and used.

In the National Health Service Nursing Home study, where care was nurse rather than medically managed, and power issues were involved in removing medical control over admission rights and the management of beds, there were obvious vested interests. The evaluation research had to take these on board while designing a study which had high scientific rigour. This scientific approach to evaluation research meant that the study was long and time-consuming and the products, in the form of scientific publications, were made available to a wide audience of different stakeholders in the provision of care, not only to the customers who commissioned the study. By the time it was concluded, policy decisions had overtaken the research.

Evaluations tend to be wanted rather more quickly than it is possible to carry out rigorous research, and the findings are generally of more local interest with publication limited to local reports. The characteristics of most evaluation projects mean that often there is little to add to a general body of knowledge or to theory building, while contributions to theory are of central importance to research. Thus evaluation research should inform theory as well as provide information which has relevance in its own right. Evaluations on the other hand, which only approximate the requirements of research, will be unlikely to contribute to theory.

The above discussion indicates why there is a distinction between many evaluations and research. However, it is possible to do evaluations which are research, so long as the study can accommodate both the rigour of research and the political and practical requirements of evaluation. Evaluation research is an endeavour which is partly social, partly political and only partly technical.

Determining the evaluation approach

While a clear specification of the reasons for undertaking an evaluation should be established at the outset, it is equally important to ascertain what kind of evaluation customers will accept as credible information. This is where the professional standards of researchers are challenged to find ways of carrying out credible work within the constraints laid down both by customers and the situation in which they are being asked to work. Nevertheless, evaluation research has itself developed the range of methods it uses to provide information since the 1960s.

Like most of social science, early evaluation looked to logical positivism to justify its method choices. Congruent with this approach was the preference for using goals articulated in advance as a basis for formulating causal hypotheses which could then be tested experimentally. This kind of thinking relies on assumptions that the implementation of a programme or policy is homogeneous across sites and unvarying over time, that goals are explicit and shared and that there are effects which are amenable to valid measurement using experimental designs. This approach to evaluation was epitomized in the classic texts of Suchman (1967) and Campbell (1969) which advocated methods approximating experiments. However, field experiments are only feasible where:

(1)   The programme under trial is a simple one with clearly defined aims.
(2)   There is a need to establish its effectiveness.
(3)   Inputs are specific and measurable.
(4)   People can agree on how outcomes can be measured.
(5)   Randomization is both politically feasible and administratively possible.
(6)   Clinical objectives do not intrude.
(7)   Non-cooperation or attention can be kept within acceptable limits.
(8)   Results are likely to be useful and timely (Booth, 1988).

Few innovative programmes and evaluation studies meet such criteria.

The assumptions of the value of experiments have come under attack not only in evaluation research but also in science as a whole. A basic difficulty lies in the nature of experiments themselves which, while probing connections between 'independent' and 'dependent' variables, cannot assign causality nor explain why a treatment is or is not effective. Quasi-experimental methods (Cook & Campbell, 1979) have also been criticised in recent years because of difficulties in interpreting treatment-related selection. Full explanation of *why* an innovation achieves its effects is extremely useful in specifying the factors which have to be present if an innovation is to be successful when transferred elsewhere (Cronbach, 1982). Together with a recognition of the need for explanatory knowledge came the recognition that it is important to let evaluation issues emerge from intensive on-site knowledge rather than formulating them prior to data collection at the outset. Innovations change in unanticipated ways, they are not stationary targets, and they are conceptualized by actors with different viewpoints, realities and meanings. Thus evaluators who came to recognize this introduced qualitative and constructivist paradigms (Guba & Lincoln, 1989). In so doing, they are prepared to use methods which take on board such different perspectives. This approach involves constructing and testing explanations of what is observed from the data, and seeking data to enable explanations to be constructed, rather than setting out hypotheses in advance and predetermining the data to be collected. They involve the participants in the innovation being evaluated more closely at all stages in the evaluation process. More recently, case study research (Yin, 1993) has gained prominence as an evaluation strategy. Multiple case studies include the collection of a range of dependent variables to assess whether there is a pattern of results.

These developments in different philosophical and methodological approaches to evaluation underscore the values of a pluralistic approach to evaluative research (Rossi & Freeman, 1993). There are merits in the different approaches, and each add in different ways to carrying out successful evaluations. While quantitative methods, particularly pragmatic randomized controlled trials (Schwartz & Lellouch, 1967), are designed and interpreted in such a way that they enable a decision to be taken about the more favourable of two treatments, such methods, despite their scientific rigour, cannot begin to uncover the sequence of intention, action, interaction and reaction which constitute the day to day implementation of a service or policy. Pragmatic trials are limited to deciding whether there is a difference between treatments, they cannot explain why such a difference is found. It is for this reason that qualitative methods have become attractive.

Smith & Cantley's (1985) evaluation of a psycho-geriatric day service, using qualitative methods, elucidated expected as well as unanticipated occurrences and developments as a new service was implemented. There is a growing respect for a diversity of approaches within one study. Because of the desirability of contributing data about structures, processes and outcomes of the National Health Service Nursing Homes, the approach taken in that research was to use a range of methods within a single complex design. This kind of research is expensive and time-consuming, but such comprehensiveness not only enables decisions to be taken about the most appropriate policy to adopt, but also contributes to understanding the means whereby the policy may be successfully disseminated to new sites. Strategies which cannot be adaptive are 'doomed to reflect only that which stood still long enough to be measured' (Rist, 1984), and evaluations must be able to cope with change. In the current National Health Service, as in many spheres of life, change is happening at an increasing rate and evaluators have to work within it.

Evaluation: a small scale example

An example may help elucidate some of these points. Let us say we are going to evaluate the impact of a seminar programme for new staff nurses. The idea behind the programme is to offer continuing education about topics which new staff nurses have themselves identified as of interest and importance to them in their new roles. These topics were obtained by a needs assessment survey of new staff nurses in the unit, carried out at a single point in time.

Since releasing staff for educational purposes involves opportunity costs – the staff or the staff replacing them could be occupied in some other activity – there is a need from managers to know whether they are cost effective.

The approach to be taken is both formative and summative. The series will be evaluated while in progress and adjustments made on the basis of what is discovered as well as an assessment of perceived benefits at the end of the series. The task has been given to a member of staff in the continuing education department in the Health Authority. How should she go about it?

The seminars have been set up during the afternoon 'overlap' – the time assumed when staff are most available. A number of lecture sessions have been arranged around an apparently sensible sequence of topics interspersed with discussion seminars. A number of targets for evaluation are immediately apparent and methods of collecting data suggest themselves. These might include some of the activities in Table 18.3.

By using formative methods it may very quickly become apparent that while the early afternoon seems an appropriate time, low attendance permits a rapid search for the reasons. It may be that staff are not available or that they feel reluctant to take time out for educational purposes or feel too tired to absorb information. It may be found that other times are more appropriate and more convenient or that,

Table 18.3 Some steps in an evaluation.

Evaluation question	Data to illuminate the questions	Method of collection
Is the timing of seminar/ discussion groups appropriate?	Proportion of target staff attending	Staff sign attendance sheet, calculate % attending
	Attention given by staff to lecturer/degree of participation in seminar groups	Observe behaviour, note and count questions asked, assess quality of debate
Is the content of the seminars appropriate?	Proportion of target staff attending	Number of staff attending different topics
	Attention given by staff to lecturer/degree of participation in seminar groups	Observation of behaviour, count questions, number dozing, rate extent of interest expressed by seminar participants
Is the method of presentation appropriate?	Proportion of target staff attending	Number of staff attending different kinds of seminar
	Attention given by staff to lecturer/degree of participation in seminar groups	Observation of behaviour, count questions, number dozing, rate extent of interest expressed by seminar participants
Is the sequence appropriate, i.e. lecture followed by discussion seminar?		Observe points brought forward from lecture to seminar
Are there important topics missing or inadequately addressed?	Opinion, behaviour on ward	Questionnaire or structured interview with staff nurses who attended
Has the seminar programme influenced the staff nurses' performance?	Behaviour on ward	Questionnaire or structured interview with staff nurses and ward sister regarding staff nurses' performance

because of the difficulty of short time release from wards, there may be more to be gained by seeking a larger block of time in whole days or a few days. New formats may be tried in successive repeats of the programme.

Moving to the end point – do the seminars influence the staff nurses' performance? Obtaining some behavioural assessment by others rather than only self-opinion would be helpful. In this kind of small study it is unlikely that direct before/after behavioural comparisons or comparison with a control group would be possible, but an indication may be obtained by asking the staff nurses' immediate manager to assess changes in appropriate categories of behaviour. Of course, there will be effects of time-in-post and maturation into the new staff nurse role which confound the efforts of the programme, but there is nothing that can be done about this except for comparison with a group which does not have the opportunity to attend the seminar programme. A larger comparison could compare two methods of trying to achieve the same objectives – self-study, peer-supported learning, and so on. To begin to do this kind of comparison and to develop behavioural measures of educational effectiveness would extend the evaluation into a much more rigorous design, endowing it with wider credibility. Knowledge would be gained not only about the effectiveness of the seminar programme, or what may replace it as a result of the changes brought about by the formative work, but also about different strategies and the development of staff nurse behaviour over time.

Some costings would have to be carried out to assess the actual and opportunity costs of the programme. These might include costing the exercise in terms of hours of staff nurses' time, replacement salaries, lecturers, seminar leaders and the administrative costs of the programme. It is unlikely that information about financial benefits will be readily obtainable, but some data may be found in changing practices, fewer duplications of work, fewer mistakes, reduced infection rates and so on.

Less formal outcomes of the seminar programme should be looked for. These may lie in improved morale, the formation of supportive professional relationships or participants finding opportunities to share local knowledge and benefit from it.

Others who are already knowledgeable about pedagogic processes and organizational contingencies may have set up their educational initiative in a very different way at the outset, basing it on different educational theories and prior knowledge of what is likely to be the most effective strategy. Nevertheless, the sound evaluation of innovations whatever their nature is crucial in deciding their worth – the more bold and radical the innovation, the more critical the need to evaluate it.

Conclusion

New services and educational initiatives are difficult things to evaluate. They are multi-dimensional, complicated, elusive and always 'on the move'. The evaluation methods employed must also be subtle, sophisticated and valid; they must be sufficiently dynamic to adapt to both the changing characteristics of clients' or students' setting and context and changing perceptions of needs. They must also be responsive to changing social, political and economic climates – as anyone doing health service research in the 1990s will be only too aware. All too often new schemes are introduced without thought to their evaluation, with consequent loss of opportunity and increased difficulty of obtaining baseline data. Nevertheless, attempting to provide as scientific and evidence based information as possible for service or educational development is an infinitely interesting – and challenging – occupation. Increasingly new services are being established with evaluation as an integral part, in recognition that it is wasteful and no longer ethical to promulgate untested innovations. So long as policy makers are willing to take account of the findings produced through evaluation research, it is potentially a very useful and rewarding activity.

To carry out evaluation research demands the application of research principles to the evaluation process. This is an activity of an entirely different order to other approaches to evaluation which lack scientific rigour, and may amount to no more than a group of professionals sitting around a table and passing opinions or obtaining a handful of opinions at the end of a course. For this reason it is important to understand the distinctions and similarities between evaluations and evaluation research, and to consider the substance of their findings for policy decisions. Unfortunately, all too often decisions are taken without evidence, before evaluations are reported or without due attention to their findings. It is worth stressing again the critical importance of involving policy-makers from the beginning of the evaluation process to gain their commitment to the implications of the findings for the decisions they make.

References

Bond, J., Atkinson, A., Gregson, B., Hughes, P. & Jeffries, L. (1989) *The 1984 and 1987 Surveys of Continuing Care Institutions in Six Health Authorities. Vol. 4, Evaluation of Continuing-Care Accommodation for Elderly People.* Health Care Research Unit, University of Newcastle upon Tyne.

Bond, J., Bond, S. & Gregson, B. (1990a) Nursing homes and continuing care – part 1. *Nursing Standard*, 4(36), 38–40.

Bond, J., Bond, S. & Gregson, B. (1990b) Nursing homes and continuing care – part 3. *Nursing Standard*, 4(38), 35–7.

Bond, S., Bond, J., Gregson, B. & Donaldson, C. (1990c) Nursing homes and continuing care – part 2. *Nursing Standard*, 4(37), 21–23.

Booth, T. (1988) *Developing Policy Research.* Gower, Aldershot.

Campbell, D.T. (1969) Reforms as experiments. *American Psychologist*, 24, 409–28.

Cook, T.D. & Campbell, D.T. (1979) *Quasi-experimentation Design and Analysis Issues for Field Settings.* Houghton Mifflin, Boston.

Cronbach, L.J. (1982) *Designing Evaluations of Educational and Social Programmes.* Jossey Bass, San Francisco.

Garety, P.A. & Morris, I. (1984) A new unit for long-stay psychiatric patients: organisation, attitudes and quality of care. *Psychological Medicine*, 14, 183–92.

George, A.L. & McKeown, T.J. (1985) Case studies and theories of organisational decision making. In *Advances in Information Processing in Organizations*, Vol 2. JAI Press, Greenwich, CT.

Guba, E.G. & Lincoln, Y.S. (1989) *Fourth Generation Evaluation.* Sage Publications, New York and London.

Herman, J.L., Morris, L.L. & Fitz-Gibbon, C.T. (1987) *Evaluation handbook.* Sage Publications, New York and London.

Parlett, M. & Hamilton, D. (1977) Evaluation as illumination: a new approach to the study of innovatory programmes. In *Beyond the Numbers Game* (eds D. Hamilton *et al.*). MacMillan, Basingstoke.

Pettigrew, A., Ferlie, E. & McKee L. (1992) *Shaping Strategic Change.* Sage Publications, London.

Rist, R. (1984) On the application of qualitative research to the policy process: an emergent linkage. In *Social Crises and Educational Research* (eds L. Barton & S. Walker). Croom Helm, London.

Rossi, P.H. & Freeman, H.E. (1993) *Evaluation: A Systematic Approach*, 5th edn. Sage Publications, Thousand Oaks, California.

Schwartz, D. & Lellouch, J. (1967) Explanatory and pragmatic attitudes in therapeutic trials. *Journal of Chronic Diseases*, **20**, 637–48.

Smith, G. & Cantley, C. (1985) *Assessing Health Care: A Study in Organisational Evaluation.* Open University Press, Milton Keynes.

Suchman, E. (1967) *Evaluative Research.* Sage Publications, New York and London.

Yin, R.K. (1993) *Case Study Research: Design and Methods.* Sage Publications, New York and London.

Chapter 19

Survey Design and Sampling

F. Ian Atkinson

The intention of this chapter is to introduce the general principles of survey research design and methods of random sampling. Broadly, survey research can be seen as either descriptive or analytical in purpose. Descriptive surveys aim to make descriptive statements about a study population. The intention of analytical surveys is to explore associations between the different variables under study. While it is useful to distinguish these two main purposes, in practice, much survey work is carried out for both descriptive and analytical reasons.

A major feature of a survey is that information is obtained from a sample of subjects who are selected from a study population and then, on the basis of this information the whole study population can be described. In other words, population parameters can be estimated on the basis of sample statistics. Already this has introduced terms which need to be defined.

The term *population* refers to all those people about which a researcher wishes to make statements. In research it is up to the investigator to define the population of interest. For example, if you wanted to make statements about the prevalence of smoking among registered nurses in a single Health Board area then the population would be all registered nurses employed in that Health Board. Populations for surveys are not always people, they may be items. If hospital managers wanted to make a statement about the quality of a consignment of disposable syringes delivered to a hospital then every syringe in that consignment would constitute the population of interest. A *sample* refers to the group of people that a researcher selects from a defined population and these are the individuals about whom information will be collected. This information can be summarized as *sample statistics* (for example the mean age of a sample). A population parameter refers to a measurable characteristic of a study population which is not known but estimated on the basis of a sample statistic in descriptive surveys.

By their very nature, descriptive survey findings do not allow statements of *fact* to be made about a population parameter. Indeed any statement about a population based on sample findings can only be a probability statement, meaning that there is a chance that it could be wrong. The challenge is to reduce the chance of this final statement being wrong to an acceptable and calculable level. This can only be achieved by giving attention to the design of surveys and the principles which need to be applied are outlined below.

At this point it might be reasonable to ask, 'If there is a chance that the final statements about a population will be wrong then why bother doing surveys at all? Why not get information from everyone, for example all the ward sisters, then statements of fact could be made about how many smoked and no one could question the findings?'

If information is collected from all individuals in a defined population this is referred to as a population census. Although the idea of carrying out a census may hold some attractions, a brief consideration of the nature of censuses as compared to sample surveys shows the latter to have definite advantages. First, it is very difficult to get information from everybody in a defined population, there are always some who either can't be contacted or decline to help with an investigation. Even in the national census where people are compelled by law to complete and return a form there are still those who refuse. As a consequence the researcher may still be unable to make factual statements about the population. Second, a census can be very expensive to carry. Third, in some instances it might be entirely impractical to get complete information from a population. In the example of a consignment of disposable syringes, if each was to be tested for contamination then none would be left for the hospital to use. Also some populations change so that they cannot be counted in any event or they may be so large or inaccessible that counting them becomes impossible.

For practical reasons survey designs and methods may have to be used in order to study populations. In Britain, much of what is known about the nation's health, social conditions, standards of living, work, education, social attitudes and behaviour is based upon survey findings (see for example, Office of Population Censuses and Surveys, 1992; Government Statistical Service, 1994).

One of the major objectives of any survey research is to achieve the highest possible degree of accuracy in the findings. Generally there are seen to be three main sources of inaccuracy, or error, in survey work. These are known as sampling error, non-response error and response error. Each of these concepts are discussed later in this chapter. The avoidance of errors is central to the design of surveys and by giving attention to the procedures employed they can be controlled.

Sample selection

The first problem for the researcher is how to select a sample which will represent the population under study. A system of selection is needed to ensure that the researcher and factors extraneous to the research, have no influence whatsoever on the selection procedure. If there is a possibility that individuals with particular characteristics might stand a higher chance of being included in a sample than do others in the population then the final sample could represent a population different from the one intended for study. Consequently the research findings could be inappropriately applied to what is essentially a different study population.

For example, imagine you needed to assess the numbers of nurses with a positive or negative view towards proposed changes in salaries and conditions of service. In order to estimate the feeling of the profession in a particular hospital it is decided to sample nurses and ask them how they will vote on the proposed changes. The population here would be all nurses both qualified and in training at the hospital. A sample might be taken by a convenient procedure involving the researcher sitting in a hospital corridor and asking the views of all who came by. Unfortunately and unbeknown to the researcher this corridor leads to an area stocked with journals and daily newspapers, all of which were publishing detailed comment on the issue. The outcome of this might be that a high proportion of nurses who answered the questions were aware of the full implications of the proposed agreement and would not support it. Had the sample been obtained by other means or in another part of the hospital then an entirely different picture could have emerged in the findings because a less well informed group of nurses would have been selected. As it was, the sample selected was biased and did not represent the whole population of nurses in the hospital.

How then can a sample that might represent a defined population be selected? In order to obtain such a sample a method is needed that will remove all biases in selection. The only way this can be achieved is by incorporating a system of randomness into the selection procedure. The term *random* does not mean haphazard or careless but refers to a precise method of selection where all individuals in a defined population stand an equal chance of being selected for inclusion in the study sample.

Simple random sample

There are many types of sample design which incorporate the principles of random selection. Here the methods of selecting a *simple random sample* are outlined to introduce the basic principles of random sampling. An easily understood and full exposition of variations in the design of random samples is provided by Moser & Kalton (1985). The procedures involved in selecting a simple random sample are illustrated here with a practical example of sampling to estimate the mean age of 100 patients who attended an out-patient clinic. The procedures involved in this exercise are identical to those which would have to be followed in real sample selection.

Sampling frame

After having defined a study population the first stage of sample selection is to obtain a list of all individuals in that population. This list is known as the *sampling frame* and from it the sample is chosen. It is essential that the sampling frame gives a complete coverage of the population otherwise it will not be adequate for its purpose. Clearly if some members of the population are not included in the list they stand no chance of being selected and the resulting sample could be biased.

Obtaining an adequate sampling frame often poses problems for research which involves human populations.

Once the sampling frame is obtained individuals are numbered consecutively starting at zero. For purposes of the practical exercise the population is represented by all the people included in Fig. 19.1. The members of this population have

The Population

38	17	42	63	41	33	34	68	7	23
.00	.01	.02	.03	.04	.05	.06	.07	.08	.09.
49	18	46	44	62	70	67	20	48	61
.10	.11	.12	.13	.14	.15	.16	.17	.18	.19.
14	48	59	28	51	71	10	30	8	27
.20	.21	.22	.23	.24	.25	.26	.27	.28	.29.
46	71	66	18	57	29	53	61	81	60
.30	.31	.32	.33	.34	.35	.36	.37	.38	.39.
53	25	40	19	11	56	18	41	29	29
.40	.41	.42	.43	.44	.45	.46	.47	.48	.49.
68	66	37	76	46	77	50	45	13	75
.50	.51	.52	.53	.54	.55	.56	.57	.58	.59.
69	28	15	86	55	81	19	29	74	21
.60	.61	.62	.63	.64	.65	.66	.67	.68	.69.
78	80	79	33	39	88	72	69	35	92
.70	.71	.72	.73	.74	.75	.76	.77	.78	.79.
64	81	72	17	9	55	42	49	87	16
.80	.81	.82	.83	.84	.85	.86	.87	.88	.89.
14	39	41	28	48	86	52	6	35	21
.90	.91	.92	.93	.94	.95	.96	.97	.98	.99.

Fig. 19.1 The population. One hundred patients who attended an out-patient clinic.

already been given consecutive numbers starting at zero and finishing at 99. The two-digit number underneath each person represents their number in the sampling frame. The number above each person represents their age.

Sample selection

Imagine a sample of 15 people is required; all that is needed is a list of 15 two-digit random numbers and the people on the list with corresponding numbers are taken for the sample. Random numbers can be obtained in several different ways but the example of the tombola drum method gives the clearest understanding of the nature of randomness. To generate random numbers using a tombola involves marking ten discs with a single digit from zero to nine. The discs are placed in the drum which is spun and a single disc picked out. The number is written down, the disc is put back in the drum and the process is repeated until sufficient numbers have been obtained to select the sample. This process ensures that all numbers have an equal chance of being selected which itself is the property of randomness. If a tombola drum was used to select a sample of 15 people from a population of 100 then the procedure would have to be repeated a total of 30 times. This would provide 15 two-digit numbers between zero ('00') and '99', therefore covering every numbered individual in the population. Such a procedure could become rather tedious if a large sample was required so random numbers are published in sets of statistical tables (Lindley & Scott, 1984) or they can be easily generated by a computer. Figure 19.2 is a table of random numbers which were generated by a computer.

For our sample, 15 two-digit numbers between zero and 99 have to be found and they are chosen in the following way. First select a point in any row and any column of Fig. 19.2. Imagine the third column along and the fifth row down is chosen, that is number 8. A two-digit number is required so two columns have to be used. The first number then is 87 and the person who has number 87 in the sampling frame (Fig. 19.1) is selected for the sample. The second number is then selected by going down the column so the next person to be included in the sample is number 81. This process is repeated until a list of 15 random numbers have been obtained. If by chance the same number is encountered twice, then that person is not included in the sample twice. Rather, selection continues until a set of unique numbers (15 for this sample) have been obtained. The sample selected in this example is shown in Fig. 19.3.

In some sample designs, a particular subject might be included in the sample more than once and this is called sampling with replacement. In social surveys this is not generally done and is termed sampling without replacement.

Having completed this procedure a simple random sample consisting of 15 individuals has been selected. A sample has no particular property which could be tested to see if it is representative of our population. All that is known about it is that it was just as likely to be chosen as any other sample. Any *test* of randomness can only be applied to the process by which the sample was selected.

28	98	16	42	02	52	11	94	58	65
07	48	17	11	90	06	44	16	83	92
44	96	27	13	38	71	70	45	61	13
96	18	84	58	25	95	37	11	12	77
75	**87**	41	62	61	85	62	35	84	02

69	**81**	00	90	65	10	96	03	27	96
40	**96**	08	06	39	39	51	43	13	59
45	**21**	62	59	92	62	57	03	02	74
14	**74**	29	57	32	57	52	12	39	44
82	**25**	38	03	30	96	74	70	86	13

59	**80**	06	78	09	29	10	43	09	68
76	**34**	36	58	48	33	86	09	31	34
37	**04**	38	11	74	28	03	79	12	52
68	**89**	13	93	80	58	75	32	40	47
74	**45**	59	62	02	15	87	95	63	44

31	**20**	12	19	74	31	71	10	51	30
53	**51**	86	80	74	48	56	06	15	30
52	**28**	71	45	61	22	01	03	47	89
57	**41**	82	32	86	09	02	01	98	12
47	43	77	34	65	32	83	34	20	36

Fig. 19.2 Random numbers. (*Note:* the 15 highlighted numbers indicate those selected for the example given in the text.)

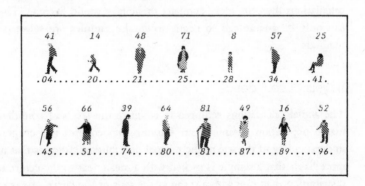

Fig. 19.3 The sample selected.

Generalization

In order to introduce the idea of how survey findings can be generalized to a whole population, in other words, how population parameters can be estimated on the basis of sample statistics, a sample mean is used to illustrate the general principles. Estimations from other types of sample statistics, for example proportions, variance and differences, are in principle similar to procedures applied to the mean and are considered by Armitage & Berry (1987).

The reason for selecting this sample was to calculate the mean sample age in order to estimate the mean age of the population. As already noted, the number above each person in Fig. 19.1 represents their age, in years, so the mean age of the sample can be calculated as 45.8 years. In real research the value of a population parameter is not known but in this case the true population mean can be calculated and it is 46.09 years. Notably these two numbers are not the same and if more samples were taken it is likely that they too would have mean values which were different from the true population mean. The difference between a sample statistic and the true population parameter is referred to as sampling error. This raises the question, 'If sample means can vary, then how can the true population mean be estimated with any confidence on the basis of one sample?'.

The answer to this lies in the fact that although the mean values obtained are determined randomly, if a large number of different samples were selected the mean values obtained begin to vary in an astonishingly predictable way. If a very large number of samples were taken from the population and the mean age of each was plotted on graph paper eventually a symmetrical bell shaped curve, approximating the profile of a *normal* distribution, would be produced. (Readers not familiar with the normal distribution should consult Chapters 27 and 28.) The curve produced by this graph is known as the sampling distribution of the mean and is very important in establishing levels of confidence in survey findings. If an infinite number of samples were taken and the mean of all the sample means calculated, the result would be exactly equal to the true population mean. In terms of the sampling distribution curve this implies that the value at its centre equals the true population mean. Further, the larger the sample size used to make these calculations then the more compact this curve would become. These phenomena can only be guaranteed to occur when the samples are selected using random methods.

Levels of confidence

The actual calculations required to estimate the levels of confidence in the estimated population parameter are outwith the scope of this chapter. However an understanding of the use of the normal distribution indicates that it is many times more likely that a sample is picked with a mean near to the centre of the sampling distribution than one with a mean at the tails of the curve. Areas enclosed by the standard normal distribution represent the probability of observing a value, in this case a sample mean, from a normally distributed variable such as the sampling distribution of the mean. Using this knowledge the chances of a sample mean falling different distances from the true population means can be calculated. It is by using these tools for analysis that levels of confidence in survey findings are estimated. Readers who wish to follow up the subject of making population estimates and calculating confidence limits are referred to Chapter 28 of this book and to Armitage & Berry (1987).

In research practice, obtaining truly random samples is extremely difficult and often impossible. The main difficulty lies in finding sampling frames which are adequate for their purpose. Consider the problems of selecting random samples of disabled people (Martin *et al.*, 1988), informal carers (Green, 1985) and injecting drug users engaged in prostitution (Rhodes *et al.*, 1994). Researchers cannot expect to obtain sampling frames for any of these populations yet, as the above authors have shown, each have been the subject of survey type research. Unfortunately, if samples are not randomly selected then the statistical model upon which descriptive surveys are based ceases to apply. This is not to say that survey research becomes invalid because of this difficulty, rather it just becomes difficult to extrapolate the findings to wider populations. Often it is the insights attained through the analysis of associations between different variables affecting a sample which prove to be the most valuable part of survey findings.

Sample size

There are no simple answers to the question of how big a sample should be recruited for survey work. There are formulae in the literature (Moser & Kalton, 1985; Armitage & Berry, 1987) which can be applied to the problem but still they alone cannot provide definitive answers. These formulae take into account factors including the levels of confidence which need to be attained in the findings, the size of the population and the variability of our measures when they are applied to the study population.

Accuracy in survey work is determined by careful design and execution of the research and large samples alone do not in any way guarantee the accuracy of findings. To illustrate this point many research textbooks describe an American survey which aimed to predict the results of a presidential election and used a sample size of ten million people. Because of the ways in which the sample was selected incorrect conclusions were drawn about the forthcoming election result.

In practice, sample size is to a large extent determined by the ways in which the data are to be anlysed. If it is intended that the information should be tabulated this means that respondents will have to be divided into different categories, for example male and female; young, middle aged and old; those who are ill or not ill (see Fig. 19.4). Figure 19.4 illustrates the rapid reduction in the sizes of sub-groups for analysis after dividing a sample of 100 people by only three variables (sex, age band and illness). In this example it would be impractical, because of the small numbers after the third division, to control for the influence of both age and sex when examining the effects of another factor on the health of the sample. In Fig. 19.4 the splitting into sub-groups is made equally at each division. In research practice this equality rarely occurs and after three divisions it may be found that some sub-groups contain no respondents at all.

The process of dividing and sub-dividing can only be continued so long as there remain workable numbers of respondents in the sub-groups and, even with a large initial sample, only a few divisions can leave such small numbers that conclusions could not be drawn from them. It is important therefore to clarify which sub-division of the sample will be the final one, and what would be the smallest desirable number of respondents to have within it for the purposes of analysis.

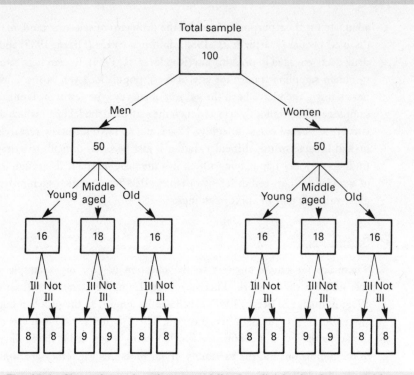

Fig. 19.4   Sizes of sample sub-groups following division by three variables.

This procedure can, of course, lead an investigator to estimate that enormous samples are required but here an unavoidable constraint thwarts these intentions – the limitations of time and resources. The process of collecting data from respondents can be costly and time-consuming so, inevitably, considerations arising from the organization and funding of research impinge upon the nature and size of research endeavours.

Sources of error

As already noted there are three major causes of error which affect survey findings. The nature of sampling error has been described and the methods for dealing with this type of inaccuracy were outlined. The problems of non-response and response error are now considered.

Non-response error

An essential part of sampling is to determine precisely who is to be included in the study. This has to be followed by ensuring that information is obtained from all those included. If some of the sample either refuse to help with the survey or for some reason cannot be contacted then there is a risk of introducing error into the findings through non-response.

To illustrate the mechanics of this type of error, imagine that for the survey of the numbers of registered nurses who smoked a simple random sample was taken, but only one half of the nurses agreed to help with the research. Their decisions to help or not might have been influenced by their own smoking behaviour. Imagine that those who did smoke felt threatened by the thought of having to answer questions on the subject while the non-smokers felt no inhibitions. As a result a high proportion of non-smokers and a low proportion of smokers would provide data for the research. The consequences for the survey findings would therefore be to underestimate the prevalence of smoking.

In dealing with respondents every effort must be made to encourage them to provide the information required. A careful choice of research topic, clear explanations as to the purpose and importance of the study, well constructed questionnaires and interview schedules all contribute towards motivating respondents to cooperate.

When faced with a non-response problem the question which has to be addressed by the researcher is 'Do those people who have responded differ from those who have not responded, in ways relevant to the aims of the research?'. Finding an answer to this question may not be easy but could be crucial for the validity of research findings.

Response error

The next source of inaccuracy is termed *response error* and this takes two forms, random error and systematic error.

Random error

Random error broadly refers to making mistakes in measurement and/or in the recording of data. This type of error always occurs in any endeavour which involves measurement of any kind and there is a well developed *law of errors*. Because mistakes in this type of error behave in a random way, in the long run they even each other out and will not unduly affect the findings of research involving groups of respondents. This can be illustrated using the example of estimating the mean age of a sample. An interviewer might inaccurately record a respondent's age because of fatigue or a lapse of concentration but the recording made is just as likely to be above as below the respondent's true age. If it is truly random error, then an equal number of overestimates and underestimates will be made in the course of collecting data from the whole sample. When the mean age is calculated the numbers will balance each other out and a correct mean age will be produced. In other words random error tends to control itself statistically.

Systematic error

Systematic error is rather different in its mode of operation and arises from problems in the way in which phenomena are measured. Using the example of age, imagine the phrasing of the question predisposed respondents to say they were younger than they really were. The outcome of this would be to systematically underestimate the age of the whole sample. Because the researcher may be unaware of the bias in the question these errors would not be accounted for in the presentation of research findings. Even if the biased question was eventually recognized, it would be impossible to make corrections to the data obtained. Consequently systematic error has to be guarded against from the outset of the research. This will involve the careful testing of questions used in interviews or questionnaires and precise calibration of all measuring instruments being used for the research.

Conclusion

This chapter has attempted to acquaint the reader with the basic principles upon which survey research is based. The main sources of error in survey findings, how they operate and how they might be controlled have been discussed. This short consideration can only offer an intending researcher an introduction to survey design and sampling, but it is hoped that it will provide an initial grounding for further study in the area. Survey research can be applied in many fields of enquiry and its principles will continue to provide an indispensable tool for planners, policy makers and all those who, for whatever reason, need to describe and analyse the characteristics of populations.

References

Armitage, P. & Berry, G. (1987) *Statistical Methods In Medical Research*, 2nd edn. Blackwell Scientific Publications, Oxford.

Government Statistical Service (1994) *Social Trends*, No 24. HMSO, London.

Green, H. (1985) *Informal Carers*. General Household Survey 1985. Office of Population Censuses and Surveys, Social Survey Division. HMSO, London.

Lindley, D.V. & Scott, W.F. (1984) *New Cambridge Elementary Statistical Tables*; 78. Cambridge University Press, Cambridge.

Martin, J., Meltzer, H. & Elliot, D (1988) *The Prevalence of Disability Among Adults*. Office of Population Censuses and Surveys, Social Survey Division, Surveys of Disability in Great Britain, Report 1. HMSO, London.

Moser, C.A. & Kalton, G. (1985) *Survey Methods in Social Investigation*. Gower, London.

Office of Population Censuses and Surveys (1992) *The General Household Survey*. HMSO, London.

Rhodes, T., Donoghoe, M., Hunter, G. & Stimson G.V. (1994) HIV prevalence no higher among female drug injectors also involved in prostitution, *AIDS Care*, 6, No 3, 269–76.

Other recommended reading

Marsh, C. (1982) *The Survey Method: The Contribution of Surveys to Sociological Explanation*. Contemporary Social Research Series No 6. George Allen and Unwin, London.

C: Data Collection

The selection of a data collection instrument offers considerable scope and choice. This section is not intended to present a comprehensive range of data collection methods, but to introduce a small variety of techniques.

Each of the data collection methods selected for inclusion has been well tested, and has been more or less widely used in health care research.

The material presented in relation to attitude measurement, interview, questionnaire, observation, the critical incident technique and physiological measurement provides a *basis* for understanding each of these methods and, for potential researchers, an overview of a number of data collection methods for consideration and further study using the references in each chapter.

What are attitudes?

Attitudes are about what is liked and disliked. The study of attitude is not, however, concerned with a transient feeling or mood but with the consistent and enduring thoughts, beliefs and feelings people have about particular attitude objects, that is, about issues, people or events. An attitude is thus a disposition to evaluate something in a particular way. This evaluative component of attitudes is generally studied in relation to the *beliefs* people hold about a particular issue and the *actions* they take towards it. Attitudes thus consist of three aspects: an evaluative component, a belief or cognitive component and an action or behavioural component. For example, a person might believe that blood donors are altruistic, that is the cognitive/belief component, and feel very positively about the idea of freely donating blood for health care, that is the evaluative component, and may freely donate blood whenever able to, that is the action/behavioural component. The emphasis placed on these three components varies greatly in both attitude theory and research. Social psychologists for several decades have investigated the links between beliefs and evaluations on the one hand and between evaluations and behaviours on the other.

Beliefs, the thoughts or cognitions we have, show a general correspondence to whether something is positively or negatively evaluated. It is perhaps not surprising that if someone holds positive attitudes towards, say, nursing staff then they will also have predominantly favourable thoughts about them, for example, that they are caring, understanding people. Conversely, if someone holds negative attitudes towards nursing staff they will have predominantly unfavourable thoughts, for example, that they are distant and unapproachable.

The relationship between evaluations and behaviours is, however, less clear cut. For many years social scientists regarded attitudes as the cause of behaviour. People with positive attitudes towards a particular object or event were assumed to engage in positive behaviour towards it, while the converse applied for people with negative attitudes. However, a review in the 1960s or work investigating the link between attitudes and behaviour (Wicker, 1969), reported that there was little more than a modest link between attitudes and behaviour. Subsequent research exploring the reasons for this poor relationship suggested that attitudes did indeed relate to behaviour, but only under certain circumstances (Fishbein & Ajzen, 1975). For example, attitudes do seem to be better able to predict behaviour if both are defined with an equivalent level of specificity or generality. Just as an attitude object can be defined very generally, for example, nursing staff, or more specifically, for example, nursing staff on ward X, behaviours too can be defined very generally, for example, all behaviours of nursing staff, or more specifically, for example, behaviours of those particular nursing staff on ward X.

It is also important to bear in mind, however, that attitudes are not the only factor predictive of behaviour. Indeed, factors such as expectations of significant others, that is, normative beliefs, in addition to issues such as perceived control over the behaviour in question, are often found to be better predictors of behaviour than attitudes themselves (Fishbein & Azjen, 1975). One might, for example, be favourably disposed toward the idea of donating blood but still not actually donate any. Factors such as general anxiety about the procedure involved, concern about the time commitment required, or lack of blood donating behaviour from family or friends may prevent a favourable attitude being turned into direct action.

Thus, while people's beliefs or thoughts may relate quite closely to whether an attitude object is evaluated positively or negatively, such evaluations do not necessarily relate to subsequent behaviour. It is clearly important to bear this in mind when measuring attitudes. The cognitive, evaluative and behavioural components of attitude systems can each be assessed and may provide results which differ from each other. While behaviours can be readily observed and quantified, for example, voting habits, or private versus state health care utilization, behaviours can only be assumed to reflect the person's tendency to evaluate the attitude object positively or negatively. Assessment of beliefs provides a clearer link with evaluative judgements, however, it is only within the last decade that researchers have attempted to systematically assess the cognitive component of attitudes (Petty & Cacioppo, 1981). The most frequently used method of assessing attitudes is by questionnaire aimed at examining the evaluative component of attitudes and it is this manner of assessment which forms the major focus of the present chapter.

Attitude scales

Several different questionnaire methods have been developed to measure the evaluative component of attitudes. These generally consist of a series of statements reflecting beliefs about the attitude object, to which the respondent indicates whether they agree or disagree. The belief statements selected are chosen to reflect certain criteria, which ensure that the statements do indeed assess favourable or unfavourable views towards an attitude object.

The four main scaling methods used to assess the evaluative component of attitudes are the Thurstone, Likert, Guttman and semantic-differential methods. Although the techniques differ they have basic assumptions in common. First, they assume that a person's attitude can be represented by some numerical score. Second, they assume that each item means the same to each respondent.

Thurstone method

The first major method of attitude measurement was developed by Thurstone (1928). He assumed it was possible to elicit statements about a particular issue which could then be ordered according to a dimension of favourableness–unfavourableness towards that issue. He also felt that it was possible to order a series of statements so that the distance, in numerical terms, between any two statements was equal.

In order to provide a reasonable spread of views about a particular issue, a Thurstone scale is generally made up of about 20 to 40 statements which have been derived from a larger pool of statements. The first step in constructing a Thurstone scale involves collecting a large number of statements about the particular issue. These can be obtained from the relevant literature, from discussion with experts in the field or direct questioning of people for whom the issue is of relevance. Any statements which are ambiguous, confusing, contain both positive and negative information or could be approved by people who hold negative attitudes are discarded.

As an example, let us consider a recent issue about which there has been some controversy – the suggested use of donated ovarian tissue (from mature women, from girls or women who have died or from aborted fetuses) in embryo research and assisted conception. In assessing people's attitudes toward this issue a preliminary set of statements might include:

- The use of donated ovarian tissue in research and treatment is morally wrong in all circumstances.
- The use of donated ovarian tissue in research and treatment should only be permitted if the tissue is obtained from mature women.
- The use of donated ovarian tissue should be for treatment purposes only.
- The use of donated ovarian tissue in research and treatment is perfectly acceptable.

The next step is to ask a number of people to judge the extent to which each statement expresses a positive or negative attitude towards the particular issue, regardless of their own particular attitude. This is generally conducted in the form of a sorting task. Each statement is written on a card and the person making the judgements is asked to sort the cards into 11 piles placed along a continuum from positive at one end to negative at the other. The two ends and the middle pile are labelled. The middle pile is used for neutral opinions with the remaining five piles on either side used to represent varying degrees of either positive or negative views towards the particular issue.

The ratings, that is the number of the pile in which each statement is placed, from all the judges, are then tabulated. From these data it is possible to calculate both the numerical scale position of each statement, that is, its average scale value, and the extent to which judges agreed on its placement, that is, its spread of ratings. Statements which have poor interjudge agreement are discarded. Finally, from the remaining statements, 20 to 40 are selected to constitute the attitude questionnaire.

Statements should cover the full range of median scores assigned by the judges and every statement on the scale should be about equidistant numerically from its neighbour. The questionnaire can then be given to any group of people who are asked to indicate agreement, disagreement or neutrality toward each statement. Given that each statement has a predetermined value as described above, each person's score, that is the mean value on all the items with which they agree, can then be calculated.

The hallmark of a Thurstone scale is that the intervals between the statements are approximately equal, this being achieved by the method in which it is constructed. One obvious drawback, however, is that it is rather laborious and time-consuming to construct. Indeed, one study suggested that it took a third as much time again to construct a Thurstone as opposed to a Likert scale (Barclay & Weaver, 1962). This no doubt explains why there are few references to the Thurstone method in recently published nursing research. Because measures made with the Thurstone and Likert techniques are highly correlated, many studies have relied upon some version of the more efficient Likert scaling procedure for attitude measurement.

Likert method

The Likert scale (Likert, 1932) consists of a series of opinion statements about a particular issue, event or person. The person's attitude is the extent to which they agree or disagree with each statement which is generally rated on a five-point scale where 1 is strongly disagree, 2 is disagree, 3 is undecided, 4 is agree and 5 is strongly agree. A person's attitude score is the total of their ratings with a higher score indicating a more favourable attitude. If strong disagreement with any item indicates a favourable attitude, scoring is reversed so that 5 always represents a positive view. Although the 1 to 5 format is widely used, a wide range of other formats have also been employed. For example, respondents have been asked to place a mark along a line labelled 'strongly agree' at one end and 'strongly disagree; at the other. In other instances they have been asked to circle a number between −10 and +10, or between some other numerical end-points, to indicate agreement or disagreement with various attitude statements. Whatever the format, the basic task remains the same, that is to indicate the extent to which the respondent accepts or rejects various statements relating to an attitude object.

The method of Likert scale construction is similar to that used for the Thurstone scale. Thus, an initial pool of statements is collected from relevant sources and edited accordingly. However, unlike the Thurstone scale there is no assumption that intervals on the rating scale are equal. Thus, the difference between 'agree' and 'strongly agree' may be much larger in the respondent's perception than the difference between 'agree' and 'undecided'. A Likert scale can thus indicate the relative ordering of different people's attitudes, but does not indicate precisely how close or far apart these attitudes are. A further implication of a Likert scale is that all the items are highly correlated with each other and with the total scale score as opposed to Thurstone's distinct and independent items.

Likert scales are widely used in research and there are numerous examples in the nursing literature. For example, Bowman *et al.* (1983) developed a 20 item Likert scale to collect information on nurses' attitudes towards the nursing process. That scale was adapted in a more recent study to assess nursing students' attitudes towards nursing models (McKenna, 1994). Ten of the items were negatively worded and ten positively. Each item was rated on a scale of 1 to 5 with 5 reflecting a positive attitude towards nursing models. Examples of questions are given in Fig. 20.1.

(1)	Nursing models improve care	SA	A	U	D	SD
(2)	Nursing models involve too much paperwork	SA	A	U	D	SD
(3)	Nursing models work well in practice	SA	A	U	D	SD
(4)	Nursing models are a waste of time	SA	A	U	D	SD
(5)	Nursing models can be used in any areas	SA	A	U	D	SD
(6)	There is not enough time to use nursing models	SA	A	U	D	SD

Fig. 20.1   Likert scale items assessing attitudes toward nursing models (SA – strongly agree; A – agree; U – undecided; D – disagree; SD – strongly disagree).

Although widely used, Likert scales are not without their difficulties. One particular problem is that while a particular set of responses will always add up to the same score, the same total may arise from many different combinations of responses. For example, a score of 30 could be obtained from 15 items scoring 2 or 10 items scoring 1 together with 5 items scoring 4. Such different combinations might actually be quite rare but it would clearly be preferable if the same total score always meant the same thing.

Guttman method

A further, though less widely used, method of assessing attitudes involves the Guttman method (1944, 1950), which was derived from early attempts to measure attitudes reported by Bogardus (1928). Bogardus was concerned with developing a social distance measure which was really a measure of attitude toward ethnic groups. People were asked to indicate, with regard to a specific group, which of seven relationships ranging from intimate, for example 'marriage', to most distant, for example 'exclude members of the group from the country', they would be willing to accept. Guttman extended this method of scaling by assuming that an attitude towards any object, situation or event can be assessed by ordering a set of statements along a continuum of 'difficulty of acceptance'. Thus, statements range from those that are easy for most people to accept to those which few people would endorse. Acceptance of one item implies that people would also accept those which are less difficult to accept. An example of such a scale is given in Fig. 20.2.

In order to construct a scale which represents a single dimension, subjects are presented with an initial set of statements and the extent to which they respond

Least difficult to accept	(1)	As long as the accommodation and care are appropriate, people with a learning disability should be able to live anywhere they want.
	(2)	There are some residential streets where it is probably better not to house people with a learning disability.
	(3)	Sheltered housing for people with a learning disability should be restricted to certain areas of any one town.
Most difficult to accept	(4)	People with a learning disability should be kept in hospitals away from the general population.

Fig. 20.2 Guttman scale items assessing attitude toward community care for people with a learning disability.

with specified answer patterns recorded. These patterns, referred to as scale types, follow a certain step-like order. The subject may accept none of the statements in the set (score 0), may accept the first statement only (score 1), the first and second statement only (score 2), the first, second and third statement only (score 3) and so on. If the subject gives a non-scale response, for example accepts the third statement but not the first and second, it is assumed that they have made a response error. By analysing the number of response errors it is possible to determine the extent to which the initial set of statements represents a uni-dimensional scale. Eliminating poor statements and retesting enables a scaleable set of statements to be developed.

One problem with such a method is that it is almost impossible to develop a perfect uni-dimensional scale. People may actually be responding to their own perceived dimension or to multiple dimensions rather than to the one assumed to underlie the scale. This may well be because both attitudes and behaviour are rather too complex to be encompassed by a uni-dimensional scale.

Semantic differential

Each of the above approaches measures attitudes by examining the extent to which people agree or disagree with various opinion statements. In contrast, Osgood and his colleagues (Osgood *et al.* 1957) focused on the meaning people give to a word or concept. A semantic-differential instrument consists of a particular object, situation or event which people then rate on a series of bipolar adjectives, such as good–bad, fast–slow, active–passive and so on.

Extensive research by Osgood *et al.* (1957) suggests that most adjectives can be grouped into three categories. The largest number of adjectives, such as good–bad and happy–sad, reflect evaluation. A second group of interrelated dimensions, including strong–weak and easy–hard, reflect perceived strength or potency. The third group, including dimensions such as fast–slow and young–old, is termed activity. The potency and activity dimensions do not relate that closely to attitude research. The evaluative dimension is one used by most other kinds of attitude scale and, as noted earlier, is the dimension that most definitions of attitude stress as distinguishing between an attitude and a simple belief. The term *semantic differential* refers to the way of measuring several different semantic dimensions, or different kinds of meaning reflected by the different adjective descriptors.

A recent example of this method used in nursing research is a study which evaluated nurses' attitudes toward patients with AIDS (Cole & Slocumb, 1993) (see Fig. 20.3). The ten bipolar adjectives expressing evaluative meaning were selected from previous research and subsequent review by nursing experts. Six of the bipolar adjectives were randomly reversed in order to provide a positive–negative/ negative–positive balance. To examine whether nurses' attitudes differed according to the manner of contracting AIDS the semantic differential scale was headed with one of four modes of a male acquiring the virus, that is, though (a) sexual activity with males; (b) sexual activity with females; (c) sharing needles and (d) a blood transfusion.

A male who acquired AIDS through sexual activity with males

(1)	good____:____:____:____:____:____:____ bad
(2)	immoral____:____:____:____:____:____:____ moral
(3)	dangerous____:____:____:____:____:____:____ safe
(4)	clean____:____:____:____:____:____:____ dirty
(5)	unjustified____:____:____:____:____:____:____ justified
(6)	victim____:____:____:____:____:____:____ perpetrator
(7)	trustworthy____:____:____:____:____:____:____ dishonest
(8)	unfair____:____:____:____:____:____:____ fair
(9)	positive____:____:____:____:____:____:____ negative
(10)	guilty____:____:____:____:____:____:____ innocent

Fig. 20.3   Semantic-differential instrument for one concept (from Cole & Slocumb, 1993).

As research has established which adjectives express evaluative meaning, semantic differential attitude scales are easy to construct. However, the task of completing a semantic differential scale may be seen as rather unusual – we do not normally rate objects, situations or events on scales such as strong–weak or hard–soft.

Assessing attitudes and normative beliefs

In thinking about attitude measurement it is clearly important to link theory with assessment. In research, the need for a clear rationale for conducting the measurement, other than that it is of an intrinsically interesting topic, is important.

Unfortunately much attitude research fails to address this issue. One such method of not just measuring but also analysing attitudes, which is referred to as the expectancy value approach, was proposed by Fishbein & Ajzen (1975). Respondents are asked to rate their beliefs about each item, that is, the 'value' component, and then the extent to which they believe each dimension applies to the issue being considered, that is the 'expectancy' component. Each expectancy is combined with its value to give an overall E–V score. This method can be used to analyse the assumption of the theory of reasoned action (Fishbein & Ajzen, 1975) that overt behaviour in a particular situation is related to the individual's intention to carry out the behaviour in question. As noted earlier, the probability that we will engage in a behaviour is related not only to our beliefs but also to other variables such as our expectations of significant others, that is, normative beliefs, and our perceived control over the behaviour in question.

This theory and approach were used in a recent study by Nash *et al.* (1993) to assess nurses' attitudes towards and intention to assess patients' pain. Different pairs of questions were used to assess attitudes, normative beliefs, behavioural intention and perceived control. Attitude was measured by subjects' responses to items concerning six identifiable beliefs and corresponding evaluations of those beliefs. Normative beliefs were similarly assessed by examining three set of beliefs about others and motivation to comply with these expectations of others. Behavioural intention was assessed by two questions concerning the likelihood of conducting pain assessments. Perceived control was evaluated by two questions concerning degree of control over and ease in conducting pain assessment. Each item was rated on a seven point scale from +3 (indicating whether the item was likely, desirable, involved complete control or was easy) to –3 (indicating whether the item was unlikely, undesirable, involved very little control or was difficult). Examples are shown in Fig. 20.4.

The main advantages of this approach are that it is clearly linked to theoretical assumptions and that it provides the possibility for analysing assumptions behind an overall score.

Other methods

As noted earlier, attitudes consist of a behavioural, evaluative and cognitive component, each of which can be measured. Discussion to this point has focused on the evaluative component. There are numerous occasions when actual behaviour can be assessed as an attitudinal indicator. For example, refusing to sign a petition or to go along with a group decision. In recent years psychologists have also grown more interested in assessing the cognitive component of attitudes. One such technique is *thought listing* (Petty & Cacioppo, 1981). After hearing or reading a message subjects are asked to write down in a specified time (say three minutes) all their thoughts which are relevant to the issue and message in question. Subsequently the thoughts are rated and categorized, for example according to whether they agree or disagree with the message or issue. From such information it is possible to learn

(1) Attitude
    (a) Behavioural belief
        A comprehensive pain assessment will permit a more accurate picture
        of the patients' situation
        likely_____unlikely

    (b) Evaluation
        An accurate picture of the patient's situation is
        desirable_____undesirable

(2) Subjective norm
    (a) Normative belief
        Other nurses think that I should conduct comprehensive pain
        assessments
        likely_____unlikely

    (b) Motivation to comply
        I do what other nurses think I should do for patients
        likely_____unlikely

Fig. 20.4 Examples of questionnaire items assessing attitudes and normative beliefs.

about the beliefs and knowledge underlying attitudes. Similar information can be obtained from content analysis of essays or group discussion.

More recently research has investigated whether specific bodily reactions reflect attitudes. Cacioppo & Petty (1987) found small but measurable changes in the activity of facial muscles around the mouth as people listen to and think about persuasive messages. One pattern emerges when the message produces a positive, agreeing response while another pattern occurs with a counter argument.

Given the variety of methods available for assessing the different components of attitudes a legitimate question to ask is whether one measure is more appropriate than another?

Which measure to use?

Given that different researchers focus on differing aspects of attitudes it seems quite appropriate that different measurement methods should be used. The emphasis in some studies might be on the belief or cognitive component of attitudes, while in others it might be the evaluative component. There are other occasions when more than one domain might be assessed, for example, evaluative and behavioural. However, as noted earlier, it is important to bear in mind that there may be a less than perfect relationship between the scores obtained in this way. The measure should suit the aims of the study. If, for example, the aim is to ultimately change behaviour then clearly a baseline assessment of behaviour is required. If it is simply to gauge how people feel about a particular issue then one of the attitudinal scales discussed could be used.

The question of which scale to use has been partly addressed in previous sections. The Thurstone method is extremely time-consuming and the Likert method may be a more appropriate alternative. The Guttman method is relatively straightforward, although it can be difficult to construct a uni-dimensional scale. The semantic-differential method may seem rather unusual to respondents but allows for the assessment of meaning rather than just opinion. As the results of using different scaling methods to assess attitudes are remarkably similar, the decision about which scale to use is likely to be based on ease of construction of the scale and ease of administering it to respondents.

However, it is important to bear in mind that a major problem with any self-report measure of attitudes is that people may wish to conceal rather than reveal their true attitudes. This may be particularly likely if their views are unpopular or extreme. It is well known that many people wish to make a desirable impression and, rather than giving their real views, may respond by giving views they believe the respondent wishes to know. As a result of this problem some researchers have used a technique referred to as the bogus pipeline (Jones & Sigall, 1971). The basic paradigm involves attaching respondents to a machine which they are told measures tiny electrical changes in their muscles and can hence assess their true opinions. Respondents are then asked attitude questions to which the experimenter knows their views (respondents having been pretested some weeks earlier) and can then 'rig' the machine so that it seems to respond to these attitudes very accurately. Respondents are then asked to express their views on a new set of issues in the belief that erroneous responding will be indicated by the machine. There is some evidence that this technique yields more accurate measures of attitudes (for example Gaes *et al.*, 1978), although not all findings have been positive (for example Cherry *et al.*, 1976). In addition, the need for equipment, pre-assessment measures for respondents and the fact that only one person can be assessed at a time clearly impose serious practical constraints on the use of such a procedure.

In conclusion, therefore, no method of attitude assessment is completely problem-free. In thinking about which scale or method of attitude assessment to use, the most important consideration is that the measure should suit the aims of the study.

References

Barclay, J.E. & Weaver, H.B. (1962) Comparative reliabilities and the ease of construction of Thurstone and Likert attitude scales. *Journal of Social Psychology*, 58, 109–120.

Bogardus, E.S. (1928) *Immigration and Race Attitudes*. D.C. Heath, Boston.

Bowman, G.S., Thompson, D.R. & Sutton, T.W. (1983) Nurses' attitudes towards the nursing process. *Journal of Advanced Nursing*, 8, 125–9.

Cacioppo, J.T. & Petty, R.E. (1987) Stalking rudimentary processes of social influences: a psychophysiological approach. In *Social Influence: The Ontario Symposium* (eds M.P. Zanna, J.M. Olson & C.P. Herman), Vol 5. Erlbaum, Hillsdale, N.J.

Cherry, F., Byrne, D. & Mitchell, H.E. (1976) Clogs in the bogus pipeline: demand characteristics and social desirability. *Journal of Research in Personality*, 10, 69–75.

Cole, F.L. & Slocumb, E.M. (1993) Nurses' attitudes toward patients with AIDS. *Journal of Advanced Nursing*, **18**, 1112–17.

Fishbein, M. & Ajzen, I. (1975) *Belief, Attitude, Intention and Behavior. An Introduction to Theory and Research*. Addison-Wesley, Reading, Massachusetts.

Gaes, G.G., Kalle, R.J. & Tedeschi, J.T. (1978) Impression management in the forced compliance situation: two studies using the bogus pipeline. *Journal of Experimental Social Psychology*, **14**, 493–510.

Guttman, L. (1944) A basis for scaling quantitative data. *American Sociological Review*, **9**, 139–50.

Guttman, L. (1950) The third component of scalable attitudes. *International Journal of Opinion and Attitude Research*, **4**, 285–7.

Jones, E.E. & Sigall, H. (1971) The bogus pipeline: a new paradigm for measuring affect and attitude. *Psychological Bulletin*, **76**, 349–64.

Likert, R. (1932) A technique for the measurement of attitudes. *Archives of Psychology*, **22**, 1–55.

McKenna, H.P. (1994) The attitudes of traditional and undergraduate nursing students towards nursing models: a comparative study. *Journal of Advanced Nursing*, **19**, 527–36.

Nash, R., Edwards, H. & Nebauer, M. (1993) Effect of attitudes, subjective norms and perceived control on nurses' intention to assess patients' pain. *Journal of Advanced Nursing*, **18**, 941–7.

Osgood, C.E., Suci, G.J. & Tannenbaum, P.H. (1957) *The Measurement of Meaning*. University of Illinois Press, Urbana, Illinois.

Petty, R.E. & Cacioppo, J.T. (1981) *Attitudes and Persuasion: Classic and Contemporary Approaches*. W.C. Brown, Dubuque, I.A.

Thurstone, L.L. (1928) Attitudes can be measured. *American Journal of Sociology*, **33**, 529–54.

Wicker, A.W. (1969) Attitudes versus actions: the relationship of verbal and overt behavioral responses to attitude objects. *Journal of Social Issues*, **25**, 41–78.

Chapter 21

Interview

Philip J. Barker

The interview is the commonest means of data collection at our disposal. Nurses interview patients and their carers routinely, as part of everyday practice. The ordinary status of the interview may suggest simplicity. In this chapter, the factors which are common to everyday interviewing and the research interview will be discussed, supported by some illustrations of the key distinctions between them.

The research interview may be used:

(1) To explore a subject area, as a preliminary form of inquiry. In the exploratory interview you identify situations, events and their relationships to one another, which form the basis of hypotheses.
(2) To collect data as part of the formal core of the study. The data collection interview measures a specific variable, or set of variables, usually by means of a carefully constructed set of questions, or schedule.
(3) To supplement other methods of inquiry.

You may wish to collect additional information, following some unexpected results, or to validate responses obtained by other means, for example mail questionnaire. Alternatively, you may wish to probe more deeply into the subject's responses to the original questions set.

The objective of the interview (data collection) will be considered at more length in Chapter 22. Here, consideration is given to the interpersonal context of the interview: what needs to take place between interviewer/interviewee, how the interview should be structured and potential problems involved in interviewing different groups across different subject areas. Brief consideration is given to the distinction between different types of research interview.

General principles

The quality of the information generated from the interview is dependent, to a great extent, on the behaviour of the interviewer. Even in a structured, or semi-structured, interview where the interviewer is guided, wholly or in part, by a set of questions, characteristics of the interviewer's behaviour can influence the outcome.

General interpersonal style

The interviewer needs to be able to engage the interviewee in a relationship involving more than a simple question and answer session. She needs to be able to show attentiveness, listening actively to what is being said, sitting an appropriate distance from the person, adopting a posture which suggests that she is relaxed and open to the interviewee's responses. Throughout the interview steady eye contact should be maintained, appropriate to what amounts to a deep conversation. These considerations illustrate the 'helping' status of the interviewer: who acts as facilitator for the interviewee's responses, helping the interviewee feel comfortable and relaxed (Keenan, 1976).

Do not have these skills

Introduction and rationale

The interviewer's first requirement is to 'set the agenda' for the interview. An explanation is given of the aims and objectives of the study in general and the interview in particular, how it is to be conducted, why the respondent was chosen, and for whom the data are being collected. A clear statement is made concerning the anonymity of the interviewee and/or the confidential nature of any information collected. It is also advantageous to invite any questions regarding the nature and objectives of the interview, before beginning.

This kind of openness is essential for dealing with three major obstacles. First, the respondent may mistake you for some other form of official. This might influence the responses given. Second, the respondent may modify his responses if an unambiguous guarantee of confidentiality is not offered. Finally, you may be seen as someone who is testing, or checking up on, the respondent. This may generate levels of anxiety which preclude appropriate responses. These obstacles are likely to prevail in the case of interviewing both staff and patients.

Establishing rapport with the respondent requires the exercise of traditional pleasantries, and the interpersonal style already noted. These features support the declaration of intent you have offered; both are designed to reduce anxiety and facilitate comfort.

Questioning

Every interview requires a plan. This will address the main subject areas for enquiry, and will include a procedure for pursuing clarification of responses to the main questions. This plan in the form of an interview schedule is discussed briefly in Chapter 22. The interview schedule serves to standardize the interview. Each respondent is asked the same questions, in the same sequence, in a similar manner. Questions are worded in such a way that they are understandable to all respondents. Where the respondent fails to understand the question, repeat the question before you try to offer further explanation. In this sense you treat the interview schedule as a scientific instrument, offering the same cues to a wide ranging population of respondents.

Where the questionnaire involves filter questions (if 'yes', move to question 26, for example), respondents can become confused over which item to answer next. The problem does not arise where well trained interviewers can move quickly from one optional question to the next; apparently asking the respondent only one series of questions. Where respondents do not understand the question, repeat or clarify the question as shown in Fig. 21.1.

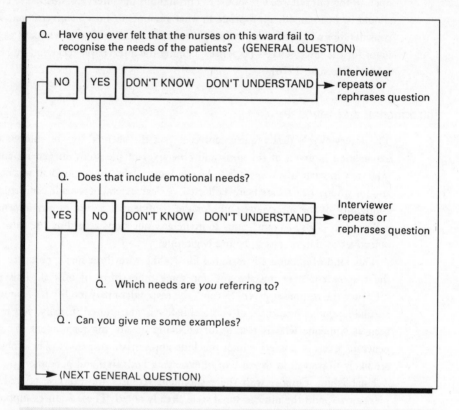

Fig. 21.1   Example of filter question.

Amplifying responses

In some situations, the interview may involve closed questions, requiring yes/no answers. Alternatively, the respondent may be invited to select a response from a range of alternatives: 'always/often/sometimes/never'. Where there are no indications to the contrary – such as illiteracy or suspected poor comprehension – such an interview schedule might be offered as a self-report questionnaire, since the facilitative presence of the interviewer seems to be redundant. The interview should be used only when the nature of the questions asked, or the characteristics of the interviewee, demand it.

Collecting data by formal interviewing involves a three-stage process:

(1)   First of all, ask the respondent the questions.

(2) Next, invite the respondent to either add further information or clarify the
initial response.
(3) Finally, reflect back the core of the response, seeking confirmation that your
understanding is correct.

Example

Interviewer: 'How do you feel about working with people with AIDS?'
Respondent: 'I'm not sure. I guess I feel a bit wary. There is so little we know.'
Interviewer: 'Can you tell me a bit more about that: what you are wary about?'
Respondent: 'Well, the virus ... I mean ... They say that we are not at risk
providing we take the right precautions. But I've read about people catching the
virus, without having full contact ... you know blood, body fluids and all that.'
Interviewer: 'So you feel as if you're at risk, in some way?'
Respondent: 'That's right. I think we focus too much attention on the patient's
welfare.'

The interviewer here tries to probe in a non–directive manner (Graesser & Black,
1985), helping the respondent to identify a response, to consider it further and
finally to confirm or revise the response. In some interviews, the respondent is
asked more direct questions, where responses are confirmed in the manner
described above. Reed's (1986) study of chemically dependent nurses employed a
structured interview schedule covering personal history, family history, educational
background, health history, drug history, attempts to cope, consequences of
addiction and relapse history. The majority of the questions required yes/no
answers or a response chosen from identified options. In some of the questions, the
respondent was invited to supply additional information (Have you ever been
arrested? Yes/No. If yes, please list charges). This format was essentially fact-
based. Most of the data collected were unambiguous and focused upon recall of
actual events. In Wray's (1994) survey of schizophrenia suffers' understanding of
their condition and satisfaction with services, the subjects were asked to identify
'their degree of satisfaction' by using a five-point scale: from 'very dissatisfied' to
'very satisfied'.

Davis's (1984, 1986) descriptions of the experience of student nurses employed a
less structured schedule. Given that the respondents in these reports were trying to
clarify what they felt about past experiences, the semi-structured approach was the
more appropriate.

The structure of the interview and the form of the questions should be linked to
the aims of the study. Where the researcher has a clearly defined objective,
involving the collection of discrete, factual information, the need for amplification
of responses will be limited. Where the interview is used as an exploratory tool, to
build hypotheses, or to canvas attitudes, beliefs or other less clear cut forms of data,
careful amplification of responses will be vital.

Training interviewers

Selection

The use of an interviewer to collect information from subjects allows for a greater degree of flexibility than would prevail through the use of a self-report questionnaire. The interviewer can clarify and modify questions to elicit a response and may also modify her presentation or approach to enhance the respondent's motivation. Interviewers often change the tone of their voice or speech rate to establish rapport with the subject. Such adjustments may keep respondents interested and responsive throughout the interview. Such flexibility, however, may be gained at the expense of a standardized interview. The researcher may be left wondering whether or not differences among respondents reflect their individual differences or those of different interviewers. Researchers are generally advised to recruit interviewers with relatively similar characteristics; after which all are trained in the use of a standardized procedure.

Personal characteristics

Personal factors such as age, sex and race of interviewers can have an effect on the interview data. Pay special attention to the recruitment of interviewers with characteristics likely to facilitate the positive relationships necessary for exploratory questioning to occur. Where possible, it is advisable to employ interviewers of the same sex as the subjects, and to use interviewers who are close to the age group of the subjects. Young people may respond to much older interviewers by either being subservient or rebellious; older subjects may feel offended by very young interviewers who might be seen as inexperienced. The ideal age range is between 25 and 45; very young people may lack tact and the necessary interpersonal skills; much older people may be unwilling to follow instructions carefully (Topf, 1988).

The interviewer's general appearance can also be important. Traditional rules about 'plainly attired interviewers' being most successful (Brown, 1937), or 'prosperous looking' or 'too glamorous' interviewers being a disadvantage (Parten, 1950), are probably no longer valid. However, despite the major cultural changes of the past two decades, it would be inappropriate to consider that 'anything goes' when recruiting interviewers. Individuals presenting with any extreme characteristic, whether of accent or dress style, are perhaps best avoided. Similarly, individuals who are extremely enthusiastic or pessimistic about the study, expressing strong political affiliations, with past negative experiences of interviewing (or a related area such as sales), or possible contaminating views about the therapeutic potential of interviewing, are at risk of prejudicing the outcome.

Training in the standardized interview

Prospective interviewers need to be aware from the outset of the importance of adhering to the interview rules. They should be discouraged from introducing new questions, all additional questions aimed at exploring or amplifying prior responses should be programmed as part of the schedule. The interviewer needs also to be aware that changing the emphasis on specific words can change the context of the question. Even changing the emphasis of the question can have a major effect, viz

from 'What makes you say that?' ... to ... 'Why do you say that?'

This represents a significant change from a challenge to a more personal inquiry (Oppenheim, 1968).

Preparation of interviewers should comprise the following:

(1) Interview rehearsal under role-play conditions, followed by feedback. Ideally, these rehearsals should be audio- or videotaped;
(2) Practice of coding the role-play subjects' responses from the recordings, comparing these codings with those of more experienced interviewers.
(3) Once the basic format is established, emphasis should be given to the dangers of adapting wording or emphasis, or to omitting questions or part-questions.
(4) Brainstorming sessions, where the interviewers anticipate problems which might occur in vivo are helpful for establishing a resolution menu.

Not least, all interviewers should be 'valued' by the researcher. Their preparation should be sensitively staged, and should be designed to enhance the interviewer's motivation to use the standardized guidelines positively, rather than serve to provoke unnecessary anxiety or irritation.

Motivation of the interviewer

The apparent simplicity of interviewing can, however, be misleading. Research assistants who are employed to collect such data require careful preparation. Interviewers need to be made acutely aware that there is more to interviewing than asking people questions and getting information from them. The interviewer needs to have an overview of the research process, identifying her/his part in the overall plan. The interviewer should also be made aware of how the sample will be drawn and how the emergent data are to be analysed. The interviewer should also gain an appreciation of why certain interview techniques have been emphasized as part of this preparation.

The interviewer also needs to be motivated by the researcher. It is inadequate to assume that the interviewer will bring enthusiasm to the job; this feeling should be instilled in the interviewer. Emphasis needs to be placed upon why the study is important and why it is necessary to pursue a particular line of questioning. Finally, emphasis must be given to the craft of the interviewer, emphasizing the importance of the interviewer's skills.

Monitoring

Attention also needs to be paid to maintaining the effectiveness of the interviewer across time, especially where the project has a long duration or interviews are widely spaced. Possible causes of interviewer drift are:

(1) Loss of the original frame of reference. Once the interviewer has ended the preparatory training, she no longer has others to compare herself with and may lose the objective criteria necessary to maintain appropriate standards.

(2) Loss of reinforcement. Under training conditions, the researcher encourages the interviewer to stay 'on target'. In the field, practical problems, or the exposure to respondents, may result in a subtle change in attitude towards the interview process.

To avoid such problems, interviewers require regular supervision to detect any significant drift (Collins, 1988). Group sessions, where the interview procedure is reviewed and the identification of problems associated with 'drift' are invited, can all be effective. Alternatively, the researcher may invite the interviewer to audiotape a selection of the interviews (where this is not part of the protocol) to allow checking for irregularities, as a quality control procedure.

Unstructured and structured interviews

The three main types of interview are

- Structured – where all the interviewer's questions are determined in advance.
- Semi-structured – where the interviewer invites the respondent to develop her/his response by asking supplementary questions of the interviewer's own choosing.
- Unstructured – where the interviewer invites the respondent to talk about a number of 'themes' or 'topics'.

Each of these types of interview produces different forms of data with different requirements for their analysis. Structured interviews tend to produce straightforward 'factual' responses which can be counted or otherwise analysed statistically. Unstructured interviews, often called focus interviews, can produce a wealth of information which may be very cumbersome and difficult to interpret without using the researcher's own value judgements.

The structured interview has the potential for the production of highly reliable data, given that each subject is studied using the same set of questions, asked in approximately the same manner by the same interviewer; this is dependent, however, upon the design of the questionnaire (Gilbert, 1993). The structured interview does limit the subject's responses. Many people often wish to 'amplify' their answer, an option which is not recognized by the structured interview.

Semi-structured interviews allow more opportunity for expansion of replies and may, in some circumstances, be used as a form of 'gentle guidance'. The semi-structured and unstructured interview are most commonly used in qualitative research studies, where discrete research hypotheses may not have been stated, seeking instead to interpret and understand the meaning of particular events (see Chapter 11). Each type of interview has its own advantages and disadvantages. The researcher must ensure that the form of interview selected is appropriate for the objectives of the study in hand.

Special considerations

As noted above, some interview situations require careful consideration in the selection of an appropriate interviewer. People with major emotional problems, mental illness or learning disabilities may demand the selection of specially trained interviewers, using interview schedules which acknowledge the cognitive or emotional disabilities of the subject (Flynn, 1986). Where highly sensitive topics are examined – as in sexual abuse – the characteristics of the interviewer and the schedule are crucial (Quinn, 1989). In this context it is worth noting that expectations of difficulty are often confounded. Rodgers' (1987) study of older people, for example, found that the subjects' recall of information was not significantly less 'faulty' than that of other age groups. The assumption that all older people are likely to encounter difficulty with interviews may be no more than an assumption.

Advantages of the interview

Collecting information through direct, face-to-face contact with the subject has some advantages over self-report questionnaires completed by the respondent independently.

(1) People are more likely to discard questionnaires or leave sections blank. When faced with an interviewer, there is greater likelihood of a fuller response to all questions.

(2) Some subjects will be unable to complete self-report questionnaires through blindness, illiteracy, poor education or limited comprehension or reasoning. Very young, older, or anxious people may also be put off by the demands of the self-report questionnaire.

(3) The interview allows areas of uncertainty or ambiguity to be clarified, avoiding the misinterpretations and possible anticipation of conclusions which might arise from use of a self-report questionnaire.

(4) Some forms of interview allow the subject to expand on their response: this is rarely possible or likely in a self-report questionnaire. The subject may talk expansively where he would be unlikely to write detailed or lengthy responses.

(5) The interviewer can control the context of the response by her presence. It is not unknown for respondents to questionnaires to seek help from friends or colleagues, thereby contaminating the results.

(6) Additional data on the performance, attitude and degree of understanding of the subject may be collected by the interviewer. The supplementary observations may be used to qualify final conclusions, or as preparation for the design of other interview schedules and research hypotheses.

Conclusion

Interviews are a costly method of data collection, but offer the promise of better returns, in terms of both the overall quality and the quantity of responses. Interviews are a more appropriate method of data collection for a wider range of populations, and the interviewer always has an opportunity to 'rescue' a respondent from confusion or fatigue, options which are not possible under self-report conditions. In addition to the standardized 'exploratory' interview discussed briefly in this chapter, interviews can employ any one of the vast range of structured measures noted in Chapter 22. These range from the use of general semantic differentials (White, 1986) to highly specific pain questionnaires (Wilkie 1990). Interviews can be unstructured, aiming to explore the subject's experience through use of a topic guide (Skidmore, 1986). At the other extreme, interviews can be conducted by telephone, allowing the participation of a wider range of geographically distant subjects.

References

Brown, L. (1937) *Market Research and Analysis*. Ronald Press, New York.

Collins, C. (1988) Interviewer training and supervision. *Nursing Research*, 37(2), 122–4.

Davis, B.D. (1984) Interviews with student nurses about their training. *Nurse Education Today*, 4(6), 136–40.

Davis, B.D. (1986) The strain of training: being a student psychiatric nurse. In *Psychiatric Nursing Research*, (ed. J. Brooking). John Wiley, Chichester.

Flynn, M.C. (1986) Adults who are mentally handicapped as consumers: issues and guidelines for interviewing. *Journal of Mental Deficiency Research*, 30(4), 369–77.

Gilbert, N. (1993) *Researching social life*. Sage Publications, London.

Graesser, A. & Black, J. (eds) (1985) *The Psychology of Questions*. Erlbaum Associates, Hillsdale, NJ.

Keenan, A. (1976) Effects of non-verbal behaviour of interviewers on candidates' performance. *Journal of Occupational Psychology*, 49, 171–6.

Oppenheim, A.N. (1968) *Questionnaire Design and Attitude Measurement*. Heinemann, London.

Parten, M.B. (1950) *Surveys, Polls and Samples*. Harper, New York.

Quinn, K.M. (1989) Influences of an interviewer's behaviours in child sexual abuse investigations. *Bulletin of the American Academy of Psychiatry and Law*, 17(1), 45–52.

Reed, M.T. (1986) Descriptive study of chemically dependent nurses. In *Psychiatric Nursing Research*, (ed. J. Brooking). John Wiley, Chichester.

Rodgers, W.L. (1987) Interviewing older adults: the accuracy of factual information. *Journal of Gerontology*, 42(4), 387–94.

Skidmore, D. (1986) The effectiveness of community psychiatric nursing teams and base locations. In *Psychiatric Nursing Research*, (ed. J. Brooking). John Wiley, Chichester.

Topf, M. (1988) Verbal interpersonal effectiveness. *Journal of Psychosocial and Mental Health Nursing*, 26(7), 8–11; 15–16.

White, E. (1986) Factors influencing general practitioners to refer patients to community psychiatric nurses. In *Psychiatric Nursing Research*, (ed. J. Brooking), Chapter 12. John

Wiley, Chichester.

Wilkie, D.J. (1990) Use of the McGill Pain Questionnaire to measure pain: a meta-analysis. *Nursing Research*, **39**(1), 36–41.

Wray, S.J. (1994) Schizophrenia sufferers and their carers: a survey of understanding of the condition and its treatment, and of satisfaction with services. *Journal of Psychiatric and Mental Health Nursing*, **1**, 115–23.

Chapter 22

Questionnaire

Philip J. Barker

The word *questionnaire* is an umbrella term for a variety of instruments, some involving straightforward questioning, with 'closed' (yes/no) answers; others inviting more 'open' responses, by use of checklists, ratings, or open-ended comments. Some questionnaires involve combinations of two or more different approaches. Where the questionnaire is employed within an interview, it may be described as an interview schedule (see Chapter 21). Where subjects provide attitudinal data, using some scaling technique, it may be described as a rating scale. It is appropriate to view these technical differences as representative only of the diversity of questionnaire design and application.

Emphasis is given in this chapter to the methodology of questionnaire construction; this is relevant both to self-report surveys (the mail questionnaire) and the use of questionnaires in direct interviewing, as described in the previous chapter. The general principles of questionnaire design are assumed to be similar in both situations.

The function of the questionnaire

The main use of the questionnaire is to collect data. In a descriptive study, these data will be used to explore themes or to develop an explanatory theory (see Chapter 11). In an experimental study these data will be used to test the hypothesis(es) of the study. Consider a study which asks the following question: 'What is the effect of "peer support" on the "mood levels" of clinicians working in terminal care?'

In such a study there exists a need to express, first of all, a relationship between the two variables: how are 'peer support' and 'mood levels' related? The resultant hypothesis is a conjectural statement about the possible relationship between two or more variables. In the null form (see Chapter 14), the hypothesis might state that peer support has no effect upon mood levels of terminal care clinicians. Peer support might involve behaviours which are defined by others as 'supportive' (in the study setting they would be perceived by the clinicians to be present or absent); and mood levels might represent internal, self-reported experiences.

A questionnaire, completed either independently (self-report) or within an interview (interview schedule) might be the most appropriate mechanism for collecting information on the clinicians' perceptions of others and related emotional experiences. Alternatively, the researcher might choose to study the experiences of the terminal care team by using unstructured interviews (see Chapters 11 and 12).

The questionnaire, in that example, might aim to study the terminal care situation, highlighting the hypothetical relationship between the experimental variables. For this reason, the questionnaire must present questions which have a direct bearing upon the variables under study: peer support and mood levels. Each of these terms must be defined in operational terms, to ensure that the respondent is in no doubt as to which perceived behaviours and personal experiences are under study. In this sense, the first requirement of the questionnaire is to be valid; it must measure what it claims to measure.

The questionnaire should collect this information with the minimum distortion. The questions should elicit, as closely as possible, the true response of the individual. Questions should not 'lead' the respondent into making responses and should be open to analysis which does not require undue interpretation of the actual answers (see Chapters 27 and 29). These general aims are pursued by giving consideration to the overall design and administration of the questionnaire. Design issues relate to language, frame of reference, information level, nature, sequence and form of questions. Administration will be discussed briefly in the case of self-report (survey) questionnaires. Chapter 21 discusses administration in some more detail.

General principles

The primary aim in designing the questionnaire is to communicate with the respondent. The respondent needs to understand the questions, and needs an appropriate structure to facilitate his response. To achieve this aim acknowledge the central role of language, and the general context in which the questions are set (the frame of reference), and the nature of the responses expected (the information level).

Language

The first priority is to choose language which allows the optimum exchange of ideas. Key words should be within the comprehension of the respondent; colloquialisms or cliches should be clarified or avoided. It seems self-evident that a questionnaire designed to elicit the respective attitudes of medical staff and patients towards 'quality of care', might differ in terms of both the question asked and the language used to define the questions. Consideration is given to the possible levels of literacy, ethnic and cultural background, as well as age and understanding of respondents. Technical language may be unintelligible to some; direct reference to sensitive subject matter, such as sexuality or sexual abuse, may be anxiety provoking. The form of language chosen will facilitate communication. Avoid patronizing people (by being too simplistic) or confusing, embarrassing or upsetting them by use of inappropriate terminology or expressions.

Frame of reference

The questionnaire needs also to introduce topics in a form which links in to the respondent's idea of what is or is not relevant to the study. As noted in the previous chapter, the respondent is given an 'agenda' for the interview, this prepares him for the line of questioning involved. Care is taken to ensure that the questions develop in a manner which fulfils the respondent's notions about reasonableness and logic. For example:

Question 1: 'Have you had a distressing emotional experience at work within the last month?'
Question 2: (If yes) 'What effect did this have upon you, personally?'
Question 3: 'Did that experience have any effect upon your work?'
Question 4   (If yes) 'In what way?'

At the same time the order of the questions should encourage, rather than discourage, threaten of confuse the respondent. It is appropriate to begin with non-threatening questions, which are general in their focus, moving gradually to more complex, and potentially more demanding questions.

Information level

The questionnaire should also take care not to assume that a specific level of information is possessed by the respondent. The respondent may feel embarrassed or resentful if a question cannot be answered; this may prejudice the rest of the interview. Alternatively, the person may pretend to have knowledge which he does not possess in order to avoid embarrassment.

Design of the questionnaire

The design steps

The development of a questionnaire involves a series of five inter-related stages, some of which are discussed in more detail.

(1) *What* kind of information is required? This represents the focus of the study.
(2) The researcher should decide on what would be the most appropriate means of *eliciting* this information; through self-report, structured or semi-structured interview. The method adopted will have major implications for the design of the questionnaire.
(3) The researcher needs next to identify the kind of questions which need to be asked and the kind of responses which might be appropriate. This will determine the format and content of the questions and answers.

(4) How the questions are *worded* is crucial to the success of the instrument. If the questions are not asked in the appropriate form of words, the necessary responses will not be forthcoming.
(5) Finally, the layout of the questionnaire must be considered, including attention to the sequencing of questions.

Once the questionnaire is designed, the instrument needs to be tested on a pilot sample and revised in the light of experience until it appears to be meeting the researcher's requirements.

Nature of the questions

The questionnaire should focus only upon those aspects of the subject's experience necessary for the study in hand. Many questionnaires begin by collecting details about the respondent such as personal characteristics, history and social context. The questionnaire should collect only as much information as is necessary to fulfil the specific aims of the study. For this reason general life histories, used as a preamble to different studies, may be time wasting by being over-inclusive, or may fail to focus on the relevant biographical or demographic data.

The questionnaire can be used to collect basic information, identifying whether or not certain events have occurred; whether people agree or disagree with specific views or attitudes; whether or not they would like to see certain events occurring in the future. Such 'closed' questionnaires are relatively simple to administer or complete, but need to be carefully designed to ensure that the questions represent the most comprehensive response to the research questions.

Alternatively, you may wish the respondents to quantify some experience, using a scaling technique as an adjunct to the yes/no question, or selecting from a range of responses to provide a measure of frequency or severity. The respondents might also provide a 'qualitative' measure of some experience or attitude, using a rating scale or drawing from a list of adjectives, in an effort to explain more specifically how they feel or what they believe. The basic nature of the questionnaire is, however, determined by the research question; what do you *need* to know?

Question form

The form of the question involves the nature of the response expected. Two forms are possible: 'open' questions are structured to allow the respondents to answer in their own words, briefly or at length; 'closed' questions invite the respondent to select from pre-assigned categories of response.

Open questions

Here, the respondents are asked to supply any kind of information they consider appropriate. Examples of open questions are:

(1) How do you feel about men in nursing?
(2) What aspects of your training did you find most rewarding?

(3)   How can we integrate research findings into clinical practice?

Such open-ended questions assume that the respondent has feelings, recollections or views on the topics addressed. The manner in which the question is asked allows the respondents time to consider their responses. These can be developed and clarified by *funnelling*, as described in the sequence section below. The main advantage of open questions is that the respondents are allowed to define, partially, their own frame of reference. Although the three examples above specify a general target area (feelings about men, rewarding aspects of training, integration of research), the respondents have a range of options open when *framing* their reply. The open question also allows you to evaluate both attitudes and information level. The respondents may be unaware of the position of men in nursing, or of specific research examples pertinent to their area of work. The open-ended question allows you to assess what the person thinks or feels, and also what the respondent 'knows' about the subject. However, if the respondent is asked to give an estimate of the number of men in nursing, or to discuss a specific research example, a perceived *information deficit* might generate anxiety, obstructing an appropriate response, perhaps even prejudicing the response to the rest of the questionnaire. The open nature of the question also allows an opportunity to collect information or to identify areas of interest not anticipated in advance.

A number of drawbacks are involved in the use of open questions. Respondents may answer at great length, making data analysis difficult. Where respondents answer in great detail in the early stages, fatigue may present a problem in the later stages. Comparison of responses to the same questionnaire across time may also be difficult, especially where respondents phrase their answers differently on different occasions.

Open questions are most appropriate where the subjects are being invited to assess a personal experience or as part of an exploratory study, aimed at developing appropriate closed questions.

Closed questions

These invite the respondent to choose from a range of possibilities. The simplest questions involve *strict alternatives* or *dichotomous* questions. Examples of closed questions are:

(1)   Are you employed at present: yes/no?
(2)   Nursing is a genuine profession: agree/disagree.

Where more freedom is required to answer other questions *alternative statements* are appropriate. For example:

How often did you meet with your preceptor?
    (   ) more than once a day
    (   ) daily
    (   ) once every two days
    (   ) every two to three days

(   ) every three to seven days
(   ) less than every seven days

Alternatively, a *checklist* or matrix question can be used, as shown in Fig. 22.1.

How important are the following people to your care and treatment?

	Not important	Some importance	Very important	Of great importance
General practitioner				
Health visitor				
District nurse				
Consultant psychiatrist				
Social worker				
Clinical psychologist				
Community psychiatric nurse				

Fig. 22.1 Example of a checklist or matrix question.

Respondents can also be asked to select from a *menu* of responses which are factual:

Are you: single, married, divorced, separated, unemployed, employed, self-employed, retired (underline)

or attitudinal:

Which of the following statements most reflects your present opinion:
benzodiazepines should never be prescribed to patients with anxiety
benzodiazepines are useful only in low dosages, over a short term
benzodiazepines are effective in short- to medium-term treatment of anxiety
the disadvantages of long-term usage of benzodiazepines are exaggerated

Finally, respondents may be asked to rank order their responses along some continuum: such as importance, preference or danger:

How important are the following personality characteristics in teaching staff?
Rank order the characteristics indicating (1) for the most important through to
(5) for the least important
(   ) humorous
(   ) creative

(   ) analytic
(   ) warm
(   ) challenging

The longer the questionnaire, the more appropriate are *dichotomous* questions which speed up the answer rate, thereby reducing the risk of respondent fatigue. The major drawback to this form of question is the *forced* nature of the response. People need to commit themselves strongly to one answer or the other. This may lead to information loss or may prove offputting to the respondent.

Any of the multiple choice options can help the respondent recall or clarify events, beliefs, or feelings. There is some danger, however, that the set of optional responses might *suggest* that such experiences have occurred or that such views have been or are held.

Length and wording

As noted earlier, the language used in the questionnaire is of central importance. Questions should be phrased with the lowest, rather than the average educational level of the target population in mind. Analysis of the comprehension level of the questionnaire is possible through use of standardized methods such as the FOG index (Gunning, 1952) or reading difficulty formula (Flesch, 1949). (For a wide-ranging discussion of issues and methods related to communicating with patients see Ley, 1988).

Questions should be as short as possible. Oppenheim (1992) maintains that the maximum length of any question should be 20 words. It could be argued, however, that it is not the number of words which is important so much as the number of ideas contained within the question. The following two examples are of similar length. The former, however, involves two questions, whereas the latter has only one:

Have you ever worked with people who abuse alcohol either in hospital or in the community?

and

Can you tell me if you have any experience of working with people who have abused alcohol?

Special attention should be paid to vague or ambiguous terms or phrases which can mislead or confuse the respondent. Terms such as *occasionally* or *often* should be defined in terms of some specific time scale or frequency; technical terms should be paraphrased in the appropriate vernacular. All questions should be worded positively, 'Does this ever happen?' rather than negatively 'This doesn't ever happen, does it?' If the respondent answered yes (or no) to the latter, it would not be clear whether this meant 'yes this doesn't happen' or 'yes it does'.

Questions which focus upon sensitive areas, such as sexual behaviour or the abuse of drugs, require careful wording. Kinsey *et al.* (1953) acknowledged that respondents might be embarrassed by questions about their sexual behaviour. The solution, which has been widely copied, involved assuming that low-valued, or unusual forms of behaviour were possessed by the respondents, thereby relieving them of the burden of denial. Respondents are more likely to give details about some negative or low-valued behaviour if the question, 'When did you first begin to feel stressed at work?' is asked. The alternative version 'Did you ever feel that you couldn't cope with work?' is more likely to be answered negatively. In this context, it should be remembered that all questionnaires and interview schedules represent an intrusion into the private life of the individual. Care needs to be taken to spare embarrassment and to promote honest responses. Where highly sensitive topics form the basis of the measure, self-report questionnaires may be more appropriate than use of the interview schedule.

Question sequence

A well designed questionnaire involves progressing easily from one question to the next, in a sequence which appears logical to the respondent. Indeed, the respondent should be able to anticipate the next question. This logical sequence might differ significantly from the order which is most pleasing to the researcher. The sequence can be determined by funnelling questions, asking the most general, unrestrictive questions first as a preamble to successively more specific questions:

Example

Question 1:   'What do you think of the present state of nursing education?'
Question 2:   'What are your thoughts about the proposals to develop wider post basic training opportunities?'
Question 3:   'What aspects of clinical nursing would benefit most from further training input?'
Question 4:   'What sort of things should we be doing differently there?'
Question 5:   'Some would say that we just can't afford such developments at present, what do you think?'

The funnel technique provides a means of access to the person's true views or opinions, avoiding distorting the answer by the contaminating proximity to answers which might be conflicting in nature. In the example above, the respondent is given a great deal of freedom on the first question, then is asked to discuss the topic more specifically. Questions 3 and 4 allow the respondent to clarify his own views about the topic, before being asked the crucial final question. If question 5 was asked alone, or even after question 2, a different response might be forthcoming.

In self-report questionnaires filter questions may be employed to guide the respondent through different groups of questions. The respondent who answers 'no' to one question may be asked to 'proceed to question 6'. It should be noted, however, that this procedure can cause confusion.

Other considerations

Take every precaution against influencing the response, whether by design or default. Leading questions or the use of loaded words can cause considerable influence. Equally, failing to cite the range of alternatives may represent a form of bias (Oppenheim, 1992): For example: 'Do you prefer working with patients of your own sex?' is less appropriate than: 'Do you have any preferences for working with men or women patients, or doesn't it matter?'

Care also needs to be taken in ordering the sequence of questions requiring yes/no answers. Cronbach (1950) described the phenomenon of response set where the same response is given repeatedly, despite the question. One possible solution is to employ multiple choice questions rather than strict alternatives. Another option is to vary the positioning of the responses. For example:

Question 1:   ... Yes/no/don't know
Question 2:   ... Don't know/no/yes

Similarly, the layout of the self-report questionnaire can affect the responses. These should be clearly worded and attractively presented. The immediate visual impact will either arouse the respondent's interest or discourage completion. All self-report measures should carry (on a separate page) a clearly written introduction, providing a general explanation of the purpose of the questionnaire. Instructions for completion should include a completed example; this should be similar in form, but should not include one of the actual items from the questionnaire.

The layout should also employ emphasis, using different type sizes, bold type or underlining, to help guide the respondent. If questionnaires are to be returned by post, the page size should allow easy folding into a stamped addressed envelope. It is generally held that a serif typeface (for example Times Roman) is easier to read than a sans-serif style (such as Helvetica) (McColl, 1994). Some studies even suggest that light-coloured paper is more attractive; in the case of postal returns, yellow, closely followed by pink, has better return rates than other colours (Eastwood, 1940).

Finally, all questionnaires should be submitted to a pre-test: this is a trial run designed to evaluate the adequacy of the tool in measuring the research variables, isolating any bias, vagueness and otherwise inadequate questions. This test should be conducted with a small sample of subjects drawn from the study population.

Scaling methods

Scales involve a set of symbols or numbers so constructed that they can be assigned to subjects, or their behaviours, indicating the subject's *possession* or *performance* of whatever the scale claims to measure. Typically, scales measure attributes or constructs; warmth, hostility, anger or dependency, for example. Subjects can rate themselves or may be judged by independent raters. A variety of scaling methods are possible.

Agreement–disagreement scales

Two main variants of this scale are in common use. In the first variant, subjects are asked to agree or disagree or indicate yes or no. In the second variant, subjects are asked to choose from three or more responses: yes/don't know/no; or strongly agree/agree/no opinion/disagree/strongly disagree.

Visual analogue

Here, subjects are invited to indicate, with a cross or tick, where on a continuum between one attribute and another they believe they (or others) lie. These scales are bipolar, inviting the respondent to provide a judgment somewhere between one end of the continuum and the other.

Example

In general, how would you define the patients in your ward? (Indicate by placing X on the line.)

Independent _____very dependent

Alternatively, the continuum can incorporate the points used to measure the respondent's score. The most common scale used is 7 points:

Independent _____very dependent

        1   2   3   4   5   6   7

Likert scales

Attitudes can be measured more specifically using *degrees* of agreement or disagreement. The Likert scale involves statements which are considered to be approximately equal. Typically, the Likert scale employs 10 to 20 statements which are considered to be approximately equal. The respondent ticks the item which most approximates their attitude or opinion. Respondents to Barker's (1988) depression locus of control scale were asked to indicate their responses to statements such as: 'Good mental health is largely a matter of good fortune' using the scale:

agree strongly	1
agree a lot	2
tend to agree	3
tend to disagree	4
disagree a lot	5
disagree strongly	6

The Likert scale uses equal numbers of positive and negative statements, avoiding a 'don't know' response. The orientation of the statement can be either positive or negative: the statement above could be rephrased: 'Good mental health has nothing to do with luck or good fortune.'

Semantic-differential scale

Here, the respondent is asked to rate a specific concept across a number of characteristics, using seven-point bipolar ratings. The semantic differential uses bipolar adjectives, such as happy–sad; good–bad. In the example below, the respondents are asked to give their views of community psychiatric nurses:

Community psychiatric nurses (CPNs) are:

Responsible _____irresponsible

7   6   5   4   3   2   1

Ineffective _____effective

1   2   3   4   5   6   7

As the example shows, characteristics should be reversed, in terms of their positive–negative values, to avoid the fixed response set discussed earlier.

Typically, the respondents' attitude towards each concept is evaluated across a number of dimensions: judging, for example, how valuable, good or fair is the concept; potency – how strong, large, effective; and activity – how active, fast, efficient. In a study of general practitioners' attitudes towards the service provided by CPNs compared with six other occupational groups, White (1986) used a 14-scale semantic differential.

Use of questionnaires

Survey questionnaire

Researchers have consistently employed mail questionnaires as a relatively economic and expedient method for collecting data from either large population samples or from subjects who are geographically inaccessible. Studies might aim, for example, to follow up subjects discharged from experimental nursing projects, or to study graduates from basic or post-basic educational programmes. In either case, direct interviewing might either be costly in terms of interviewer time, or impossible in terms of travel restrictions.

Self-report format

The survey questionnaire can take a number of forms. Biographical (demographic) data are a common constituent, serving to identify key characteristics of the population surveyed. The rest of the questionnaire can employ either yes/no or either/or questions, multiple choice questions, ratings or open-ended comments.

Examples

(1) During your stay in hospital were you given information about your condition? Yes/No

(2) All long-stay residents should be transferred to alternative facilities in the community. Agree/Disagree

(3) When you were admitted to hospital, were you given information about:
     your condition Y/N
     your nursing care Y/N
     visiting arrangements Y/N
     your medical treatment Y/N
     other hospital services Y/N
     Please circle yes (Y) or no (N)

(4) How do you think your training affected your subsequent professional practice or attitudes? The 1–5 scale indicates 1 = very negative effect; 3 = no effect; 5 = very positive effect.

clinical practice	1 2 3 4 5
management skills	1 2 3 4 5
development of your service	1 2 3 4 5
patient/client involvement	1 2 3 4 5
staff support	1 2 3 4 5

(5) What aspects of the programme did you find unsatisfactory? Describe briefly.

     _____

     _____

     _____

The design of the mail questionnaire is also important. Shorter formats produce better response rates than longer questionnaires. As noted earlier, care needs to be taken over the presentation of the questionnaire, including typing, lay-out and language. A clear, concise and friendly accompanying letter, supported by a stamped, self-addressed envelope, can also enhance response rates. Care needs to be taken over the wording of items, to avoid leading the respondent, or confusing through use of vague or ambiguous terms. Some studies provide small financial incentives contingent upon completion. Even where funding is available to offer such an incentive to complete the questionnaire, the researcher needs to carefully consider ethical issues and the risk of offending some respondents.

Despite their practical advantages, where mail questionnaires are employed alone, a number of drawbacks have consistently been cited: poor response rates, inability to check accuracy of responses and difficulty in making valid generalizations from the resultant unrepresentative sample (see Warwick & Linninger, 1975; Williams, 1987). Robinson (1989) noted that methods of improving response rates, and reducing sampling bias, remain elusive. Most authorities suggest that the selective nature of the responses calls any conclusions into question. In White's (1986) study of the attitudes of general practitioners employing the semantic differential (see above), despite the brevity of the questionnaire, a response rate of only 72% was achieved. In Kerlinger's (1986) view, returns of at least 80–90% should be sought. Failing this, non-respondents should be studied to learn something of their characteristics.

Summary

The various questionnaire formats described in this chapter are designed to collect information from the subject. The information can be facilitated by an interviewer (using the interview schedule) in a face-to-face or telephone interaction. More often the information is elicited through self-report, where the questionnaires are either mailed to the respondent or delivered and collected at a later date by the researcher. The former is more appropriate for larger samples, distributed widely; the latter for smaller, local samples. As with all methods of data collection, it is necessary to evaluate the potential usefulness of any instrument or method prior to its use within the formal study. As with other methods, estimates of validity and reliability will indicate the extent to which the instrument will usefully measure the research construct.

In designing any of the questionnaire formats described in this chapter, much emphasis should be given to the importance of rigorously testing the formats (Oppenheim, 1992). There is a need to establish that the tool reduces to a minimum errors of comprehension or completion, whether committed by interviewers or respondents.

The advantages of the use of questionnaires, within an interview schedule format, were described in the previous chapter. Researchers who elect to employ self-report questionnaire methods are likely to be influenced by the following factors:

(1)   They are less costly than interviews, in terms of time and energy.
(2)   They facilitate access to larger samples.
(3)   They are appropriate for subjects geographically distant from the researcher.
(4)   They are more anonymous than direct interviews.
(5)   They are less threatening, especially where 'taboo' material is under review.
(6)   They are less prone to bias, evident in the interviewer interpretation.

These advantages need to be balanced, however, against numerous disadvantages associated with such formats. The key difficulty involves the often blunt refusal of respondents to complete, and/or return, the questionnaires. In a related vein, some subjects may ask friends or relatives to assist, or even complete the questionnaire for them, thus prejudicing the sample. Similarly, people with handicaps may be restrained from completing self-report measures, while other subjects may fail to comprehend the meaning of specific questions. This potential problem demands significant rigour in the construction and pilot testing of the format. Finally, questionnaires can often only address the research themes superficially. It is clear, however, that the constraints of time, money and availability of support workers will make self-report measures an attractive proposition to many researchers (Parahoo, 1994).

References

Barker, P. (1988) *An evaluation of specific nursing interventions in the management of patients suffering from manic depressive psychosis.* PhD thesis, Chapter 11, Dundee Institute of Technology.

Cronbach, L.J. (1950) Further evidence on response sets and test design. *Educational and Psychological Measurement*, **10**, 3.

Eastwood, R.P. (1940) *Sales Control by Quantitative Methods.* Columbia University Press, New York.

Flesch, R. (1949) *The art of readable writing.* Harper, New York.

Gunning, R. (1952) *The Technique of Clear Writing.* McGraw-Hill, New York.

Kerlinger, F.N. (1986) *Foundations of Behavioural Research*, 3rd edn. CBS Publishing Japan, NY.

Kinsey, A.C., Pomeroy, W.B. & Martin, C.E. (1953) *Sexual Behaviour in the Human Male.* W.B. Saunders, Philadelphia.

Ley, P. (1988) *Communicating with Patients: Improving Communication, Satisfaction and Compliance.* Croom Helm, London.

McColl, E. (1994) Questionnaire design and construction. *Nurse Researcher*, 1(2), 16–25.

Oppenheim, A.N. (1992) *Questionnaire Design, Interviewing and Attitude Measurement*, 2nd edn. Pinter Publishing, London.

Parahoo, K. (1994) Questionnaires: use, value and limitations. *Nurse Researcher*, 1(2), 4–15.

Robinson, D. (1989) Response rates in questionnaires. *Senior Nurse*, 9(10), 25–6.

Warwick, D. & Linninger, C. (1975) *The Sample Survey: Theory and Practice.* McGraw-Hill, New York.

White, E. (1986) Factors influencing GPs to refer patients to community psychiatric nurses. In *Psychiatric Nursing Research*, (ed. J. Brooking), Chapter 12. John Wiley, Chichester.

Williams, C.A. (1987) Research by mail and other distractions. *Journal of Professional Nursing*, 3(6), 327; 376.

Recommended reading

Bircumshaw, D. (1989) A survey of the attitudes of senior nurses towards graduates. *Journal of Advanced Nursing*, 14(1), 68–72.

Carr, E.C. (1990) Post-operative pain: patient's expectations and experiences. *Journal of Advanced Nursing*, 15(1), 89–100.

Fenton, M.V. (1987) Development of the scale of humanistic nursing behaviours. *Nursing Research*, 36(2), 82–7.

Flagler, S. (1989) Semantic differentials and the process of developing one to measure maternal role competence. *Journal of Advanced Nursing*, 14(3), 190–7.

Gulick, E.E. (1987) Parsimony and model confirmation of the ADL self-care scale for multiple sclerosis persons. *Nursing Research*, 36(5), 278–83.

Holmes, S. (1989) Use of a modified symptom distress scale in the assessment of the cancer patient. *International Journal of Nursing Studies*, 26(1), 69–80.

Humphris, G.M. & Turner, A. (1989) Job satisfaction and attitudes of nursing staff on a unit for the elderly severely infirm, with change of location. *Journal of Advanced Nursing*, 14(4), 298–307.

Chapter 23

Observation

Philip J. Barker

Introduction

All data collection methods involve extensions or consolidations of the researcher's everyday behaviour. This is most true of observation; everyone uses their senses to collect information about their world, interpreting such data to make sense of their experience of their world. Observation could be defined as a heightened form of such everyday sensation; the systemic use of the researcher's sensory mechanism, within a rigorous framework. In everyday observation we test the evidence collected by our senses. In the research setting, observation is characterized by doubt. Take nothing on trust, but aim to define, clarify, redefine and measure objectively the events which occur.

Why be objective?

The use of observational methods can be arduous. The researcher who selects an observational framework will have considered alternatives and found them wanting. Interviewing people (Chapter 21), or inviting them to complete self-report rating scales or questionnaires (Chapter 22), gives the following information: what the subjects think they do, or how they feel about their own or others' actions. The attitudes people have towards themselves or others, or their experience of their own lives, is a laudable object of study. Such personal *subjective* experience, however, tells us little about what actually happened. The researcher who selects an observational framework wants to know what really did take place, between whom and to what end. In some cases you may also be interested to extend this awareness through direct measurement. How often did this take place, or for how long; in effect, what was the magnitude of the event? In all cases, however, a similar aim is expressed, to describe, if not also to explain events in the research setting (Sackett, 1978).

The limits of objective reality

Shakespeare observed that 'all the world's a stage and all men and women merely players'. This observation reflects the difficulty over attempts to measure what is really going on in any given situation. Indeed, for some decades – ever since the discovery of quantum physics – traditional assumptions about the objective world have been challenged (Casti, 1992). Increasingly it is accepted that our interaction with the world, for example through observation, has an effect on what we observe. As a result, when we say that through observation we shall establish what is really taking place, we must add the caveat: what is taking place when under the conditions of observation.

What to observe?

Observational methods may be used to collect data from across a wide spectrum. The following represent the most commonly selected target areas.

Individual characteristics

Information which defines either the constant characteristics of the study population, such as apparently enduring or, alternatively, more temporary patterns of behaviour, physical states, or physiological reactions, are a key feature of many observational studies. In nursing research, data which define the health or illness characteristics of the individual, and gross or subtle fluctuations in their presentation, will have a major bearing upon the definition of nursing needs and measures of nursing 'outcomes'. Similarly, the defining characteristics of nurses may provide the most important form of data for educational or managerial studies, investigating anything from the experience of training to sickness and absenteeism.

Non-verbal communication

Facial expression, gestures, body postures and interpersonal distance are key elements in the communication process, and represent an important area for nurse researchers. Some theorists would argue that these behaviours often define the meaning of the communication more clearly than verbal behaviour, which can be deceptive and misleading. How nurses interact with patients, other staff or one another may be of as much significance as what they say to one another (Wolfgang, 1979).

Verbal behaviour

The content and structure of communication is an accessible, if difficult, area for observers. The ways in which nurses interact with patients, relatives, other professional groups, or each other, are important areas of research. How such verbal interactions take place under specific conditions such as in emergencies, or under emotional conditions, provides a sharper focus to the research goals.

Everyday living skills

The activities which patients perform as part of their everyday routine provide another important research target. Patients' engagement in self-care, social and recreational activities, tells the researcher much about their needs, progress of deterioration, if not also about the effects of the nurses' intervention (Smith *et al.* 1987).

Nursing skills

This group represents a parallel set of observations, focused more specifically upon technical aspects of the nurse–patient relationship. How nurses admit patients to hospital, complete specific assessments, conduct tests or other procedures, or prepare and complete care plans, are typical examples of observational subject matter.

Environmental characteristics

Information concerning the stimulus conditions under which all of the above behaviours take place provides the definition of the scenario in which nursing care takes place (Owens & Ashcroft, 1982).

Direct (non-participant) and indirect (participant) observation

Observation can be employed in two ways. Direct observation is characterized by objectivity, a systematic framework and the use of formal recording technologies. In participant observation the observer collects information from within the research setting. In the former, the observer tries to remain apart from the study situation, aiming to collect objective data uncontaminated either by the observer's presence or her value system. In the latter, the researcher aims to become a member (albeit temporarily) of the group under study. In such participant observation the researcher becomes involved with the object of study, such as a group of nurses or patients, and collects data through logs or field notes (Patton, 1987; Samarel, 1989).

All observation is dependent upon the quality of the data recorded. In participant observation, overt recording materials may represent an obvious intrusion and formal recording methods are often dispensed with. Instead, mental notes are translated afterwards into log or field note form. Proponents of participant observation argue that more unstructured methods allow a deeper insight into the 'workings' of the research setting, and often eschew more structured methods on the grounds that they are mechanistic, offering only a superficial, if not artificial, account of the research setting. Alternatively, critics of participant observation are concerned about the extent to which such a method may be prone to observer bias or *observer effect*. How does the observer retain objectivity if she is part of the study situation, and how can the study group fail to be affected by an observer living in their midst?

Participant observation is most commonly associated with the qualitative approach discussed in Chapters 11 and 12. Some methodological conflict may be involved in mixing qualitative and quantitative methods. For this reason participant observation is not featured specifically in this chapter. However, many of the general principles governing observation cover both approaches to the collection of data by observation.

The observer

The ideal observer of any social situation would be a machine programmed to recognize and monitor those aspects of social behaviour of interest to the researcher. Human observers may be expected to follow the research protocol, but may end up being influenced by their own instincts or prejudices. Kerlinger (1979) has observed that scientific objectivity has little to do with the presumed objectivity of scientists themselves but is, rather, a quality of the methodology. This view is important for the selection and training of observers. Few are likely to be objective by nature, but all must be prepared specifically to use the research methodology which has been confirmed as an objective procedure.

The world of objective observation

What is objective observation?

All methods of observation have some objectivity. The extent to which any method of observation can be called objective depends on the degree of agreement between two observers using the observational method. The methods discussed in this chapter do not possess any monopoly on objectivity. The only difference between the methods here and, for example, participant observation procedures, lies in the extent to which any two observers using the procedure might agree on what is taking place. Objective observation, like other forms of observation, involves inference. Judgements and decisions concern *what* to observe, and *what* different variables might *represent*. These involve assumptions about the meaning of behaviour if not about the whole world. All methods of observation end up classifying and categorizing variables. Each involves assumptions about the meaning of the events which have been observed (Jones & Nisbett, 1987). Direct observation may be defined as more objective, but no less inferential, than other methods to the extent that different observers will end up with a similar *picture* of the observed setting, providing that they employ the same observational procedure (Weick, 1985).

Naturalistic observation

Studies which elect to use an observational method tend to focus upon the natural environment, for example caring behaviours actually performed in a specific clinical setting. Naturalistic observation draws heavily upon the principles and methodology of ethology. Naturalistic observation can be defined as the practice of noting and recording facts and events in accordance with, or in imitation of what has been called, 'the essential character of the thing' (Jones *et al.*, 1974).

Before you can record this essential character, a clear definition of the things must be developed. This should allow all observers to recognize the phenomenon when they see *it*. Although direct observation involves a specific focus upon events occurring under specific conditions, this does not obviate the need for clear definition of the events and conditions. At some stage in the research process, you will make inferences about the relationship between the actual behaviour of the subjects and related environmental events. Such inferences depend upon empirical evidence, which must be as free of ambiguity (and inference) as possible. The defining features of naturalistic observation, therefore, are:

(1) Recording of behavioural events where they occur.
(2) Emphasis upon operational definitions of the observed behaviour and related environmental events.
(3) Recording of events when they occur.
(4) Recordings conducted by impartial, reliable observers (Boice, 1983).

Observational targets

Observational units: large or small?

Observational targets are commonly divided into molar or molecular targets. Molar behaviour involves large units of activity, such as *co-operativeness*, *interaction*, *aggression*, *helping*. Molecular behaviours involve small, often highly specific, units of behaviour: 'nodded head (in agreement)', 'made eye contact', 'hit other', 'supported patient's arm'. Researchers are often divided ideologically between the value of either of these approaches. Proponents of the study of molar behaviour suggest that this represents a *real* event, which becomes lost in the minutiae of molecular examples, which are often not valid representations of the area of inquiry. Molecular advocates suggest that molar studies often fail to attain adequate levels of reliability, as observers cannot agree as to whether or not these ill-defined events have occurred. You need to carefully consider the balance between both approaches. A highly reliable observational method can be developed if you define all the components of the target behaviour operationally. Helping could be defined as:

'holding patient's arm; supporting cup; giving instructions; making encouraging statements; pointing; opening doors; holding part of patient's clothing . . . and so on'.

Observers using such molecular definitions might attain a high degree of agreement on their occurrence. In the process, it could be argued that the pursuit of reliability has led to the loss of validity of the observational procedure. Were all the occurrences of these behaviours representative of helping? It is possible that on some occasions some of these molecular actions had other functions?

Molar definitions, which involve broader *natural* definitions, may appear more valid. Helping might alternatively be defined as:

'giving physical support; listening attentively; interacting harmoniously to assist the attainment of the patient's own goals'.

Such definitions allow the observer to capture something of the 'flavour' of the event. Because of their inherent ambiguity, these definitions might lead to interpretation, probably resulting in a lowering of reliability.

Item pool

The so-called item pool may be determined in advance or may require a preliminary descriptive study of the research environment. Typically, a *running narrative* might be employed to describe in some detail the activities of the subjects in relation to a variety of environmental effects. The researcher may decide to devote a period of time to continuous direct observation, recording as much of the general activity in the research setting as possible, afterwards abstracting behaviours and setting events which appear congruent with the research aims.

Operational definitions

The study which elects an observational methodology is likely to be concerned with the discrete, or *actual*, relationship between sets of variables. Such a relationship is often assumed to be causal. It should not be forgotten, however, that although it is helpful to think causally, causal laws cannot be demonstrated empirically (Blalock, 1961). It is sufficient to demonstrate the strength of a relationship between two sets of variables. This does not demonstrate, however, that p causes q.

The researcher has a large universe of actions, events and situations available which might define the subject area. From this universe, specific patterns of behaviour, and specific setting conditions, need to be identified to narrow the focus of the study and to make observation viable. Once identified, these must be defined operationally, to provide the researcher, and more importantly the observers, with a working definition of each behavioural response or setting event which might comprise the observational target.

The item pool is defined first, either by pre-selection, or by a preliminary *journalistic* description of the study setting. In some studies, the item pool may be almost *self-selective*; a study of the nursing care of people suffering from incontinence might elect to observe the frequency of micturition in different situations. Given that micturition involves voiding urine, the researcher may define some forms of micturition as *continence* (when the subject urinates in a toilet facility), others as *incontinence* (urinating in bed). These behaviours are defined not in terms of what the subject does, but in terms of the stimulus conditions under which the behaviour occurs.

If you wish to explain some aspect of the study environment which is presently unclear, every effort should be made to define both the social behaviour of the subjects and the environmental stimuli under which these behaviours might appear.

Stimulus conditions

Bijou & Baer (1968) define three stimulus sources:

(1)   The physical environment: Any aspect of the physical world of the subjects. The details required in an operational definition of this class would involve size, colour, texture, weight, and so on, of objects within, or of, the environment itself. Other sensory stimuli which might be incorporated within this environment, such as sounds (music, bells, birds) or light (flickering neon, bright sunshine) should also be included.

(2)   The social environment. This would include details of the number, status and geographical relationship to the subject of others, and will provide basic data. Additional stimulus classification would involve defining the behaviour of significant others towards the subject; this might involve single class stimuli (nurse prompts subject to drink from cup) or multiple stimulus classes (nurse talks to subject; guides subject's arm; nurse holds plate on table).

(3)   The internal environment of the subject. In field studies undertaken in the natural environment, it is probably impossible to monitor this class of stimuli. Examples include hunger, thirst, pain and visceral activity. In a seminal study, Bijou *et al.* (1968) suggested that contemporary research methods were inappropriate for measuring such 'biologically anchored variables'. It is clear that in many settings, nurse researchers must work towards incorporation of such variables in an effort to provide a more satisfactory explanation of the interactions between nurses and patients. In some nursing research studies, contemporaneous monitoring of some internal variables may be possible through use of physiological and biophysical measures.

Subject behaviour

Operational definitions of behaviour should contain sufficient information to measure the occurrence of the event reliably. The definition should not be overly complex: cry might be defined as:

'repeated, usually low pitched, vocalizations, for example "waah, aaah-hah" '.

The definition serves only to help the observer classify the occurrence and to distinguish, where possible, one behaviour which might be confused with a pattern. Clearly, subjects might be crying with frustration . . . in despair . . . or with joy. The 'meaning' of the behaviour may emerge by identification of complementary behaviours (such as gestures or body posture) or by recording environmental context (stimulus conditions).

Observer effect

Many researchers who are unused to direct observation fear that the presence of the observer will be a major, and continuing, disruptive influence. Although the entry of an independent observer to the research setting can have an initial disturbing effect, providing that certain considerations are applied this disruption will be short-lived (Heyns & Lippit, 1954). Subjects could be observed discreetly from a distance, by audio or video recording or through viewing screens. These methods involve no disruption of the natural behaviour of the study group but do represent a major intrusion of a potentially unethical nature and should be rejected from consideration. The observer needs to have a clear view of the research territory, while remaining unobtrusive. Direct observational data are often collected by research assistants who, initially, explain in full the purpose of their presence in the setting and ask for the consent of the group to be observed.

Observational methods

The two main classes of observational method are automated and pencil and paper. Automated methods allow the observer to monitor single or multiple responses in real time (event recorders). However, the advantage of sensitive, real-time recording may be outweighed by considerations of cost and the level of sophistication and training required of observers in their use. Less complex automated devices, such as tally counters, hand held or worn or the wrist, pedometers and stopwatches, are used as an adjunct to pencil and paper methods. In some situations audio or audio visual recording may be appropriate, these recordings allowing more discreet analysis by pencil and paper methods later. Situations which might justify the use of such observations are:

(1) When the action is so rapid that other methods of observation are inadequate.
(2) When the action is complex.
(3) When distinction between one behaviour (or behaviour of one subject) and another is difficult.

In any of these situations, replay, pause and slowing of the recorded action allow more detailed analysis. Unless such automated devices are used unobtrusively, however, they are also likely to represent a major source of observer effect. The disruptive influence of such devices with children has long been reported (Hutt & Hutt, 1970). This may be the case with other sensitive populations, such as hospital patients and the nurses caring for them. Pencil and paper methods embrace a wealth of possibilities. In principle, all forms of observing and recording would be included under this heading. For the sake of simplicity, only formal methods of observing and recording possessing a high degree of objectivity will be addressed here.

Observational rating scales

Observers can measure the subject by use of rating scales which are similar to the self-report measures described in Chapter 22. The most commonly used methods are:

(1)   The category rating scale

Here the observer is asked to quantify the presence of specified behaviours. The observer is asked to select a category, from a menu, which best characterizes the behaviour or characteristics of the subject. The observer then rates the degree of category present. The category item 'empathic' might be:

How empathic is the nurse? (tick one only)

very empathic   (   )
empathic   (   )
not empathic   (   )
not at all empathic (   )

Alternatively, the item could be defined further:

How empathic is the nurse? (tick one)

always very empathic; can predict the patient's emotional state (   )
mostly empathic; shows understanding of patient's feelings   (   )
rarely empathic; often fails to acknowledge patient's feelings   (   )
mostly unempathic; ignores patient's feelings   (   )

(2)   The numerical rating scale

This format is similar to the Likert scales described in Chapter 22. Here the observer gives a numerical rating, or score, according to the perceived presence of some attribute, characteristic, or pattern of behaviour (Downing & Brockington, 1978). The observer might be asked to rate a range of characteristics or behaviours 'using the following scale':

0:   absent; not performed
1:   minimal; performed infrequently or to limited degree
2:   moderate; performed intermittently or to some extent
3:   considerable; performed consistently or to great extent

(3)   The graphic rating scale

This is similar to the linear analogue scale (Chapter 22) and employs a line or bar, with accompanying descriptive statements:

Describe the subject's presentation between 8 am and 12 noon:

very	quite	a little	not
depressed	depressed	depressed	depressed

These scales can be presented in several ways: continuous lines, unmarked lines with two extreme definitions, identified intervals (as above) or segmented lines. Their key feature is that they fix a continuum in the observer's mind, suggesting intervals or degrees of the characteristic or behaviour. In Guilford's (1954) view, their virtues are many and their faults are few.

Observational rating scales can be used to measure virtually any variable which can be defined operationally by the researcher. In addition to behaviours, or behavioural characteristics, such scales might measure, for example:

(1)   The quality of nursing assessments.
(2)   Nurses' handwriting in care plans.
(3)   Student nurses' use of theoretical concepts in written assignments.
(4)   Nurses' emotional state under interview conditions.

Despite their potential, or perhaps because of their apparent widespread 'usefulness', a word of caution is appropriate. Even where scales are well designed, they are prone to bias. One form of bias is the *halo effect*. Rugg (1921) defined this as a 'general mental attitude' towards the personality of other people which dominates our attitude towards their particular qualities. In research terms, this means that the observers' measure of some specific quality, behaviour or other attribute of the person may be dominated by their overall view of the person.

A further problem with ratings is the tendency of observers to err on the side of severity or leniency – observers may be too critical and tough or they may 'feel sorry' for the subjects. Another dimension of this problem is the error of central tendency, where (usually) novice observers avoid all extreme judgements and consistently give the subjects an intermediate rating. All such problems indicate the need for rigorous preparation and monitoring of observers.

Direct observational methods

Actions which are short-lived and have a discrete beginning and end can be counted, using a frequency record. This is known as a frequency count. Any event which can be expressed appropriately as a number can be measured in this way. For example, how often (within a stated time frame) subjects:

(1)   Are reported absent.
(2)   Speak to patients.
(3)   Are called out of meetings.
(4)   Request analgesic medication.

These can all be expressed as numerical frequencies. The major criterion for selection of this method is that the observer can identify the beginning and end of each event precisely.

The frequency count is most useful when the events occur at a moderate rate, neither too often nor too infrequently. Where high rates of occurrence exist, hand-held tally counters or more sophisticated automatic recording devices can be used as an adjunct. The major failing of this method is that, except where automated devices are used, the resultant measure gives no indication of distribution across time. Measure of the frequency of some event, per hour, day, week, and so on, is possible but, without the use of automated devices or an alternative recording format fluctuations in rate across time are lost.

Duration

The duration record measures the elapsed time of a given behaviour during a specific observation period. This is appropriate for behaviours of variable duration, such as talking, watching television, changing a catheter, for example. The observer needs to be able to identify the beginning and end of the behaviour, and must acknowledge all temporary cessations in the performance. The major drawback is that it is almost always confined to single-subject observation. It may, however, be incorporated easily with other methods into a multi-method observational format.

Latency

How long subjects take to respond to a given stimulus provides an alternative temporal dimension. For example, how long nurses take to:

(1) Respond to a patient's call for assistance.
(2) Locate emergency resuscitation equipment.
(3) Reach agreement on a specific issue of ward policy.

In some cases, the measure involves the time taken to begin the behaviour. In others, the measure involves the time taken, from the cue, to complete the action.

Sampling behaviour

Two major methods of sampling behaviour are possible. These give an estimate of the frequency of some specified behaviour across time. This approach is used when the straightforward frequency count is found wanting.

The interval record

This method determines whether or not the behaviour has occurred within a specific time interval. Three variants are possible.

(1) In the first, an arbitrary time interval is selected, such as one minute. Any occurrence of the behaviour within the interval is recorded. A checklist of behaviours is commonly incorporated, and the serial occurrence of the different behaviours is recorded using serial numbers. This provides a total frequency for each behaviour, and an illustration of the temporal relationship of one behaviour to another. It provides only a crude estimate, however, of the time spent engaged in each behaviour.

(2) Alternatively, the time interval selected may be short enough to accommodate only one occurrence of the behaviour. If the observer determines that the behaviour to be observed lasts, on average, 20 seconds, this time interval is used to monitor its frequency. The common rule is that the behaviour is recorded as having occurred only if it occurs during most of the time interval. This method allows an estimate of the frequency of the behaviour, its rate across time and the approximate amount of time spent engaging in the behaviour.

(3) Where the observer tries to measure more complex patterns of behaviour, including their relationship to the environment, the interval recording method requires further modification. In Fig. 23.1 (Barker, 1977), the observer is collecting data on the behaviour of a young child in a playroom. Given the number of categories of behaviour and location included, a 10-second time interval is used – 5 seconds to observe and 5 seconds to record. The observer enters only the code for the location or behaviour in each time cell.

		1	2	3	4	5	6
Location	W: Wall D: Door F: Floor C: Chair T: Table	F	F	F	C	F	T
No object	ST: Standing SI: Sitting W: Walking C: Crawling SP: Spinning	SI	SI	ST	SI	W	ST
With self	B: Blowing V: Vocalizing R: Rocking H: Hitting WA: Waving arms WL: Waving legs RH: Rubbing hands RF: Rubbing face	R	R	WA	RH	V	H

Fig. 23.1 Example of data collection sheet: observation.

Time sample

This method involves brief observations, usually momentary, designed to identify whether or not a specific behaviour was occurring at a particular point in time. This may be used for single behaviours with single subjects, or with multiple behaviours across groups. This format allows a rough estimate of the frequency of patterns of behaviours across time, requiring no special equipment and limited training of observers (Weick, 1985).

General considerations

Narrow or broad focus?

The major differences between recording methods, apart from those already noted, lie in their specificity or generality.

Specific observational systems measure either single or multiple classes of behaviour:

(1) Single response classes focus upon one behaviour to the exclusion of all others.
(2) Multiple class responses focus upon several behaviours. Typically, these are divided into mutually exclusive categories (behaviours which cannot occur at the same time as others in that class) and concomitant behaviours (behaviours which can be contemporaneous with others).

General observational systems involve recording not only the subjects' responses but also the setting stimuli, for example the behaviour of other people in the environment, and other events which might be related to the subjects' actions. This form of observation is most valuable since it allows an opportunity to infer connections between the relative frequency of responses and their temporal relationship to other stimuli.

Training observers

A well developed observational method is only as good as the skill of the observer. Observers require the following preparation:

- *Orientation to the study.* Observers need to know how the observation format has been developed and why specific behaviours and/or settings have been selected. These boundary considerations are important if the observer is to develop an unusual perception of perhaps familiar patterns of behaviour.
- *Unstructured observation period.* Observers should be offered an opportunity to study the research setting without the aid of the observational schedule. This exercise should provide the observers with an awareness of their need for clear definitions and a formal observational structure.
- *Formal introduction.* Even the simplest recording tool is likely to appear daunting at first glance. For this reason the observers should be guided patiently through the observational method, and should be provided with clear instructions as to the researcher's expectations.
- *Role play.* Initial training should be conducted under role play conditions, perhaps using a video recording or group of actors, the action being stopped at strategic intervals to allow questions and clarification.
- *Pilot observation period.* The observers should spend a period of time completing the measures under full research conditions. Data from this pilot are discarded following critical analysis of the experience of the observers and the establishment of inter-observer reliability. This period can also be used to *acclimatize* the subjects to the observer's presence, thereby reducing the potency of observer effect when formal data collection begins.

Reliability and validity

The use of formal means of direct measurement and clear operational definitions is not always sufficient to guarantee reliable data collection. Agreement between observers is essential if the measures are to be described as objective. Disagreements between observers can occur for the following reasons:

(1) The operational definitions may be inadequate.
(2) The observational code may be inadequate.
(3) The observers may be inadequately trained.
(4) The procedure for calculating reliability may be faulty.

The pilot observation phase is used to investigate these first three possibilities. At least two observers should study the same situation independently; their data are subsequently analysed to assess the degree of agreement. The most commonly used statistical method for computing reliability is the correlation coefficient (see Chapters 27 and 28). The acceptable degree of agreement between observers is a moot point. Commonly, however, a reliability coefficient of less than 0.8 may be unacceptable.

The validity of observational methods has largely been neglected in the social science research literature due in part to the absence of external criteria to validate the kind of variables studied. Reliability and validity are closely connected. Clearly, an observational method which is not reliable cannot be valid. However, it can be reliable without necessarily being valid. Validity is concerned with the extent to which the observational method measures what it claims to measure. Does the interval measure illustrated in this chapter (Fig. 23.1) actually measure 'free play', or is it measuring something similar, but not identical. (For further discussion see Boice, 1983; Brink & Wood, 1989.)

Summary

Observational methods are appropriate for nursing research studies, given that nurses spend much of their professional lives observing patients. Many nursing research questions may best be answered by collecting data from 'outwith' the research setting rather than by interviews or use of self-report measures. This applies equally to descriptive and experimental studies of nursing care, as well as to studies of the organizational context of nursing and the function of nurse education environments. Observational methods have a special appeal since they offer an opportunity to collect data 'at first hand', studying what actually takes place in any given setting.

Despite this appeal, observation presents many ethical and practical problems. It was noted in the introduction that unless subjects agreed to being 'studied', any observational system, no matter how innocuous, would be unethical. It is clear that many people, patients, and nurses themselves, find observation too intrusive. Weick (1985) observed that people have strong needs not to examine their lives and observers may threaten this avoidance. Even if consent is gained, the emotional state of the observer can bias the resultant data. Although steps can be taken to prepare and monitor observers, it seems unlikely that many observers will adopt a 'camera like' persona. Despite these reservations, it is clear that many problems and issues in nursing will only be understood further by use of observational methods. Researchers are required to develop the necessary rigour central to the design of valid instruments and the accompanying discipline needed to ensure their reliability.

References

Barker, P. (1977) The ABC of ABA: observational method in applied behaviour analysis. In *Observational Methods in Nursing Research*, (ed. R. Dingwall & M. Colledge). Department of Health and Social Security, London.

Bijou, S.W. & Baer, D.M. (1968) *Child Development: A Systematic and Empirical Theory*. Appleton-Century Crofts, New York.

Bijou, S.W., Peterson, D. & Ault, S. (1968) A method to integrate descriptive and empirical field studies at the level of data and empirical concepts. *Journal of Applied Behaviour Analysis*, **2**, 175–91.

Blalock, H. (1961) *Causal Inferences in Nonexperimental Research*. University of North Carolina Press, Chapel Hill, NC.

Boice, R. (1983) Observational skills. *Psychological Bulletin*, **93**(1), 3–29.

Brink, P.J. & Wood, M.J. (eds) (1989) *Advanced Design in Nursing Research*. Sage Publications, London.

Casti, J.L. (1992) How real is the 'real' world? In *Paradigms Lost*, Chapter 7. Abacus, London.

Downing, A.R. & Brockington, I.F. (1978) Nurse rating of psychotic behaviour. *Journal of Advanced Nursing*, **3**, 551–61.

Guilford, J. (1954) *Psychometric Methods*, 2nd edn. McGraw Hill, New York.

Heyns, R. & Lippit, R. (1954) Systematic observational techniques. In *Handbook of Social Psychology*, (ed. G. Lindsey). Addison Wesley, Baltimore, MA.

Hutt, S.J. & Hutt, C. (1970) *Direct Observation and Measurement of Behaviour*. C.C. Thomas, Springfield, Illinois.

Jones, E.E. & Nisbett, R.E. (1987) The actor and the observer: divergent perceptions of the cause of behaviour. In *Attribution: Perceiving the Causes of Behaviour*, (ed. E.E. Jones). Lawrence Erlbaum, Hillsdale, NJ.

Jones, R.R., Reid, J.B. & Patterson, G.R. (1974) *Naturalistic Observation in Clinical Assessment*, (ed P. McReynolds), Vol. 3. Jossey Bass, San Francisco.

Kerlinger, F. (1979) *Behavioural Research: A Conceptual Approach*. Holt Rinehart and Winston, New York.

Owens, G. & Ashcroft, J.B. (1982) Functional analysis in applied psychology. *British Journal of Clinical Psychology*, **21**, 181–9.

Patton, M.Q. (1987) *How to use Qualitative Methods in Evaluation*. Sage, California.

Rugg, H.O. (1921) Is the rating of human characteristics practicable? *Journal of Educational Psychology*, **12**, 425.

Sackett, G.P. (1978) (ed.) *Observing Behaviour*, Vol. 2. University Park Press, Baltimore, MA.

Samarel, N. (1989) Caring for the living and dying: a study of role transition. *International Journal of Nursing Studies*, **26**(4), 313–26.

Smith, D.W., Hogan, A.J. & Rohrer, J.E. (1987) Activities of daily living as qualitative indicators of nursing effort. *Medical Care*, **25**(2), 120–30.

Weick, K.E. (1985) Systematic observation methods. In *Handbook of Social Psychiatry*, (ed. G. Lindsey & E. Aronson), Vol. 1. Random House, New York.

Wolfgang, A. (ed.) (1979) *Nonverbal Behaviour: Applications and Cultural Implications*. Academic Press, New York.

Chapter 24

The Critical Incident Technique

Desmond F.S. Cormack

The critical incident technique is a set of procedures for collecting direct observations of human behaviour in such a way as to facilitate solving practical problems. An incident relates to any observable human activity that is sufficiently complete in itself to permit inferences to be made. This data collection technique was popularized by Flanagan (1954), an American psychologist, who wrote one of the earliest comprehensive descriptions of it.

The use of this technique by war-time researchers demonstrates how it was applied during the early stage of its development. Although the situation and problems described below are clearly not related to nursing, the same principles apply irrespective of the situation being researched. The problems facing the researchers towards the end of the 1939–45 war related to establishing those factors (incidents) which enabled United States Army Air Force crews to achieve success during their combat flying missions. Following each mission, crew members were asked to report incidents observed by them which were effective or ineffective in terms of achieving a successful flying mission. The questions put to the crew members related specifically to the activities of the officer leading the mission; they were asked, 'Describe the officer's action' and 'What did he do?'. Analysis of several thousand responses (critical incidents) from crew members enabled the researcher to describe what the officer leading such a mission would have to do to achieve success and what he should not do to avoid failure.

It is possible to see how such a technique might be used in nursing to establish the factors that relate, for example, to giving a good report. In this example, respondents such as nurses who receive reports may be asked to describe activities (critical incidents) which result in an effective report being given by the nurse in charge of the ward. Examples of what nurses might say in response to that question are, 'The ward sister gave *all* nurses a report', or 'She gave us a report on *all* patients', or 'The report was very clear and specific'. A question relating to ineffective reporting might get replies such as, 'Sister is very vague when she tells us about the patients', or 'She occasionally forgets to tell us really important things', or 'Only the staff nurse gets the report'. Analysis of respondents' responses will enable the researcher to compile a description of effective and ineffective report-giving.

The use to which the researcher puts the information collected using the critical incident technique depends on the purpose of the research. For example, the analysed critical incidents may be used when teaching nurses how to give reports, or they may be used when assessing the ward sister's ability to give a report. The teacher or assessor is able, as a result of having effective/ineffective report-giving analysed in this way, to have specific and critical elements of the report-giving process in mind when teaching or assessing. In short, they will no longer teach and assess in terms of what they *think* is important from a highly personal and often biased viewpoint. Rather, they will teach and assess in terms of specific criteria arrived at as a result of having applied this technique. Figure 24.1 shows how the critical incident technique may be used to improve the quality of report-giving.

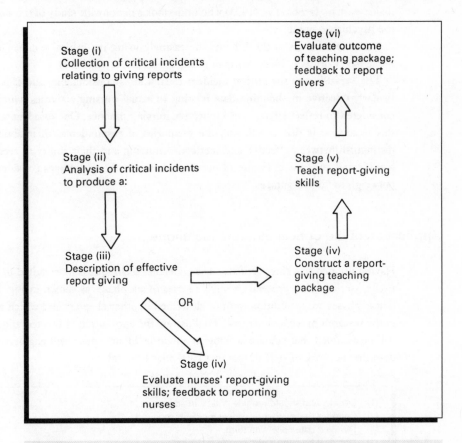

Fig. 24.1 Example of application of critical incident technique.

A major advantage of the critical incident technique is that it depends on descriptions of *actual* effective events, rather than on descriptions of things as they should be. Thus the technique is more concerned with the real, rather than the imagined world, and is able to take account of the constraints and limitations under which we all live and work. Critical incidents have been described by Clamp (1980) as

'... snapshot views of the daily work of the nurse ... the advantages of this technique are that they provide a sharply focussed description in which opinions, generalisations and personal judgements are reduced to a minimum'.

Use of the critical incident technique in nursing

The critical incident technique, as a means of collecting nursing research data, has been widely used in the USA for more than 20 years. It has been used, for example, to identify the role of the private duty nurse, to identify criteria for the evaluation of student nurses and to develop an evaluation procedure for assessing staff nurses. Two important reference works on the use of the technique in the USA are those by Fivars & Gonsell (1966), who used it to identify problems in nursing, and the major work by Jacobs *et al.* (1973) who undertook a nationwide study of the work of the psychiatric nurse.

Nurse researchers in the UK are increasingly using the critical incident technique (see Cormack, 1983; Norman *et al.*, 1992; Cox *et al.*, 1993).

The versatility of the critical incident technique is considerable, and it is particularly effective in obtaining data relating to actual nursing activities which are considered to reflect effective or ineffective nursing practice. One disadvantage of this technique is that it relies on the memories of respondents, their ability to distinguish between effective and ineffective nursing and their ability to recollect specific and concrete examples of nursing. However, the advantages considerably outweigh the disadvantages.

Application of the critical incident technique

Having decided that this particular data collection technique is most suited to your needs, you can then proceed through a series of six phases as shown in Fig. 24.2. These phases are in addition to those described in other chapters and which relate to the research process in general. To illustrate the application of this technique, it will be assumed that you are seeking to obtain incidents which will enable you to describe the work of staff nurses in a particular hospital.

---

(1) Decide who should provide critical incidents.
(2) Consider the number of critical incidents required.
(3) Design a data collection form.
(4) Decide where to collect critical incidents.
(5) Collect critical incidents.
(6) Analyse critical incidents.

Fig. 24.2 Application of the critical incident technique.

Decide who should provide critical incidents

First, identify the group or groups of people who will be able to give an informed description of effective/ineffective nursing. It is often useful to include a range of respondent groups who are close to the work of the nurse. Bearing in mind that the work of nurses may include patient care, relating to other staff members, communicating with relatives and working with other staff groups, all of these may be considered as potential respondents.

Clearly, the range of respondent groups will vary considerably from setting to setting. It may be impossible to include patients who are extremely ill, but possible to include those who are relatively well. Similarly, in those settings where the work of nurses takes them into contact with other staff groups such as physicians, occupational therapists, physiotherapists, social workers and psychologists, it may be appropriate to invite those groups to contribute. In short, decide which groups to include on the basis of their knowledge of the work of the nurse, and which groups to exclude because of their lack of contact with, or knowledge of, them.

Consider the number of critical incidents required

There is no way of knowing in advance how many incidents need to be collected to answer the question being researched. As a general guide, the less complex the subject being researched, the smaller is the number of incidents required, and the more complex the subject, the greater the number of incidents required. For example, if you are only concerned with the work of the nurse as it relates to student teaching, far fewer will be required than if you are concerned with all work carried out by the nurse. Even so, there is no way of predetermining the number of required incidents.

As a general rule, begin by collecting critical incidents without having any specific number in mind, and collect the minimum number which will provide an answer to the question being asked. This can be achieved by continuing to collect and analyse critical incidents until the last one hundred incidents fail to provide new information about the work of the nurse. Only then can you be reasonably sure that the collection of further incidents would add nothing new, and that the incidents already collected contain a reasonably comprehensive description of the subject being researched.

Design a data collection form

The data collection form is used to give instructions to respondents and to record their responses. It may also be used to contain additional information such as the grade of the respondent and the grade of nurse being described in the incident. As with all data collection tools, only information which is needed should be collected.

The form on which the critical incident is to be written will, in most instances, be accompanied by written information giving the respondent additional information such as the purpose of the study, the promise of anonymity and confidentiality, or both. An example of a data collection form relating to effective incidents is shown in Fig. 24.3.

In most instances, it is also of value to collect critical incidents which describe activities which are ineffective, that is the behaviours which should be avoided in order to achieve effective functioning. Figure. 24.4 presents an example of a form for collecting examples of ineffective critical incidents.

Please recall a time when a nurse did something which you think should be ENCOURAGED because it seemed to be very EFFECTIVE. Please give your answer in five parts as follows:

A. Grade of nurse being reported on. _____

B. What were the events leading up to the activity? _____

_____

_____

_____

C. What did the nurse do that seemed so EFFECTIVE? _____

_____

_____

_____

D. Why was the activity so EFFECTIVE? _____

_____

_____

_____

E. Grade of respondent. _____

Fig. 24.3 Sample form for collecting effective critical incidents.

Decide where to collect critical incidents

The setting in which incidents will be collected depends largely on the purpose and scope of the study. If you are concerned only with the work of nurses within a single ward of one hospital, then only incidents from respondents who are familiar with the work of nurses in that particular ward are collected. Alternatively, to describe the work of nurses in six surgical wards within a hospital, the source of critical incidents must be extended accordingly. Finally, if you are interested in describing the work of nurses in a group of hospitals, a sample of respondents who are familiar with the work of nurses in that group of hospitals will be recruited.

Collect critical incidents

Two methods of collecting critical incidents, which resulted in very different response rates, were used by Cormack (1983). First, groups of potential nurse respondents were personally given appropriate forms and instructions and asked to

Please recall a time when a nurse did something which you think should be DISCOURAGED because it seemed to be very INEFFECTIVE. Please give your answer in five parts as follows:

A. Grade of nurse being reported on. _____

B. What were the events leading up to the activity? _____

_____

_____

_____

C. What did the nurse do that seemed so INEFFECTIVE? _____

_____

_____

_____

D. Why was the activity so INEFFECTIVE? _____

_____

_____

_____

E. Grade of respondent. _____

Fig. 24.4 Sample form for collecting ineffective critical incidents.

use the internal mailing system to return the completed critical incidents to him. The response rate using that method was 2.45%. Second, groups of nurse respondents were given the appropriate form and instructions and asked to complete them in his presence. The response rate using that method was 79%.

It is probably best to gather potential respondents in small groups and to ask them to participate by giving appropriate information about the study, what is required of them, and to answer questions they might have. Cormack (1983) asked his nurse respondents to provide two effective and two ineffective critical incidents.

Analyse critical incidents

Although all critical incidents will relate to the same general subject, the work of the nurse for example, they will describe differing aspects of that work. Some incidents may relate to administrative tasks, others to patient care or to teaching, for example.

Analysis of data usually takes the form of inductive classification of incidents. This means that a classification system is constructed as the data are being analysed, rather than before. If the first incident relates to 'physical nursing care', then one part of the classification will relate to 'physical nursing care'. If the second incident relates to 'teaching learners' this clearly does not fit into the only existing part of the classification system, therefore a second part must be created. This process continues until all incidents have been classified within the system which is being created as a result of the classification.

The incidents may well be classified using a two- or three-tier system which starts with a fairly general description and progresses to an increasingly more specific one. The classification system may contain a number of general areas, one of which is 'nursing care', a category of which may be 'physical nursing care', and which contains a sub-category such as 'gives bed bath'. In using critical incidents to describe the work of psychiatric nurses, Cormack (1983) created a classification system with four major areas, each with a number of categories, with each of these having a number of sub-categories. An adaptation from that classification system (shown in Fig. 24.5) will demonstrate its structure.

If the critical incidents relate to the work of the nurse, you now have a description of the work of that group, and can proceed beyond this point according to the purpose of the research. If a description of the work of the nurse is all that is required, the analysis need go no further. If the aim is to establish what nurses require to be taught in order to be effective nurses, the description of the work of that group might be converted into an in-service or continuing education syllabus which will form the basis of the nurses' continuing/in-service education.

A full description of the application of the critical incident technique, and the means of analysing and classifying data, is given in Cormack (1983).

Conclusion

As with all data collection techniques, the collection of critical incidents requires careful preparation, planning and practice. It is heavily dependent on the ability of respondents to provide specific examples of the activity or work being researched, and their ability to distinguish between effective and ineffective practice. These are skills which may not come easily to potential respondents, particularly some nurse respondents who may have little recent experience in examining and describing their work in this way. However, the researcher who chooses this data collection technique can, with sufficient effort, skill and understanding, minimize the problems which respondents will undoubtedly have.

The provision of ineffective critical incidents, crucial to understanding some aspects of effective nursing, may be difficult for some respondents. Some may be afraid that by describing examples of ineffective nursing, they may be seen as 'telling tales' or 'letting the side down'. Bearing in mind that an understanding of what a work group should not do is as important as the knowledge of what it should do, it is essential that you enable the respondent to provide critical incidents without fear of reprisal or criticism from colleagues or senior staff. In this respect there is much to be done to ensure that the responses are confidential and provided anonymously.

AREA A: STAFF INITIATED THERAPEUTIC INTERVENTION
Categories
(1) Uses self as a therapeutic tool
   Sub-categories:
   (i) Makes self available to patients
   (ii) Provides opportunities or encourages patients to talk about their problems,
      etc. etc.
(2) Makes therapeutic use of the environment
   Sub-categories:
   (i) Encourages patient-patient understanding and relationships
   (ii) Encourages or facilitates patients playing an active part in their treatment,
      etc. etc.
Note: AREA A had a total of 5 categories

AREA B: ADMINISTRATIVE ACTIVITY
Categories:
(1) Ensures availability of non clinical patient data
   Sub-categories
   (i) Is aware of identity of patients
   (ii) Is familiar, when necessary, of the location of patients,
      etc. etc.
(2) Protects and secures patients' property
   Sub-categories:
   (i) Arranges for, or offers, security of patients' property
   (ii) Shows respect and concern for patients' property,
      etc. etc.
Note: AREA B had a total of 3 categories

AREA C: PROVIDES, PLANS FOR OR MONITORS PHYSICAL CARE
Categories:
(1) Administers medication
   Sub-categories:
   (i) Administers medications carefully, accurately, and as prescribed
   (ii) Ensures, by observation or assistance, that medications are taken,
      etc. etc.
(2) Gives physical care
   Sub-categories:
   (i) Monitors physical health of patient
   (ii) Selects or initiates appropriate physical care,
      etc. etc.
Note: AREA C had a total of 2 categories

AREA D: PERSONNEL FUNCTION
Categories:
(1) Maximizes staff contribution
   Sub-categories:
   (i) Encourages, accepts, and uses appropriate staff suggestions
   (ii) Arranges work load or routine to maximize staff effectiveness and/or patient
      care,
      etc. etc.
   Note: AREA D had a total of 2 sub-categories

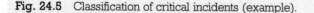

Fig. 24.5 Classification of critical incidents (example).

References

Clamp, C. (1980) Learning through incidents. *Nursing Times*, **40**, 1755–8.

Cormack, D. (1983) *Psychiatric Nursing Described*. Churchill Livingstone, Edinburgh.

Cox, K., Bergen, A. & Norman, I.J. (1993) Exploring consumer views of care provided by the Macmillan nurse using the critical incident technique. *Journal of Advanced Nursing*, **18**, 408–15.

Fivars, G. & Gonsell, D. (1966) *Nursing Evaluation: The problem and the process*. Macmillan, New York.

Flanagan, J.C. (1954) The critical incident technique. *Psychological Bulletin*, **51**(4), 327–58.

Jacobs, A., Gamel, N. & Brotz, C. (1973) *Critical Behaviors in Psychiatric Mental Health Nursing*, Vols 1, 2 and 3. American Institutes for Research.

Norman, I.J., Redfern. S.J., Tomalin, D.A. & Oliver, S. (1992) Developing Flanagan's critical incident technique to elicit indicators of high and low quality nursing care from patients and their nurses. *Journal of Advanced Nursing*, **17**, 590–600.

Further reading

Andersson, B. & Nilsson, S. (1964) Studies in the reliability and validity of the critical incident technique. *Journal of Applied Psychology*, **48**(6), 398–403.

Callery, P. & Smith, L. (1991) A study of role negotiation between nurses and the parents of hospitalized children. *Journal of Advanced Nursing*, **16**, 772–81.

Dachelet, C.J., Wemett, M.F., Garling, J., Craig-Kuhn, K., Kent, N. & Kitzman, H.J. (1981) The critical incident technique applied to the evaluation of the clinical practicum setting. *Journal of Nursing Education*, **20**, 15–31.

Grant, N.K. & Hrycak, N (1985) How can you find out what patients think about their care. *The Canadian Nurse*, **81**(4), 51.

Sims, A. (1976) The critical incident technique in evaluating student nurse performance. *International Journal of Nursing Studies*, **13**, 123–30.

Wilde, V. (1992) Controversial hypotheses on the relationship between researcher and informant in qualitative research. *Journal of Advanced Nursing*, **17**, 234–42.

Woolsey, L.K. (1986) The critical incident technique: an innovative, qualitative method of research. *Canadian Journal of Counselling*, **20**(4), 242–54.

Chapter 25

Physiological Measurement

Paul Fulbrook

Introduction

Measurement

To measure is to determine the size or range of something. The result is a measurement which is accorded numerical significance to characterize the quantity of the object or thing measured. The tools which are used for measuring are described as instruments and are standardized to enable accurate comparison of measured things.

Physiological data

The measurement of physiological data may be performed for many reasons in nursing research.

Description

Data may be collected for statistical analysis in order to provide statistics about a group of patients being studied. Mean body weight or blood pressure might be appropriate measurements to make. This type of information helps to give the reader of the research a clearer picture of its relevance to their own practice. In other words it assists with the reader's judgement of the generalizability of the findings.

Relationship

Physiological statistics might be further analysed in relation to other data collected and the group of patients studied. For example, a group of 40-year-old men might be studied over a period of several years in relation to heart disease. By analysing body weight and blood pressure in relation to those who do eventually develop heart disease it might be possible to identify an *at-risk* group on the basis of either their weight or blood pressure, or a combination of the two.

Response

Often physiological features are measured as a means of indicating the response to a controlled action. For example, heart rate and blood pressure changes might be measured in response to a standardized period of rest and used to indicate levels of relaxation. In a *controlled* situation the rest period would be described as the independent variable and the heart rate and blood pressure changes as the dependent variables (because they depend on the independent variable to produce a change).

Comparison

Physiological measurements may also be used to enable comparison of 'like with like' which would be necessary if, for example, control groups were required for a clinical trial. Using the same examples of body weight and blood pressure – this time as a measure of success – a researcher might compare an innovative nursing strategy with a conventional nursing practice. An example is Cerny's (1989) research with cystic fibrosis patients. He compared conventional bronchial therapy of postural drainage with chest percussion and vibration, with an exercise pro-gramme as a stimulus for sputum expectoration. He evaluated the effectiveness of the two regimes by measuring pulmonary function and was able to demonstrate that both therapies were equally beneficial.

A similar, hypothetical example would be a nurse on a medical ward caring for patients following myocardial infarction who felt that her ward's rehabilitation programme lacked adequate dietary information. Although it may only be a 'hunch', a dietary information booklet might be introduced to the rehabilitation programme of an experimental group of ten patients with high blood pressure and obesity. Its effect might be measured and compared to a control group of ten patients with statistically similar blood pressure and weight undergoing the con-ventional rehabilitation programme only. The degree of success of introducing the dietary information booklet would be judged according to the ability of statistics to suggest that the addition of the booklet had a greater effect.

Controlled situations

It is important to note that the nursing setting rarely produces a controlled situation, since there may be many other phenomena which may be occurring at the same time. For example, during a period of rest in a ward environment such as that described in the earlier hypothetical study, there may or may not be a lot of noise, the patient in the next bed might be using a commode, or the subject may have slept very badly the night before. All of these factors might affect the person's psy-chological status, possibly affecting their cardiac response. Unless the researcher collects an inordinate amount of *possibly* relevant environmental data it is impossible to state that heart rate and blood pressure changes were in response to the rest period alone. Thus the scientific approach is to remove the subject from a relatively uncontrolled setting to a situation, such as a laboratory, where the environment can be better controlled. This approach is also limited, since the fact that something

·works under laboratory conditions does not prove that it works in other circumstances. Thus, laboratory findings may or may not be generalized.

Assumptions

Similar to the point made regarding environmental factors, there is a danger when making physiological measurements that the researcher fails to measure all relevant physiological parameters. It is possible that the findings of the rehabilitation study were that the booklet was effective in producing a more significant weight loss. However, patients having lost weight might also be suffering from lethargy and general weakness as a result of eating much less. But since there was no mechanism in the research design to account for these phenomena they were not measured and might therefore go unnoticed.

There are clearly many research situations which require the measurement of physiological parameters. The importance of considering the environmental factors has been outlined, but equal importance should be accorded to both the method of measurement and the instruments of measurement. The researcher needs to know that the measurement procedure is appropriate and that the instruments used are accurate and measure what they purport to measure.

Measurement procedures

This section details with the process of making physiological measurements.

In vitro and in vivo measurements

Physiological measurements may be made either in vitro or in vivo. In vitro measurements are made away from the subject. An example of an in vitro measurement is given by Fehring (1990) whose subjects measured luteinizing hormone from a sample of urine to predict ovulation time. The urine sample was tested after it was obtained. In vitro measurements are frequently made in a laboratory.

An in vivo measurement is made directly from the patient, and a value obtained at the time of measurement. Engstrom & Chen's (1984) study was based on in vivo measurements. They recorded several extrauterine measurements of pregnant women of at least 36 weeks gestation, from which they were subsequently able to predict infant birthweight with reasonable accuracy.

The issues raised in this chapter are generally relevant to both in vitro and in vivo measurements. However, most nurses are likely to be more familiar with in vivo measurements, and may therefore be drawn to these types of measurements in their research. Some common examples of in vitro and in vivo measurements are given in Fig. 25.1.

There are several research aspects in relation to in vitro measurements of which the nurse researcher should be aware. In vitro measurements usually involve the taking of a sample from a patient for analysis under laboratory conditions, although

Physiological parameter	Measuring instrument	Type of measurement
Blood pressure	Sphygmomonometer/stethoscope	In vivo
	Arterial catheter/transducer	In vivo
	Automated cuff machine	In vivo
Blood sugar	Glucose stick/glucometer	In vitro
Urine volume	Jug/weighing scales	In vitro
	Ultrasound	In vivo
Oxygen saturation	Pulse oximeter	In vivo
	Arterial blood gas machine	In vitro
	Indwelling arterial oximeter	In vivo
Tidal volume	Wright's spirometer	In vivo
Sputum culture	Culture plate/microscope	In vitro
Calf girth	Tape measure	In vivo
Nerve conduction	Peripheral nerve stimulator	In vivo
Plasma potassium	Laboratory machine	In vitro

Fig. 25.1   Some common examples of physiological measurements.

many such measurements may be made within the clinical area. Frequently the researcher will be taking samples of body fluids such as blood or urine, therefore all necessary precautions should be taken to reduce the risk of infection and cross-infection to both the researcher and the patient, and possible contamination of the sample by the researcher.

The integrity of the sample must also be safeguarded. Samples should be taken according to a standardized protocol, correctly labelled and stored, properly transferred and correctly tested (see Ware *et al.*, 1993 for an example of such a procedure). Each step of the journey from patient to laboratory has the potential to render the sample useless for research, due either to deterioration or contamination.

Once the sample has arrived at the laboratory the researcher must frequently place trust in the laboratory technicians who handle and test the sample. This trust may also have to be extended to the reliability of the laboratory equipment since researchers may be denied access to the laboratory. To overcome potential problems in the laboratory it is advisable to seek advice and support from the laboratory manager who can ensure that samples are carefully managed and that measuring instruments are accurate and properly calibrated. He should also be able to provide information regarding the specifications, reliability and validity of the measuring instruments which should be quoted in the research write-up.

Many potential problems can be avoided by maintaining control of samples taken for in vitro measurement. As soon as the sample passes from the researcher's hand it is out of her control and the potential for error becomes greater. To ensure the integrity of the sample the researcher should take responsibility for as much of the process as possible. This should include transporting samples to the laboratory and, where possible, testing them herself.

It should not always be assumed that laboratory equipment is the most accurate and it is well worth the researcher investigating alternative measuring instruments which can be used at the bedside. For example, there are many *dipstick* products which could be used as an alternative to sending samples to the laboratory. Many bedside instruments have been researched and validated and a frequent bonus, such as that found by Newman (1988) researching blood sugar levels, is that such instruments are more cost-effective than laboratory services.

The basic steps of making physiological measurements are summarized in Fig. 25.2.

```
IDENTIFY:      Variables
               •  dependent
               •  independent

DESCRIBE:      Operational definition
               •  measurement procedure
               •  protocol to be followed

DETERMINE:     Timing of measurements
               Frequency of measurements

CONTROL:       Controlling the environment
               •  can the environment be controlled?
               •  have environmental factors been considered?
```

Fig. 25.2   Making physiological measurements.

Variables

When considering the design of a research project it is vital for the researcher to consider all the independent variables which might affect the physiological parameter being measured. This is particularly difficult when conducting research within the clinical setting of nursing practice because there are so many factors (independent variables) which have the potential to influence the dependent variable. Examples of independent variables frequently recorded by researchers are subjects' age and gender. These are attributes of the research subjects which cannot be changed. However, when a researcher introduces an independent variable (such as the information booklet in the hypothetical cardiac rehabilitation study), its content or the frequency of its use might be varied.

A good research example which illustrates the value of recording multiple variables is Ware *et al.*'s (1993) study of illicit drug-taking mothers. In their study drug-taking was assessed by measuring drug levels in the urine of neonates. Age, race, residential area, type of delivery, prior number of pregnancies, gestational age of the neonate and several other factors were also recorded. Analysis of the data enabled the researchers to develop a profile of drug-taking mothers which subsequently helped to identify at-risk neonates.

Operational definition

When the researcher has decided which physiological measurements to record, the next stage is to give each one an operational definition. An *operational* definition is one which, for the purpose of the research study, describes what is meant by the variable term and how it is to be measured. An example of an operational definition might be (Fulbrook, 1993):

> **'Axillary temperature** – that temperature which is recorded 4-hourly, inter-mittently and is obtained by placing the bulb of a standard "normal range" mercury thermometer into the centre of the axilla, and left in place for a period of not less than 12 minutes with the arm firmly positioned to the side.'

Operational definitions are then used as a framework to guide the research process and to ensure a standardized approach. As such they are also very important for subsequent researchers wishing to replicate the study, and to enable readers of the research to apply the findings to their nursing practice. If, for example, the duration of thermometer insertion had been excluded from the above operational definition, neither would be possible.

Timing and frequency of measurement

When taking both in vitro and in vivo physiological measurements it is vital to ensure that they are taken at the appropriate time and frequency.

Timing of measurement

It is particularly important to consider the measurement of the dependent variable in relation to the independent variable. For example, in the hypothetical study above which measured physiological parameters following a period of rest, there may well be an effect measurable in the cardiac response, but the duration of the effect is unknown. It might be that following a one hour period of rest, heart rate and blood pressure do indeed fall. However the duration of this effect might only be 20 minutes, after which the heart returns to its pre-intervention status. All measurements recorded after this time will therefore show no change. A faulty research design which specifies physiological measurements 30 minutes following the rest period will fail to identify any effect. In this respect the importance of a pilot study cannot be over-emphasized. A pilot study can save time and energy by helping to identify the appropriate timing of measurements.

A whole range of factors could affect the validity of physiological measurements if inadequate consideration is given to the timing of their recording. Additionally it may also be necessary to take repeated measurements over a period of time in order to demonstrate consistency of findings.

Frequency of measurement

The frequency with which physiological measurements are taken may itself affect the range of responses obtained, particularly if the research subject finds the measurement stressful. The recording of blood pressure is a familiar example, since blood pressure might be temporarily elevated during a stressful event. Gruber's (1974) study is a similar example. Because there was a documented potential for parasympathetic slowing of heart rate in response to rectal thermometer insertion, she undertook a study of rectal temperature measurement. Contrary to expectations she found, in fact, that her subjects' heart rates tended to increase, probably in response to the embarrassment and anxiety caused by the procedure rather than the procedure itself.

Frequency of physiological measurements should also be planned so that they do not coincide with other events which could affect them. It would be unwise to measure respiratory rate, peak flow and tidal volume on an emphysemic patient only five minutes after he has walked back from the bathroom, unless the walk back from the bathroom was the independent variable under investigation.

Sometimes physiological measurements are taken to compare the accuracy of a variety of measuring instruments, or possibly to compare a physiological parameter measured at different sites. The researcher, for example, might wish to compare the accuracy of blood pressure measurements using a conventional sphygmomanometer with an indwelling arterial line and a non-invasive automated instrument (see Norman et al., 1991 for a comparable example). Similarly, she might wish to compare the relationship between the rectum, axilla and mouth as sites for measuring temperature using a single instrument such as a mercury thermometer (see Nichols et al., 1966, for example).

Ideally such measurements should be performed simultaneously to ensure that the conditions under which all measurements were taken were identical. It is also ideal to repeat measurements over a period of time. This enables the researcher to demonstrate reliability of findings and adds to the validity of the research.

Another reason to take repeated measurements is to demonstrate that the findings are consistent under a variety of conditions such as sleep and wake or day and night patterns. In particular, many physiological parameters are known to be affected by circadian variations. A single cluster of measurements taken in isolation has little validity compared to repeated measurements taken over a period of time.

Controlling the environment

As described in the introduction, it is very difficult to control the environment when nursing research is carried out within a non-laboratory setting, such as a clinical ward area. The scientific approach is to reduce the potential for unpredictable factors which may affect the research findings. Therefore the easily controlled environment of the laboratory is deemed the most suitable. However, within the nursing setting it is often more appropriate to try to consider all the factors which may impinge on the phenomenon which is being investigated. When designing a research study the nurse researcher must therefore make a decision in this regard, and the number of variables which require measurement or recording should be determined in advance.

Since nursing is a profession which concerns itself with caring for patients it is very difficult to remove patients from the health care setting and study them in isolation. Most nursing research is likely (and indeed desirable) to be carried out in the context of the situation in which it is likely to occur. As such the nurse researcher, rather than attempting to control the environment, should attempt to take into account the environmental factors which might affect the measurement of physiological parameters.

There are many environmental factors which could affect the physiological variable being measured. For example, ambient temperature will affect skin temperature, as might recent exertion. Also, intrinsic psychological stressors such as anxiety or extrinsic psychological stressors such as those produced by excessive noise and other noxious stimuli such as strong smells might induce a degree of stress which affects the cardiac parameter being measured. Simple investigations such as pupil diameter may vary in response to changes in light intensity. Thus it is important for the nurse researcher, who is most likely to be found investigating phenomena within the health care setting, to consider environmental influences on the variable being measured. Because it is rarely possible to standardize the environment of nursing practice, variations in environmental factors should be noted at the time and subsequently taken into account.

The potential for environmental influence on a dependent variable is given in the following hypothetical example. Cardiac output in shocked patients has been shown by some researchers to correlate with great toe temperature (for example Joly & Weil, 1969). An intensive care nurse decides to do a more up-to-date study and records the great toe temperature of a series of clinically shocked patients. She is careful to ensure that her research design is sound and does in fact make very accurate recordings of both cardiac output and great toe temperature. Subsequent statistical analysis indicates a relationship between the two variables whereby great toe temperature falls when cardiac output falls. The nurse is quite pleased with her findings and is considering trying to get her research published. A colleague asks whether she recorded room temperature and also points out that some patients' feet were covered by blankets whereas others were not. The nurse is suddenly aware that there were other factors which might have influenced great toe temperature. Unfortunately she omitted to record them and realizes that, because she cannot categorically state that the temperature changes were solely as a result of cardiac output changes, the validity of her findings is severely limited.

There is clearly a potential for environmental factors to influence both the accuracy and the meaning of physiological measurements. The nurse researcher should attempt either to negate their influence or to ensure that their presence is recorded and considered with respect to the data analysis.

Measuring instruments

This section describes issues related to the use of measuring instruments, and is summarized in Fig. 25.3. The strength of measuring instruments lies in their accuracy and objectivity, that is their ability to quantify a phenomenon. Arguably machines reduce the potential for human error. Therefore when two or more researchers use the same instrument of measurement, they are likely to obtain highly similar results.

CHOOSE:	Measuring instrument(s)
EVALUATE:	Reliability • does the instrument consistently give true readings? • are the units of measurement sensitive enough? • do the readings remain consistent over time and under different conditions?
EVALUATE:	Validity • does the instrument measure what it is supposed to measure? • does the instrument measure what you want it to measure?
CHECK:	Previous researchers' use of the instrument Manufacturer's specifications
TEST:	Standardize Calibrate
COST:	Cost • equipment hire/purchase • laboratory time

Fig. 25.3   Measuring instruments.

Reliability and validity

There are two main issues to consider with regard to the use of instruments for the measurement of physiological parameters: reliability and validity. Reliability is concerned with the instrument's accuracy of measurement, whereas validity is concerned with its ability to measure what it is supposed to measure.

Reliability in physiological measurement

Reliability is a measure of the instrument's sensitivity, in other words its precision of measurement. Precision is important in terms of the accuracy and consistency of measurement. A measuring instrument must be sensitive enough to measure a physiological parameter in question to a satisfactory degree of precision. If, for example, babies' weight gains in response to either breast or bottle feeding were to be measured with a set of scales whose smallest increment of measurement was a kilogram they would quite clearly be of no use to the researcher. Similarly, if a set of scales were used for the same study, but were found to have a variance of plus or minus 5% when a standard weight is placed on them, then they too are *unreliable* and of little use.

The reliability of an instrument is determined by many factors and the researcher would be unwise to accept a manufacturer's specifications regarding the accuracy of an instrument, since specifications are usually quoted on the basis of standardized laboratory conditions. Some instruments become inaccurate with prolonged use or wear and tear, whereas others may be more prone to errors caused by the local environment. Electronic instruments in particular are prone to errors caused by electrical interference.

Prior to commencing a research study it is advisable to test the measuring instrument to ensure that it is accurate when in use. A pilot study will usually highlight any errors or inconsistencies. Some instruments are supplied with their own testing instruments and, whenever possible, these should be used. Occasionally it is not possible to test equipment before use, for example sterile equipment. In such circumstances the reliability must be accepted from the manufacturer's specifications.

Validity in physiological measurement

Just because an instrument is reliable does not mean that it is valid. A researcher might obtain a highly accurate measure of body length using a tape measure but it would not be *valid* if the researcher wishes to know the weight of the person.

The researcher needs to address the issue of how appropriate the measuring instrument is for measuring the physiological parameter in question. Some instruments do not actually measure the parameter for which they give a value. For example, tympanic thermometers *predict* core body temperature on the basis of infra-red light emitted from the tympanic membrane. It may not therefore be as reliable in measuring as an electronic temperature sensor placed in the pulmonary artery measuring *actual* core body temperature.

It is frequently helpful to refer to previous research studies which have either used the same instrument or evaluated its reliability and validity. A lot of time and energy can be wasted trying to test instruments which have already been scrutinized by previous researchers.

Cost

Another issue to consider with respect to measuring instruments is that of cost. Electronic machines in particular are very expensive, both to purchase and maintain. It is always worth trying to enlist the instrument manufacturer's support for the research study. Because it is in their interests to promote their products they are frequently amenable to lending or even donating equipment for research purposes.

In summary, the nurse researcher must carefully consider the appropriateness of any instrument used to measure physiological parameters for a research study. Whilst the issue of cost must be considered, it should not be at the expense of instrument reliability and validity. Finally, it should not be assumed that a machine is any more capable of measuring a physiological parameter than is a human. The more complicated a measuring instrument is then the more potential there is for both researcher handling error and internal malfunction.

For an excellent overview on reliability and validity of measuring instruments see Gassert (1990).

Data collection

Sampling

Sampling procedures are described in Chapter 19. The important factor regarding a sample is that it should be representative of the population being studied. In the context of physiological measurements, sampling merits some consideration.

Data collectors

If, for example, the nurse researcher wishes to know the mean weight and blood pressure of patients admitted to a medical ward she has a choice: either she can measure the above parameters of *all* the patients admitted over a certain period of time or she can select a sample. What decision she comes to in this regard may depend on what is most convenient for her to do, since time is often a major factor. Should she decide to take measurements from all patients then her presence, or that of other data collectors, is required throughout the 24–hour period for the duration of the study, which is not usually a practical option. Whilst ensuring that all patients are included, this does introduce the potential for variation in the measurements recorded due to slightly different techniques. The advantage of the nurse researcher taking all the measurements herself is that she is sure, and can therefore state, that a uniform technique was used on every occasion.

Standard technique

If colleagues are enlisted to gather data it is vital to ensure that they are all briefed in the measurement technique required and are fully conversant with the operation of instruments used to obtain measurements. Such a procedure is described by Chan (1993), who compared ultrasound estimation of bladder urine volume with its actual measurement following catheterization. In order to ensure that the method was correct, nurses had first to be trained in the use of ultrasound techniques.

Pilot study

A pilot study is necessary prior to commencing the main study to test the ability of the research assistants to obtain accurate data.

It is all too easy to assume that nurses, by virtue of their everyday role, are more than capable of taking physiological measurements. Even a simple procedure like taking a patient's blood pressure is fraught with potential problems which may lead to inaccuracies and inconsistent techniques between data collectors. For example, was the patient sitting up or lying down, how long had they been in this position, where was the sphygmomanometer placed in relation to the patient, where was the cuff placed on the upper arm, was the cuff the correct size, was the cuff correctly applied, how was the degree of cuff inflation determined, was the rubber tubing in good condition, was the fourth or the fifth Korotkov sound used to determine diastolic pressure and was the patient relaxed? The list may be very long, but each step of the procedure should be considered to ensure standardization.

Ethical issues

In any research study there are many ethical issues which require consideration, which are addressed in detail elsewhere in this book. However there are some specific ethical issues which should be considered in relation to the measurement of physiological variables.

Foreseeable harm

No foreseeable harm should come to the subject as a result of physiological measurement. The researcher must therefore make a judgement in this respect. Virtually every procedure imaginable carries with it a degree of risk, however small. This degree of risk must be balanced with the need to carry out the research, but always with the balance tilted in favour of the research subject. It should also be remembered that it is not just physical harm that might be caused but psychological. This might be as simple as embarrassment or loss of dignity.

Abnormal findings

The researcher must also consider in advance what she will do if her findings are such that there is a threat to the patient's health. For example, what course of action should she take if she finds that one of her subjects has an abnormally elevated blood pressure? Again, the principle is that the patient should not come to any harm as a result of the research study. Quite clearly, in such instances, the researcher's priorities must be with the research subjects. All decisions must be made in their best interests, even if it means modifying or abandoning the research study.

Summary

Physiological measurements may be taken by nurse researchers for a variety of research purposes, and provided that several basic rules are followed, highly reliable and valid data will be obtained for analysis.

In the first instance the researcher should determine what measurements are necessary for the study. This should be considered from the point of view of both independent and dependent variables and in the light of the potential for environmental factors to affect their reliability and validity. The measurement technique should be carefully thought through and standardized. This is particularly important if more than one researcher is collecting data. Any instruments used to measure physiological parameters should be carefully considered in terms of reliability and validity and ideally should be tested for accuracy prior to commencement of the main study. As with all research, ethical issues must be carefully thought through in advance and permission obtained as appropriate.

References

Cerny, F.J. (1989) Relative effects of bronchial drainage and exercise for in-hospital care of patients with cystic fibrosis. *Physical Therapy*, **69**(8), 633–9.

Chan, H. (1993) Noninvasive bladder volume measurement. *Journal of Neuroscience Nursing*, **25**(5), 309–12.

Engstrom, J.L. & Chen, E.H. (1984) Prediction of birthweight by the use of extrauterine measurements during labor. *Research in Nursing and Health*, **7**(4), 314–23.

Fehring, R.J. (1990) Methods used to self-predict ovulation: a comparative study. *Journal of Obstetric, Gynecologic and Neonatal Nursing*, **19**(3), 233–7.

Fulbrook, P. (1993) Core temperature measurement: a comparison of rectal, axillary and pulmonary artery blood temperature. *Intensive and Critical Care Nursing*, **9**(4), 217–25.

Gassert, C.A. (1990) Reliability and validity of physiologic measurement. *Critical Care Nursing Quarterly*, **12**(4), 17–20.

Gruber, P.A. (1974) Changes in cardiac rate associated with the use of the rectal thermometer in the patient with acute myocardial infarction. *Heart and Lung*, **3**(2), 288–92.

Joly, H.R. & Weil, M.H. (1969) Temperature of the great toe as an indicator of the severity of shock. *Circulation*, **39**, 131–8.

Newman, R.H. (1988) Bedside blood sugar determinations in the critically ill. *Heart and Lung*, **17**(6), 667–9.

Nichols, G.A., Kucha, D.A., Glor, B.A.K. & Kelly, W.H. (1966) Oral, axillary and rectal temperature determinations and relationships. *Nursing Research*, **15**(4), 307–10.

Norman, E., Gadaleta, D. & Griffin, C.C. (1991) An evaluation of three blood pressure methods in a stabilised acute trauma population. *Nursing Research*, **40**(2), 86–9.

Ware, S., Liguori, R., Jamerson, P., Weiner, V. & Joubert-Jackson, C. (1993) Prevalence of substance abuse in a midwestern city. *Journal of Pediatric Nursing*, **8**(3), 152–8.

D: Data Handling

The preceding phases of the research process will have taken full account of the need for data to be stored, analysed, presented and reported and disseminated. When planning a study, particularly when considering data collection methods and the quantity and type of data to be collected, the researcher will have taken account of how the collected data will be handled. The handling of data collected during the pilot study will determine whether or not the data can be successfully handled; if there are problems, then the data collection methods can be adjusted in a further pilot study.

Data handling has four distinct elements: storage (see Chapter 26), analysis (see Chapters 27 to 30), presentation (see Chapter 31) and the reporting and dissemination of the research (see Chapter 32).

Chapter 26

Data Storage

Desmond F.S. Cormack and David C. Benton

The preceding six chapters have presented a selection of means of collecting research data. As the data are being collected, or at the end of their collection, they will have to be stored and subsequently analysed. Data storage has two basic related purposes: first, to enable information to be contained in a way which makes it reasonably accessible; second, to enable you to analyse the data.

Nurses are no strangers to information collection and storage, much of their time being used to record and store clinical data. Usually, however, it is stored in a way which would make an analysis of large quantities difficult. For example, in relation to each of the 600 patients in a given hospital, information relating to all patients' clinical status will be recorded daily, if not more frequently. However, if a nurse, clinician, administrator or researcher wishes to establish how many patients had been incontinent each day during a specific one week period, this may prove difficult if not impossible to ascertain. The reason for this difficulty is that episodes of incontinence, if they are recorded, are recorded in relation to individual patients and not in a way which would allow easy access, or which would enable overall calculations to be made. Alternatively, a researcher may well collect a large amount of data which, in its original form, is difficult to store and analyse. For example, in relation to the national census, the original data would consist of many millions of census forms. Clearly, it would be difficult although not impossible, to analyse it by making a manual count of the many millions of forms involved. However, a better approach is to store the data in such a way as to make such analysis easier – for example, in a computer.

The purpose of this chapter is to illustrate three commonly used methods of storing data: storage in original form, the Copeland Chatterson card (Cope Chat card) system and the computer. As with all phases of the research process, those stages which precede data storage must take account of the proposed data storage method. Similarly, the choice of data storage method will have implications for the next phase of the process, data analysis.

The means and ease by which data can be stored partly depends on whether they are of a qualitative or quantitative nature. Qualitative data are not readily transferable into a numerical format; in addition, they are often generated as a result of open questions. An example of an open question is, 'what do you find interesting about nursing?'. Responses to this question may include a verbal reply lasting up to five minutes. Such responses recorded on paper may occupy two to three pages and are relatively difficult to store in anything other than its original form. However, technology has advanced to a stage whereby various computer programs can take such dialogue and analyse for the presence of common words and concepts (more information is given on this in Chapter 30). In contrast, quantitative data, which are often generated as a result of closed questions, are relatively easily stored in a non-original format. An example of a closed question is, 'Are you a registered nurses?', responses being 'yes' or 'no', or 'don't know'. The data generated as a result of such a question, answered by 100 respondents might be:

'Yes   24
'No'   75
'Don't know'   1

Storage in original form

Data are usually recorded initially in writing and occasionally by means such as tape or video recordings. Invariably, but not necessarily, data collected by means other than in writing are transferred into written form. It is appropriate for some forms of data to remain (and to be stored) in writing and subsequently to be analysed directly from that format. For example, if data are qualitative in nature, they might be difficult to store in any other than the written form. One instance might be when the data were produced as a result of semi-structured interview in order to determine patients' perception of 'being hospitalized', and you feel that analysis is best done by reading and re-reading transcripts of the interview; maintaining data in their original form might then be the preferred option. Alternatively, the data might be sufficiently compact to require analysis in the original form, for example a single case study. Finally, data may be of the quantitative type but be of a small enough volume to be handled manually – for example, in the case of 100 questionnaires, each with five questions. A limiting factor is, however, often the level of analysis to be carried out. If complex analytical processes are to be undertaken then the advantages of using computer technology as opposed to manual calculation become self-evident. Not only is time saved but invariably accuracy is increased when large data sets are involved.

Data, therefore, can be legitimately stored in, and subsequently analysed from, their original format. Storage of data in anything other than their original form is only undertaken if there are advantages in using some other means of storage and subsequent analysis. When storing data in their original format, ensure that each piece of data is clearly recorded. For example, long-hand notes taken hurriedly during an interview might have to be rewritten and possibly typed. Second, ensure that each answer, or the reply from individual subjects, is discrete and you can clearly identify and separate each respondent's response generally, and individual questions in particular. Third, ensure that the response from each respondent is clearly labelled, for example nurse number one, two, three and so on. Fourth, scan all data immediately after recording and ensure that the record of responses is complete. Finally, seriously consider making a second copy of all data, storing each copy in a separate location. Occasionally something catastrophic, such as a fire, can occur and without a duplicate copy many weeks, months or even years of work can literally go up in smoke. Thus, data can be, and frequently are, stored in their original form. Many perfectly adequate pieces of research do not require any other means of storage.

The remainder of this chapter will be concerned with storage of quantitative data. However, bear in mind that qualitative data can be converted into quantitative data by counting the number of occasions that a particular item appears in the qualitative data. For example, you might count the number of times respondents refer to 'working with people' when describing what they find interesting about nursing.

Two further commonly used means of storing data are Cope Chat cards and a computer system; each will be discussed using data collection on a four question questionnaire as an example. The content of the questionnaire is as shown in Fig. 26.1. For the purpose of illustration, the questionnaire in Fig. 26.1 has been completed in order to demonstrate how the data collection can be stored on Cope Chat cards.

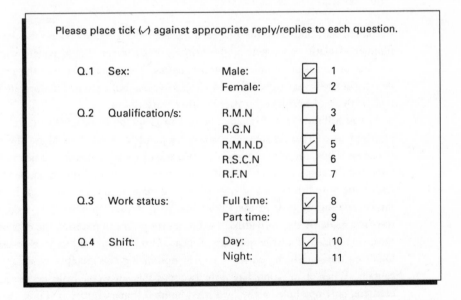

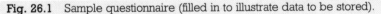

Fig. 26.1   Sample questionnaire (filled in to illustrate data to be stored).

Copeland Chatterson (Cope Chat) cards

The blank Cope Chat card must first be adapted to suit the data which are to be stored on it. Figure 26.2 demonstrates how the responses to the four questions on the completed questionnaire can be stored on the card. With a short questionnaire, you will experience few problems in designing the card to contain the data. With large questionnaires, make optimum use of the available space on the card in order

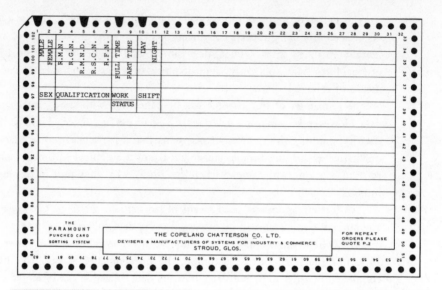

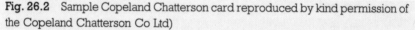

Fig. 26.2   Sample Copeland Chatterson card reproduced by kind permission of the Copeland Chatterson Co Ltd)

to contain the data. Once the first card has been designed to contain the data, the number of blank cards sent to the printing department should equate with the number of actual or completed questionnaires. The whereabouts of the printing department will vary depending on circumstances, but may include private prin-ters, or those of health authorities or other work places.

As you will note from Fig. 26.2, holes 1 to 11 on the Cope Chat card have been prepared to contain responses which correspond to boxes 1 to 11 on the ques-tionnaire. Thus, for question one, sex, two responses were possible; a tick in box 1 indicated the respondent to be male, a tick in box 2 indicated the respondent to be female. Because this particular respondent was male, as indicated by a tick in box 1, the corresponding hole in the Cope Chat card is used (punched) to record the response made by the individual. An alternative means of entering the data on the card, particularly if a large quantity of data are to be contained on it, is to use the following device which has the effect of optimizing the quantity of data it will contain. When a question has only two possible answers, male or female for example, only one hole on the card need be used (binary options). Thus, the hole may be punched if the respondent is male, and not punched if the respondent is female.

In some instances when the researcher or a research assistant is collecting data, it may be possible to make an entry directly onto the Cope Chat card. If, instead of asking nurse respondents to complete a questionnaire, you personally interviewed them and asked the same four questions, you could easily then punch pre-printed cards during the interview.

Retrieval of data from the Cope Chat system for the purposes of analysis is demonstrated in Fig. 26.3. The stack of cards is taken from their box (one box may hold up to 500 cards). A needle is pushed through the hole relating to the question

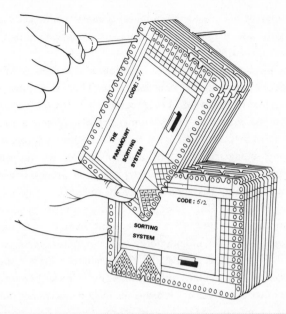

Fig. 26.3 Sorting Copeland Chatterson cards (reproduced by kind permission of the Copeland Chatterson Co Ltd).

you wish to answer, the cards are shaken and those which have been punched will fall from the stack. These are then counted and the results subjected to descriptive or inferential statistical analysis. Repeated sorting of the stack of cards can answer more complex questions such as 'How many full-time male staff with RMN and RGN qualifications work on day shift?'.

The Cope Chart data storage system comes in various sizes and degrees of complexity; fairly comprehensive systems cost only a small part of even a relatively modest research budget. A basic kit consists of: Cope Chat cards, storage box, needle and card punch (a manual tool similar in size to a set of pliers).

This inexpensive and easy to use data storage system is ideal for the new researcher working on a limited budget. Although Cope Chat cards represent a manual data storage and data retrieval system, the system can help greatly in relation to both of these aspects of the research process. While it is of little assistance in the application of inferential statistics to the data, it can be valuable in relation to reducing the data to a form which is referred to as descriptive statistics (for discussion on inferential and descriptive statistics, see Chapters 27 and 28).

For larger quantities of data, perhaps in excess of 500 questionnaires, and for data which will be analysed using inferential statistics, the use of a computing system becomes rather more necessary, although still not absolutely essential.

Computers

At least two major types of computing systems may be available to facilitate storage and analysis of data: the mainframe computer and the personal computer. Both types may be likened to very sophisticated electronic calculators, with computers having the added ability to store data and accept new programs to enable them to function in a variety of ways.

The physical components of a computer, the parts which can actually be seen and touched, are referred to as hardware. Thus, if you purchase a computer, you are purchasing hardware. The programs which exist within a commercial computer, or are written by a programmer and placed on it, are referred to as software. Computer users can either write their own software (programs), buy them from a company selling specialist software packages or use the services of a computer programmer. The languages used by computer programmers are many and varied and may only be of passing interest to the researcher since most researchers will use existing programs. Only if you wish to write your own programs will it be necessary to learn this skill and, therefore, become familiar with one or more computer languages. Examples of commonly used computer languages are COBOL, FORTRAN, PASCAL, C and BASIC. For a general overview of computing, computer languages and computer applications in nursing see Benton (1990). Although the option of writing programs is available, most researchers would not choose to do so since the time required to do so is, for most researchers, excessive. With this point in mind it is important to remember that it is not necessary to understand how a computer works, or how to write programs, in order to make full use of computers. However, if you do not personally have appropriate computer skills and knowledge, you must have access to someone who does.

Mainframe computers

These are large, extremely expensive machines which may be found at Health Authority headquarters. At a cost which usually runs into several hundreds of thousands of pounds, they will clearly be beyond the budget of all but very large scale, long term research projects. However, access to mainframe computers should be considered, even in relation to the most modest piece of research. In principle, researchers employed within the National Health Service have reasonable access to mainframe computers, as do staff working in universities and other higher education institutions.

In addition to access to the computer, nurse researchers should also negotiate access to computer programming staff and to NHS employed statisticians who may be required to give advice regarding data analysis. Thus, the nurse researcher should negotiate, where appropriate, the same access to computing and related facilities as is available to other researchers: medical staff and psychologists, for example.

Personal computers

An average personal computing system can now be bought at relatively low cost, which is invariably within the range of even the modest research budget. Figure 26.4 illustrates the normal system configuration which includes:

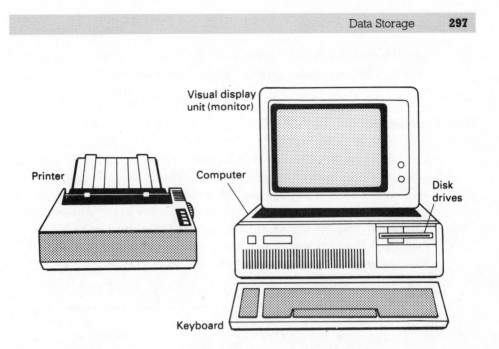

Fig. 26.4 Schematic diagram of personal computer hardware.

(1) A personal computer with visual display.
(2) A typewriter style data input facility (key board).
(3) Printer and supply of print-out paper.
(4) Disk drive and supply of disks.

At present, an increasingly large range of personal computer systems are available, and you will profit from consulting someone experienced in computing systems before buying one.

The advantage of a personal computer lies in its relatively low cost, its portability and the ease with which it can be installed and maintained in any domestic style environment that has an electricity supply. The storage capacity of the system, although smaller and less flexible than a mainframe one can, with today's technology, be in real terms as capable for all but the largest studies which involve national data sets. Even in these circumstances, with the advent of the compact disk storage systems that hold phenomenal amounts of data, personal computers are in effect the preferred choice. For example, some single compact disks can contain the equivalent of about twenty feet of library shelving. For smaller studies, disks which may be as small as three and a half inches in diameter can hold considerable quantities of data. They are easily stored and can be marked in order to identify the data which they contain.

As with the mainframe system, commercial software packages are available, and these will enable you to make full use of the personal computer, even if you have limited or, as is usually the case, no programming skills and do not have access to specialist programmers. Such programmes include some which enable descriptive and inferential analysis and specialized data presentation. For a full description of the application of computers to data analysis, turn to Chapter 30.

Use of computers

Computers have been designed to enable large quantities of data to be stored and quickly analysed. Not all data, however, are suitable for computer application, but most can be converted into a form which is suitable. Data of the quantitative type are most suitable; qualitative data are less suitable but may be converted into a form suitable for computer storage and analysis (see Baker, 1988, and Chapter 30). Figure 26.5 illustrates how a four question questionnaire might be constructed in order that the resulting data can be stored in a computer.

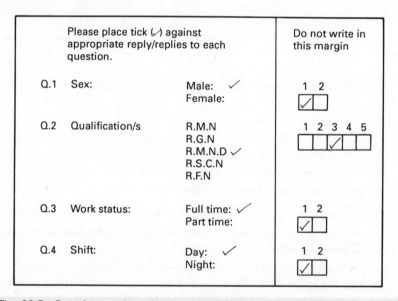

Fig. 26.5 Sample questionnaire (prepared for transfer to punch card).

The sequence of events in the collection of data on the questionnaire – which would obviously be accompanied by detailed instructions and a letter of explanation – is as follows:

(1) The respondent places a tick in the boxes which correspond to his answer.
(2) On receipt of the questionnaire, you record each of the four answers on a selected single box located at the right margin of the questionnaire.
(3) Responses are transferred to a means by which the data can be placed into a computer.

Data for both mainframe and personal computer systems can be entered in a wide number of ways. For example, for both mainframe and personal computer systems data can be typed in using a keyboard similar to that on an ordinary typewriter; some systems can use bar codes that can be scanned in a similar way to the systems used in some supermarket checkouts; flatbed scanners which look like an automatic feed photocopier can also be used if large quantities of data are to be entered. In relation to a mainframe computer, there are a number of methods used to insert data; these include entering the data via magnetic tape or punch paper tape, or by using punch cards. The latter means of entering data, although now less frequently used, will be discussed in detail in order to demonstrate how you might collect data in a form which is suitable for storage in a mainframe computer system.

Punch cards

Punch cards are seven inches by two inches, with 80 columns of possible hole positions (see Fig. 26.6). A special machine, used by a trained operator, is used to punch a hole at the appropriate point in each column. After the cards are checked, they are then placed in a card reader, which enables data from the cards to be transferred into the computer. Cards can be retained by the researcher for use in relation to further data analysis, or as back-up in case of the unlikely event of the computer accidentally losing the data.

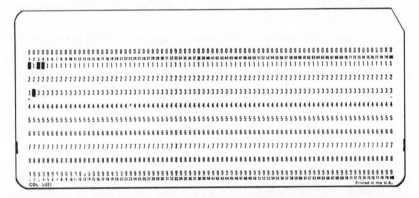

Fig. 26.6   Punch card (reproduced by kind permission of Control Dataset Ltd).

Once it has been established that the research data should be stored in a mainframe computer, consult a computer programmer and establish the form the data should take in order to facilitate their transfer to the machine. An example of how data might be coded has already been shown in Fig. 26.5, a similar system being used for storage on Cope Chat cards (Fig. 26.2). For example, in relation to question one of the questionnaire (sex), the answer is 'male', indicated by a tick in box 1.

The answer to question one is subsequently punched into the first column of the card, this being done by punching a hole where 'No 1' appears (No = 1 is male; No = 2 is female). Similarly, the answer to question two is recorded in column two of the card and a hole would be punched in No 3 in this case. Each punch card can contain up to 80 coded answers. As an example of how this works, the punch card in Fig. 26.6 has had the answers to the four questions given in Fig. 26.5 punched in. In collecting data for storage and subsequent analysis on a computer, the important point is to collect the data in a format which is suitable for transfer to a computing system. Provided that this is done – usually with advice from someone with an understanding of computing systems – the data can then be transferred into the computer by someone with the requisite specialist knowledge. Thus, if you ensure that data are in a computer-compatible format, then using the computer to store and analyse them will not present problems. The essential points are:

(1)   Give each subject an individual code number, e.g. 001, 002, 003, etc.
(2)   Give each question an individual code number, e.g. 1, 2, 3, etc.
(3)   Give each potential response an individual code number, e.g. male = 1, female = 2; yes = 1, no = 2, don't know = 3.

State of the art solutions

Before deciding which method of data storage to use, consider available alternatives and the relative strengths and weaknesses. The advice of researchers who have used data storage techniques, and of those with experience of computing systems, should be obtained during the planning phases of the research. Although punched cards are rarely used nowadays, the principle discussed can be applied to the integrated software and hardware systems now available. For example, a questionnaire can be designed on screen using software that will then generate a data storage structure capable of receiving the information from individual respondents. Respondents may, for example, sit down at a portable personal computer such as a laptop and type in the answers to the questions posed. These can then be automatically coded ready for analysis. Alternatively, if a large sample of subjects that may be geographically dispersed is being researched the questionnaire can be printed out and distributed via the mail. Returned questionnaires that have been clearly completed, usually using a soft pencil or black ink pen, can be read into the computer using a flatbed scanner. The scanner essentially locates the ticks made and codes them automatically. The advantage of this approach is that the risk of error resulting from having to have a data entry clerk or the researcher code, transpose and enter the data is significantly reduced.

Although not readily available, some systems can now use electronically generated speech to ask questions. Provided the responses are limited and the respondent answers clearly, they can be recorded and coded by the computer. Speech recognition is currently progressing rapidly but as yet is only able to deal practically with quantitative data collection. Often it is necessary for the respondent to pronounce a series of words or phrases so the computer becomes familiar with the subject's speech pattern (accent). Although this is very much tomorrow's technology, some of it is already here today and may well be available to a researcher who cultivates links with higher educational establishments.

Conclusions

Various approaches can be used for the storage of research data. These range from manual records both in original and semi-processed form (Cope Chat cards) to a variety of computer-based solutions. The choice of approach should be informed by careful consideration of the relative advantages and disadvantages of storage technique, the volume of data involved and the resources available. Whichever approach is used the researcher must be confident that the storage will enable the timely and accurate analysis of the data collected.

References

Baker, C.A. (1988) Computer applications in qualitative research. *Computers in Nursing*, 6(5), 211–14.

Benton, D. (1990) Information technology. In *Developing Your Career In Nursing*, ed. D.F.S. Cormack. Chapman and Hall, London.

Chapter 27

Quantitative Analysis (Descriptive)

Peter T. Donnan

This chapter and the chapter that follows discuss the quantitative analysis of data. The amount and nature of the data collected in a study will depend on the purpose of the study. A small or large number of cases may have been collected. The purpose of the study may be either simply descriptive or concerned with comparison of groups. In any case, numerical information on a number of individuals is collected and these form the data set.

It would be unwieldy to try to present all of the data every time the study is considered. Instead, descriptive statistics are used to summarize and present the data, extracting the salient points from the results. Descriptive statistics will form the subject matter of this chapter.

Inferential statistics, on the other hand, are concerned with making judgements and extrapolating results, testing hypotheses about the population of interest based upon the information obtained from a sample of that population. This will be explored more fully in Chapter 28. In practice both approaches are often used as they provide complementary views of the results.

Good design = good statistics

Good statistics start with good design. A study needs to be well designed in order to provide useful results and conclusions. It is thus important to consider all aspects of the statistics at the outset. It is not efficient to consider statistics only after the research has been carried out. Instead, it is necessary to set out the study in such a way that the research is more likely than not to provide the answer sought. The most important part of the design is therefore to state clearly the *aims* of the investigation.

If the aims are stated clearly (see Chapter 6), then all other aspects of design will follow, such as:

(1) The nature of the data.
(2) How the data are to be collected (Chapters 20–25).
(3) The appropriate analysis (Chapter 28).

Assuming a well designed study, with adequate data collection, the next step is to consider ways of presenting the results. Communication of the results is a vital aspect of any research. The appropriate use of statistics can provide a systematic means of assessing, summarizing and presenting the findings of such research. As already stated, this can be done in two main ways (not mutually exclusive): using descriptive and/or inferential statistics.

In most research it is usually not possible to obtain all the information from the population of interest because of resource constraints. A *population* is not only a group of people but, more exactly, is a collection or set of measurements. For example, you might be interested in the proportion of HIV positive patients who develop full-blown AIDS after a certain period of time. The population consists of all patients who are HIV positive. The data acquired (using the methods of Chapter 19) form a *sample* of this population – one from a single hospital, for example – which it is hoped has characteristics similar to the population from which it was drawn, that is, it is representative of that population. Simple random sampling (Chapter 19), is used to aid the collection of a representative sample.

Importance of sample size

The size of the sample collected may be outside the control of the researcher. For example, the researcher may be interested in a rare disease and so the number of patients with the disease (those whose records are available) will form the sample. However, in most cases the researcher will have some choice in the size of the sample to be used. If the questions posed by the study involve the comparison of groups, it is especially important to have an adequate sample size. This is estimated at the design stage. It would be wasteful of resources to sample more than is required, but a more usual error is when the sample is too small, such that the data acquired are not adequate to fulfil the aims of the study. Consider also the ethics of the latter case, especially if the research involved includes an intervention trial of a new treatment. The topic of sample size is a factor of major importance, although it will not be pursued further here. Textbook formulae are available for use in the calculation of sample size (see Armitage & Berry, 1994), and these should be consulted with the aid of a statistician prior to data collection.

Types of data

It is necessary to consider the type of data being dealt with in your research since the statistical methods used and the presentation of the data will depend on this. There are basically two types: qualitative (or categorical data) and quantitative data. The qualities and quantities measured are known as variables; height, for example, is a continuous variable; degree of pain is an ordered categorical variable. The term *qualitative* refers to a *type of data* in categories and as such is open to statistical or quantitative analysis. This should not be confused with *qualitative analysis* which is a different approach and method of analysis (see Chapter 29).

Qualitative of categorical data arise whenever individuals are classified into groups such as sex (male/female), marital status (married/divorced/separated/single) or blood group (A/B/AB/O). There is no numerical relationship between these categories and hence this type of data is known as nominal (Table 27.1). A special case arises whenever there are only two categories, such as male and female, which form a binary variable. The outcome of an intervention study is often expressed as a binary variable, for example satisfied/unsatisfied, hypertensive/not hypertensive. On the other hand, there is sometimes a natural order to the groups, for example degrees of pain in the categories of none/slight/moderate/severe, and this is referred to as an ordered categorical or ordinal variable. Degrees of agreement with a statement are often found in questionnaires to assess attitudes and feelings on particular topics (Likert scale, see Chapter 20) and these can be treated as ordinal variables.

Table 27.1   Types of data.

Type	Description	Examples
Qualitative (categorical)	(1) Nominal: data in separate classes which have no numerical relationship	Types of burn: thermal, chemical, electrical; absence/presence of pain (binary)
	(2) Ordinal: data in separate classes with order relationship	Degrees of pain, social class, degrees of agreement with statement
Quantitative	(1) Discrete: arise from counts or scales	Number of hospital beds, score on visual analogue scale
	(2) Continuous measurements: can take any value in range	Height, weight, haemoglobin level, cholesterol level

Quantitative data (Table 27.1) can arise from counts such as the number of hospital beds or the number of angina attacks in a specified time period. These can only have discrete values. Finally, quantitative data come in the form of continuous measures such as weight or blood cholesterol level, and these can take any value in a specified range. These values are only limited by the accuracy and precision of the measuring instrument. Note that there are many variables which lie somewhere between ordinal categorical and quantitative. If the number of ordered categories is large (say 10+) this variable could be treated as quantitative. Values from visual analogue scales or semantic differential scales (Chapter 20) could also be treated as quantitative, where patients are instructed to mark on a line between two extremes how they perceive their pain (Fig. 27.1), which is then given a score using a template.

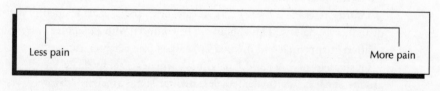

Less pain   More pain

Fig. 27.1   Visual analogue scale.

As well as being useful for presentation purposes, this classification also moulds the way in which the data can be analysed. Discrete and categorical variables lend themselves to comparisons of proportions in different groups.

Continuous data tend to be summarized by some form of average, the mean or median along with a measure of spread, and these terms will be described fully later. In a nutritional intervention intended to reduce blood cholesterol in one group compared to a control group, for example, the comparison would be made in terms of the difference in mean reduction in cholesterol between both groups.

The distinction made between qualitative (categorical) and quantitative, although essential in deciding how to present and analyse data, is not completely clear-cut. It is possible to convert a quantitative variable into a categorical variable by dividing the range of values into groups. If this is carried further, a variable with two categories can be produced, known as a binary variable. For example, let us initially consider age as a quantitative variable (Fig. 27.2). Note that at each step from left to right information is lost, that is, the measure becomes more coarse. All of these age variables may be useful; the form of the variable chosen depends upon the question the study wishes to address. It would be possible to transform in the reverse direction only if the original data were available.

Age (0 to 50)	→	< 20, 20–30, 30 +	→	< 25, 25 +
Continuous		Ordered, categorical		Binary
Quantitative		Qualitative		

Fig. 27.2   Age as a quantitative and categorical variable.

Aids to the description of data

Having decided upon the type of data to be collected, and then having collected the data (Chapters 20–25), the initial step in any data analysis is to look at the data themselves. In fact, this may be the main purpose of the study: to provide a description of a situation if this is unknown, for example, the extent of knowledge amongst the nursing profession regarding the condition of AIDS. Even when more sophisticated analyses are planned, looking at the data and the relationships between variables is extremely valuable in deciding what analyses would be appropriate. It is also useful as an aid to interpretation after the analyses have been carried out.

The main ways of describing data are in the form of tables, pie charts, bar charts/ histograms, scatter diagrams and line graphs. Tables and histograms together can convey the same information, with tables emphasizing particular numerical values, while histograms show overall patterns. All of these can be produced using statistics/graphics computer packages such as SPSS (Norusis, 1993), but although the computer will do most of the tedious work, the researcher needs to consider the purpose and format of these visual presentations, and perhaps more importantly, the relevance of the medium to the presentation.

Tables

A simple table is often all that is required to convey information from a study. Thought should be put into the format, the number of tables and the type of values to go into the body of the table: counts, totals and percentages. Note that if percentages are to be presented, the number and the total should be stated.

For example, whenever a survey is reported, the first table presented often shows the characteristics of the sample. Table 27.2 shows the characteristics of the caregiver/elder pairs in a study of the use of community services following hospital discharge (Bull, 1994). Such a table is a formal presentation of a number of descriptive statistics such as the mean with a measure of spread (standard deviation) or counts and percentages in groups (which will be described in detail later).

Be wary of any table which only gives percentages, especially if small numbers are involved; a 100% increase from an initial value of 1 is 2! Huff (1988) explores in a light-hearted way some of the more common misuses of statistics in tables and plots.

Table 27.2   Sample characteristics ($n = 185$ caregiver/elder pairs).

Characteristic	Family caregiver	Elder
Age (years)		
mean (SD)	59.3 (14.45)	73.2 (8.36)
range	20–87	55–97
Education score		
mean (SD)	12.96 (2.59)	11.87 (2.78)
range	3–20	5–20
Gender (% female)	75.7	52.3

SD = standard deviation

Line graphs

Line graphs are most frequently encountered in displaying the changes in variables over time. Figure 27.3 shows the percentages of children with high anxiety at different stages of their surgical treatment and, more importantly, the differences between those receiving the usual preparation compared to those receiving the new programme (Ellerton & Merriam, 1994).

Pie charts

A pie chart consists of a circle representing the total data or 100%, with each slice of pie being proportional to the percentage in a particular category. Thus, a pie chart

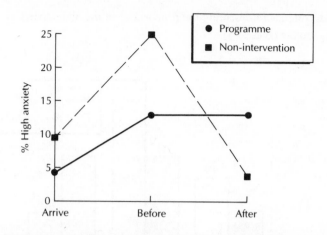

Fig. 27.3 Percentage of high child anxiety in programme group ($n = 23$) and non-intervention group ($n = 52$) (Ellerton & Merriam, 1994).

can convey the information in a table at a glance. Figure 27.4 shows the proportion of time spent by a support group for patients following discharge with 36% of the group's time taken up with after-care and treatment (McCann, 1993).

Beware of three-dimensional pie charts which, because they show volume, are misleading in that it is the size of the slice in two dimensions which represents the proportion.

Histograms

Histograms can display the percentages in particular categories in different groups and changes over time. The data in Fig. 27.3 can also be presented as a histogram

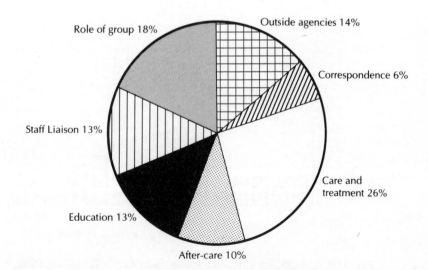

Fig. 27.4 Support group time spent on issues (McCann, 1993).

with columns representing the proportions in the high anxiety groups at different time points (Fig. 27.5)

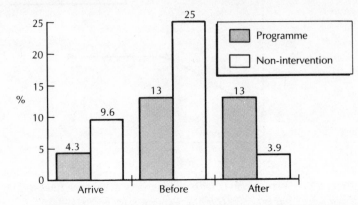

Fig. 27.5 Percentage of high child anxiety in programme group ($n = 23$) and non-intervention group ($n = 52$) (Ellerton & Merriam, 1994).

Histograms are also an effective way of presenting the counts of the number of cases in each category of a qualitative (categorical) variable showing the *distribution* of the data. The count in each category is known as the *frequency* of that category. Histograms, as well as displaying qualitative (categorical) data, can also be used to display continuous variables, such as age, by dividing the range into equal-sized intervals.

Figure 27.6 shows the distribution of patient satisfaction scores following discharge from hospital of a group of patients (Pound *et el.*, 1993). The area of each column represents the absolute count in each category. The frequencies in different categories can be directly compared if the size of each interval is equal. However,

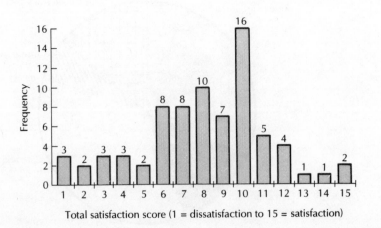

Total satisfaction score (1 = dissatisfaction to 15 = satisfaction)

Fig. 27.6 Distribution of total satisfaction scores ($n = 75$) after discharge from hospital (Pound *et al.*, 1993).

the frequency in each category is meaningless in itself; instead the *relative frequency* or proportion in each category is calculated by dividing the number in each group by the total number in the sample. If the proportion in each category is calculated, the full set of possibilities is known as a *frequency distribution*.

The histogram of this would be the same as that shown in Fig. 27.6, except that the vertical axis would be the relative frequency or percentage. For this histogram, the total area of the columns must represent 100%, assuming that all possible categories are described, and so the area of each column must represent the proportion in each category, or the *probability* of being in that category. Since the proportion in the satisfaction category of 12 is 5.3%, the probability of a member of the sample being in that category is 5.3% or 0.053. This combined set of probabilities is also known as a *probability distribution*.

For continuous data, the actual size of interval is arbitrary; trial and error will show which is most appropriate for a particular data set, although between 10 and 20 intervals are generally used. Most computer packages will plot histograms with the facility of adjusting the interval width (e.g. SPSS). A histogram can also be computed by hand for small sample sizes by tallying the data.

Normal distribution

As stated above, the set of all probabilities forms a probability distribution. This example was from a sample, so let us assume that we have a complete population. This would also form a probability distribution and if the size of the interval for the histogram were to become smaller and smaller, a curved line would eventually be produced. We would then have the *probability density function* of the population. The probability of lying between any two values can then be calculated as the area under the curve between the two values and, as for the histogram described above, the total area under the curve represents the probability of 1.0. Thus, if you wanted to know the probability of, say, having a systolic blood pressure of 130 mm Hg or above, you could calculate the area above this value from the frequency distribution of blood pressures. It would, however, be difficult to calculate the area under a curve each time this was required. Expressed mathematically, you would have to know the equation for each distribution and use integration to obtain the probability of lying between two values. Fortunately, there is one particular probability distribution which approximates to reality in a large number of cases and for this reason the areas under the curve have been tabulated extensively – this is known as a *Normal* or *Gaussian* distribution.

The Normal curve is bell-shaped with most of the values clustered around a central value, with smaller and smaller frequencies moving further and further from the centre. The distribution is symmetric with equal proportions on either side of the centre. The property of symmetry is extremely useful. As noted above, the probability of lying between any two values can be calculated as the area under the probability density curve between these two points and since the Normal distribution is symmetric, if the probability of one area in one half is known, the total probability for the two tails is twice this value. The Normal distribution is often a useful approximation to reality. Returning to the distribution of the sample of satisfaction scores, a Normal curve has been superimposed on the histogram (Fig. 27.7) showing a reasonably close fit, despite the anomalous peak at a score of 10.

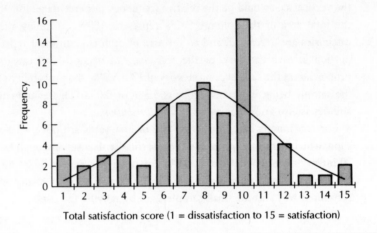

Fig. 27.7   Normal curve superimposed on distribution of satisfaction scores.

The shape and location of a Normal distribution is characterized by two values known as *parameters*, the mean and the standard deviation. The mean gives the central point of the distribution while the standard deviation determines the spread; the larger the standard deviation, the more spread out will be the distribution. A special case is when the mean is zero and the standard deviation is one: the *standard Normal* distribution. Figure 27.8 shows that, for this distribution, 95% of the observations will lie between 1.96 standard deviations on either side of the mean. The mean satisfaction score for Fig. 27.7 was 8.1 with a standard deviation of 3.2, so that 95% of the satisfaction scores lie between 1.8 and 14.4 on this scale, assuming a Normal distribution.

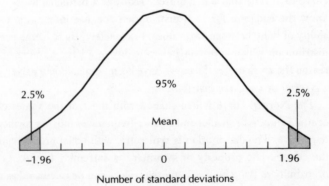

Fig. 27.8   The standard Normal distribution.

Skewness

Whenever a greater proportion of cases falls at one end of the tail, the distribution is said to be skewed. Positively skewed data are often found in research. For example, the number of units of alcohol consumed per week is usually positively skewed (Fig. 27.9). A negatively skewed distribution is the opposite of this, with most of the data to the right of the centre. The Normal distribution is clearly *not* a good approximation to these distributions.

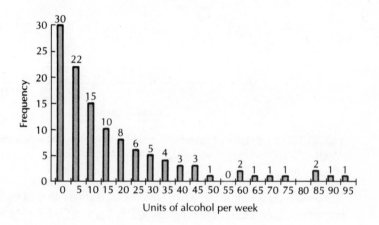

Fig. 27.9   Histogram of positively skewed data (theoretical data).

Scatterplots

These are used to represent the relationships between pairs of quantitative variables. They consist of one axis for each variable and usually a point (although any symbol will do) representing each data value; this is placed a distance along each axis corresponding to the values in these two dimensions. The ways in which these relationships can be explored will be discussed in Chapter 28. Figure 27.10 shows the relationship between gestational age and mandible length in a scatterplot from a study of 158 fetuses (Chitty *et al.*, 1993)

Summary statistics

In presenting results, it is unwieldy for the reader to have to consider all the data each time the evidence is examined. It can be more helpful to be given a few numbers which concisely convey the gist of the results, in other words, *summary statistics*. The most common of these are measures of the centre of the distribution of the data, or measures of central tendency, such as the *mean*, *median* and *mode*. The use of the common term 'average' is not advised as it is often not clear what is meant. Often these are presented along with measures of spread or variation such as the standard deviation, semi-interquartile range and range.

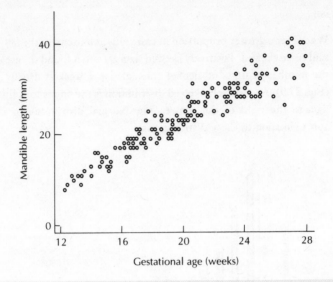

Fig. 27.10   Scatterplot of mandible length and gestational age (Chitty *et al.*, 1993).

The mean ($\bar{x}$) is simply the sum of all the observations divided by the number of observations. The mean of the numbers 6, 5, 8, 5 is (6 + 5 + 8 + 5)/4 = 6. The mean is most useful when the histogram of the distribution looks symmetrical. It has useful mathematical properties and is incorporated into many analyses. The formula for the mean is written thus:

$$\bar{x} = \frac{\sum x}{n}$$

where n is the total number of observations and the Greek capital letter sigma (Σ) indicates the sum of all values of x. The mean is a very useful summary statistic. For example, the mean age for the caregivers in Table 27.2 was 59.3 years. The mean has the disadvantage that it is very sensitive to extreme values or outliers and so would not be used to summarize positively showed distributions such as the number of cigarettes smoked, for example.

The *median* is the centre of the distribution whenever the observations are placed in order or *ranked* so that 50% of the observations lie above and below it. This measure is most useful whenever the distribution of the data is skewed, but it can also be used with a symmetrical distribution. In fact, it is highly misleading to quote the mean when the data are skewed. Consider a report stating that the mean salary for nurses is £12 000! This is misleading if the population of nurses includes clinical nurse managers, and so the distribution of salaries is therefore skewed; the median salary may be much less than this. The main drawback of the median is that it is not so easily mathematically manipulated as the mean.

If the number in the sample is odd, the median is simply the middle value when they are placed in order. It is the $(n + 1)/2$ th value. If there are five values, the median will be the third value when the data are ranked.

If the number in the sample is even, the median is the average of the two middle numbers. It is the $(n/2$ th $+ (n/2 + 1)$th$)/2$ th value. This looks complicated but is actually straightforward in practice. The median of four values is the average of the second and third values when the data are ranked, so, for example, the median of 6, 5, 8, 5 is $(5 + 6)/2 = 5.5$.

The mode is the most frequent value and is represented by the tallest column of the histogram of the distribution, and is of limited use. In terms of the normal distribution, it should be noted that the mean, median and mode all coincide, forming the central point of the distribution. Hence, one way of assessing whether a sample is approximately normal, is to compare these three measures of central tendency.

Percentiles

The median was calculated as the value above and below which 50% of the data lie if placed in order. A percentile is a value below which a percentage of the observations lie. In terms of percentiles, the median is the 50th percentile. The most commonly used percentiles are quartiles. There are three quartiles, in other words, three values which divide the data into quarters. The first quartile (Q_1) is the value below which 25% of the data lie, the second quartile is the median and the third quartile (Q_3) is the value above which 25% of the data lie. For example, if heights were recorded for a sample of nurses, then 25% of these nurses would have heights which are greater than the third or upper quartile. These measures are also useful to assess the shape of the distribution of a sample. One visual method of exploratory data analysis consists of the representation of the distribution of a variable in the form of a *boxplot*. In a basic boxplot (Fig. 27.11), the median is represented by a plus, the ends of the box are the upper and lower quartiles, while the maximum and minimum are the ends of the hinges if there are no extreme values (indicated by asterisks). Most statistical packages, such as SPSS (Norusis, 1993) and MINITAB (Ryan & Joiner, 1994) can produce boxplots.

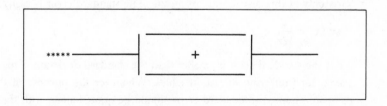

Fig. 27.11   Boxplot (theoretical data).

Measures of variability

As well as these measures of central tendency, some measure of the spread of the data about these points is necessary to fully describe a distribution. The most commonly used measures of variability are the standard deviation, standard error, range and semi-interquartile range.

Standard deviation

This is a measure of the average spread of the data about the mean, assuming that the sample has an approximately Normal distribution. The standard deviation is calculated by squaring the difference between each data point and the mean, summing these squared differences, and dividing the result by one less than the sample size. This is the sample *variance*, denoted by s^2. Finally, taking the square root of this value gives the standard deviation, s. In mathematical notation, this is written:

$$s = \sqrt{\frac{\sum(\bar{x} - x)^2}{n - 1}}$$

For the following data, 6, 5, 8, 5 which have a mean of 6, the standard deviation is calculated as the square root of $\left((6-6)^2 + (6-5)^2 + (6-8)^2 + (6-5)^2\right)/3 = 2$. Hence the standard deviation is 1.41.

Figure 27.8 shows the most used percentage point of the Normal distribution, with 95% of the observations lying between 1.96 (often rounded to 2) standard deviations above and below the mean. The main drawback of the standard deviation as a measure of spread is that, like the mean it is affected by extreme values.

Standard error

The standard error (se) of the mean is often encountered in the literature in tables and should not be confused with the standard deviation. They are however, related, but while the standard deviation measures the variability of the *observations* about the mean, the standard error measures the variability of the *mean* of the sample as an estimate of the true population from which the sample was drawn. They are both measures of variability, but of two different distributions. If more samples were taken from the population and the mean calculated for each sample, a distribution of means would be obtained and the standard error would be the measure of variability of this distribution of means. The standard error is easily calculated as

$$se(\bar{x}) = \frac{s}{\sqrt{n}}$$

Thus the standard error is smaller than the standard deviation. This is not a good reason for preferring its use in tables. Whenever the purpose of the table is to compare means, the standard error should be quoted along with the mean. However, if the purpose of the table is to compare the spread of the observations, then the standard deviation should be used. The standard error and the standard deviation, along with the mean, are also used for the purposes of statistical inference and this will be discussed in the next chapter.

Range and semi-interquartile range

The range is simply the difference between the maximum and the minimum data values. As such, the usefulness of the range is rather limited and is unduly affected by extreme values, unlike the semi-interquartile range, which is half the difference between the first and third quartiles. It is calculated as

$$1/2(Q_3 - Q_1)$$

All of these summary statistics give slightly different information concerning the characteristics of a distribution and are available in the common statistical packages.

Summary

This chapter has described the most commonly encountered ways of describing and summarizing data. The importance of looking at the data in as many ways as possible has been stressed, not only as an end in itself, but also as a means of aiding further analysis.

The chapter that follows moves on to the next step, that of generalizing the results from the sample to the larger population of interest by the application of inferential statistics.

References

Armitage, P. & Berry, G. (1994) *Statistical Methods in Medical Research*. Blackwell Scientific Publications, Oxford.

Bull, M.J. (1994) Use of formal community services by elders and their family caregivers 2 weeks following hospital discharge. *Journal of Advanced Nursing*, **19**, 503–8.

Chitty, L.S., Campbell, S. & Altman, D.G. (1993) Measurement of the fetal mandible – feasibility and construction of a centile chart. *Prenatal Diagnosis*, **13**, 749–56.

Ellerton, M.-L. & Merriam, C. (1994) Preparing children and families psychologically for day surgery: an evaluation. *Journal of Advanced Nursing*, **19**, 1057–62.

Huff, D. (1988) *How to Lie with Statistics*. Penguin, London.

McCann, G. (1993) Relatives' support groups in a special hospital: an evaluation. *Journal of Advanced Nursing*, **18**, 1883–8.

Norusis, M.J. (1993) *Statistical Package for the Social Sciences (SPSS) Release 6*. SPSS Inc, Chicago Il.

Pound, P., Gompertz, P. & Ebrahim, S. (1993) Development and results of a questionnaire to measure carer satisfaction after stroke. *Journal of Epidemiology and Community Health*, **47**, 500–5.

Ryan, B.F. & Joiner, B.L. (1994) *MINITAB Handbook*. Wadsworth, Boston.

Chapter 28

Quantitative Analysis (Inferential)

Peter T. Donnan

In Chapter 27, various ways of describing the data in a sample were discussed. This is fine as far as it goes, but usually the researcher will wish to say something more general concerning the wider target population from which the specific sample was drawn. This is achieved through the use of *inferential statistics*.

Consider a survey carried out to discover the satisfaction of mothers with midwifery care in a particular city. The results of this survey will be most useful if the results can be applied to the entire city and so inform the decision-makers of provision of midwifery care in that city. From this sample, one may wish to say something about the population of mothers in the city, that is, inferences are made about the population based on the sample. If the sample is biased, then statistical procedures will not rectify this problem and hence the need for good design in the first place.

Consider also if a midwifery intervention is to be compared to the usual service or if the effect of the new service is to be assessed in relation to social class, age or parity. Statistical inference helps to answer these questions.

The answer to these types of questions involve the use of various inferential statistical methods. Before expanding on particular methods, it is worth discussing the use of computer packages. Nowadays it is not essential to know the mechanics of calculations since computers are more efficient at this task, as well as being faster. However, some calculations are presented in this chapter, first as an aid to understanding; secondly, because computers are not always available and, finally, for those who are interested in the mechanics of the calculations. Although computers are more efficient, the widespread availability and use of computer packages creates a danger of using inappropriate methods, coupled with a lack of understanding of the output. Computers follow the maxim 'rubbish in, rubbish out!'. What is therefore required is the intelligent use of computers and the ability to know when to seek expert advice.

There are many user-friendly packages available for use on microcomputers as well as main frame computers. Two of the most commonly used are SPSS (Norusis, 1993) and MINITAB (Ryan & Joiner, 1994). (See also Chapter 30.)

In selecting statistical methods, what is essential is an understanding of when particular methods are appropriate, what assumptions are being made – and whether these assumptions are valid – and how to interpret the output. Often you will have access to a statistician or find one is a member of the research team, in endeavouring to manage this part of the research process, it is always worth consulting a statistician.

Inferential statistical methods

There are two main types of inferential statistical methods, known as *parametric* and *non-parametric*. Parametric methods, not surprisingly, centre around estimating parameters of the population – such as the mean – based upon the sample. These methods depend heavily upon making distributional assumptions about the population. On the other hand, there are what are known as non-parametric (or sometimes distribution-free) methods. These methods are applicable to estimation or hypothesis testing when the population distributions are not rigidly specified, that is, they do not have to belong to specific families such as the normal distribution. The pragmatic difference is that non-parametric methods are based upon the ranking of data rather than the actual data itself. For example, the following measurements of haemoglobin levels: 13.3, 10.5, 12.6, 14.1 have ranks 3, 1, 2 and 4 respectively.

Faced with a bewildering array of methods, it is tempting to churn out results from as many programs as possible in a statistical package in the hope that some will be useful. A more systematic approach would be to decide initially between parametric and non-parametric statistical methods.

In deciding between parametric and non-parametric methods the main considerations are:

(1) *Distributional shape.* Parametric tests depend upon the assumption of normally distributed data for the population of interest. This is often assessed visually from a histogram of the sample. For example, in Chapter 27 the histogram of satisfaction scores (Fig. 27.7) indicates that the assumption of normality would be reasonable. On the other hand, Fig. 27.9 which is highly positively skewed, suggests that this assumption would be unwarranted and non-parametric methods are indicated. An alternative would be to transform the data such that the transformed data are approximately normal. For the data in Fig. 27.9 a log transformation is appropriate and parametric methods could be applied to the transformed data. Sometimes there is no simple transformation which *normalizes* the data and non-parametric methods should be used.

(2) *Power.* For non-normal data, the power of non-parametric tests may be superior (the power of a test is in the chance of detecting a significant difference if it is present in the population).

(3) *Ease of calculation.* This is greater for non-parametric tests with small sample sizes without calculators or computers.

Since there are many excellent textbooks devoted to non-parametric methods I will not describe these here. If these methods are indicated, a classic textbook is that of Siegel (1988), which is recommended for the details of any test. For a basic introduction the work by Sprent (1981) is useful.

Since parametric methods are those most commonly encountered, this chapter will concentrate on these methods. Having decided on parametric methods, the choice of method is dependent on the nature of the study and the data collected.

Parametric methods

As discussed earlier, information is obtained concerning the population of interest from a smaller sample. From this sample you may want to say something about the whole population, that is, inferences are made based on the sample.

Assuming an unbiased study, statistical methods can help you to assess whether the result is spurious or not (hypothesis testing). In other words they evaluate the role of chance as an explanation of the results. In addition, statistical methods also allow calculation of the precision of a given sample estimate such as a proportion (confidence interval approach). In practice, both are used simultaneously to give a comprehensive analysis of the data. For a detailed discussion of the relative merits of these approaches, see Gardiner & Altman (1989).

Confidence interval approach

Consider a proportion or mean, which are population parameters estimated from the data obtained from the study sample. A *confidence interval* is defined as a range of values within which it is reasonably certain (often 95%) that the population value lies. For example, if a painkiller was administered to a random sample of female patients and it was recorded that 60% no longer felt any pain after one hour, the researcher would like to know the precision of this estimate if the painkiller were to be applied to the population in general, that is, to all female patients of the same age range with the same condition. If the confidence interval suggests that the population value could be as low as 20% or as high as 100% then the value of 60% is very imprecise and of little use. If, on the other hand, the confidence interval is from 55% to 65%, then this is a more precise estimate and also more meaningful. You could then make a stronger inference about the effect of the painkiller on the population at large than in the former case.

Confidence intervals are concerned with precision, that is, by how much the sample estimate is likely to differ on average from the 'true' population value. Thus we require an interval defined by two values which has a reasonable chance of containing the 'true' value. This can be represented pictorially as an interval on a number line (see Fig. 28.1). The constant is a number taken from the appropriate percentage point of a probability distribution (often the Normal distribution) and the two values calculated are called confidence limits. This defines a confidence interval with a specified chance (often 95%) of containing the 'true' value. Note that this does not mean that the 'true' or population value cannot lie outside the limits; it means that this is less likely. The 95% confidence interval is the one most

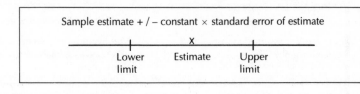

Fig. 28.1   Representation of a confidence interval.

commonly encountered, but any percentage point is possible; others often used are 90% and 99%.

In Chapter 27 the standard error of the mean was introduced. This can be generalized to any parameter estimate so that if the standard error of a parameter estimate is known, then a confidence interval can be calculated using the equation shown in Fig. 28.1. See Appendix 28.1 for details of calculations for confidence intervals.

The size of the confidence interval depends on the size of the standard error and the size of the constant in this equation. In order to emphasize that confidence intervals are concerned with the precision of point estimates, Fig. 28.2 illustrates an estimate with precise and imprecise confidence intervals.

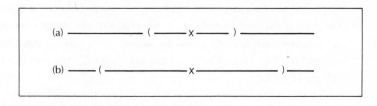

Fig. 28.2   (a) Precision and (b) imprecision.

Hypothesis testing

The previous section dealt with the calculations of confidence intervals to estimate the precision of a parameter estimate. This section deals with testing whether or not a particular value of the parameter is consistent with the data, the idea underlying *hypothesis tests*. The outcome of this approach will be a statement to say whether a particular value is *statistically significant* or not.

An hypothesis is a statement about the population; it is made prior to data collection and the validity of this hypothesis or assertion is then tested, based upon the evidence from the sample.

The hypothesis to be tested (denoted by H), for example whether or not a new intervention is better in the preparation of children for surgery, is couched in neutral terms. In other words a *null hypothesis* is proposed (the effect of the new intervention is the same as the old regime), and a test is carried out on the sample data. The null hypothesis is analogous to the assumption of innocence of the defendant before a legal trial (Fig. 28.3) and is noted by H_0. Denote the alternative by H_1. On the basis of this test (examination of the evidence), the null hypothesis is

Legal trial	Significance test
Defendant assumed innocent until proved guilty	Null hypothesis assumes no difference in effect between intervention and non-intervention
Examine evidence	Calculate test statistic based on evidence from sample
Either: (1) Accept evidence proves guilt (2) Accept evidence does not prove guilt: 'not proven' (Note: not the same as innocence)	Either: (1) Accept significant difference and reject null hypothesis (2) Accept evidence not sufficient to reject null hypothesis: not significant (Note: not the same as no difference but evidence failed to demonstrate a difference)

Fig. 28.3 Legal analogy to hypothesis testing.

either rejected or not rejected. If rejected, the alternative hypothesis, H_1, is accepted (the new intervention is better or worse than the standard procedure). Note that if the null hypothesis is not rejected, this simply means that there is insufficient evidence to reject the hypothesis, analogous to a *not proven* verdict in Scottish law (Fig. 28.3). This is not the same as *no difference* or, in terms of the legal analogy, *innocence*.

All tests are based on a number derived from the sample values; this is the test statistic. The test statistic often consists of a parameter estimate minus the value according to the null hypothesis divided by the standard error of the estimate, thus

$$\frac{\text{Parameter estimate} - H_0 \text{ value}}{\text{Standard error of the estimate}}$$

For example, the test of the null hypothesis that the mean $= 0$ is carried out by dividing the sample mean by its standard error and comparing the resultant test statistic with percentage points of the Normal distribution (assuming a large sample size). In summary, the ordering of this procedure is:

Null hypothesis → Data collection → Calculate test statistic → Accept or reject the hypothesis

The details of the test involve calculating a test statistic and comparing the calculated value to theoretical values from a probability distribution such as the Normal distribution. This comparison indicates whether or not the observed value of the test statistic would have been likely to occur if the null hypothesis had been true. If the probability of this happening by chance is sufficiently low (i.e. less than a specified small value called the *significance level* (e.g. 5% or 0.5), the null hypothesis can be rejected and the sample statistic is said to be significantly different from the hypothetical value.

Significance level

Three significance levels or p-*values* (5%, 1%, 0.1%) are in common use, although this is only a convention because of ease of presenting tables (computers now calculate *p*-values exactly), reflecting generally agreed cut-off points for strength of evidence against the null hypothesis. It is normal practice to quote the lowest of these levels at which one can reject the null hypothesis; for example, the statement 'p < 0.05' means that you can reject at the 5% level but not at the 1% level. If you cannot even reject the null hypothesis at the 5% level the result is not significant, and so this procedure is often called a significance test.

Types of error

In making any inference about a population there will always be uncertainty. In setting a significance level for the test of the null hypothesis, we are putting a value on the size of that uncertainty. The significance level is the chance of rejecting the null hypothesis when it is true and so represents the probability of an error – a Type I error. With a significance level of 5%, we are accepting a one in 20 chance of rejecting the null hypothesis when it is in fact true. Obviously, we wish to render the probability of this error as small as possible, so that the lower the significance level, the lower the probability of obtaining a result by chance.

However, there is another type of error, that of not rejecting the null hypothesis when it is in fact false. This is called a Type II error and is related to the Type I error already mentioned. Often this is larger than the Type I error. It is generally assumed that it is more acceptable to have a higher Type II error than a Type I error. In terms of the intervention trial, we are saying that it is less acceptable to conclude the intervention has an effect when in fact it does not, than to conclude that there is no effect when it fact it does. Often, instead of presenting the Type II error the *power* of a test is quoted. The power is simply 100% minus the probability of a Type II error, and so is the probability of rejecting the null hypothesis given that it is false. Hypothesis tests are often carried out at the 5% level with a power of 90% (or 10% Type II error). The power of any test is a function of the size of the sample; small samples will produce tests of lower power. Hence the power of any test is decided at the design stage whenever the size of the sample is chosen.

Comparison of two unimpaired means: *t*-test

In an experimental study comparing directed pushing to non-directed spontaneous pushing during labour, a significant difference in the duration of labour was found between the two groups (Thomson, 1993). The data were later re-analysed as it was suspected that the difference between the two groups could be due to differences in pethidine use for analgesia (Thomson & Hillier, 1994). The data were reorganized into 'pethidine' and 'no pethidine' groups in order to assess whether the difference in duration of labour was a chance finding or represented a real difference (Table 28.1).

Table 28.1   Length of the first stage of labour according to whether pethidine had been administered (Thomson & Hillier, 1994).

	No pethidine group ($n=14$)		Pethidine group ($n=18$)	
	Mean	SD	Mean	SD
Duration of first stage (hours)	7.7	3.7	11.7	4.4

The null hypothesis to be tested in this case is that there is no difference between the two means, or the difference between the means is zero. In other words, is the difference of 4 hours statistically different from zero? A test of this null hypothesis is given by:

$$t = \frac{\text{Estimate} - \text{estimate (if } H_0 \text{ true)}}{\text{standard error (estimate)}}$$

$$t = \frac{(\bar{x}_1 - \bar{x}_2) - 0}{s_p \sqrt{1/n_1 + 1/n_2}}$$

where the pooled standard deviation is given by

$$s_p = \sqrt{\frac{((n_1 - 1)s_1^2 + (n_2 - 1)s_2^2)}{n_1 + n_2 - 2}}$$

The t-distribution is used in this case, which has a similar shape to the Normal distribution but is more spread out, as the combined sample size is less than 100. This value of t is then compared to the theoretical value from t-tables (Table 28.2) with $n_1 + n_2 - 2$ degrees of freedom. Initially, the calculated value of t is compared to the 5% point of the t-tables, and if the value exceeds the tabulated value, the result is said to be significant at the 5% level. The result obtained is unlikely to have occurred by chance and so the difference is statistically significant. If it exceeds the 1% tabulated value the result is significant at the 1% level, and so on. If the value does not exceed the 5% point, it is said to be not significant (NS). The assumptions being made in this test are that both samples come from a Normal distribution and hence have the same standard deviation or variance. This would be checked before carrying out the test by plotting the histograms of the variable in each group. In the example above t is calculated as follows:

$$t = \frac{(\bar{x}_1 - \bar{x}_2) - 0}{s_p \sqrt{1/n_1 + 1/n_2}} = \frac{(11.7 - 7.7) - 0}{4.11\sqrt{1/14 + 1/18}} = 2.73$$

Table 28.2   Critical values for the *t*-distribution.

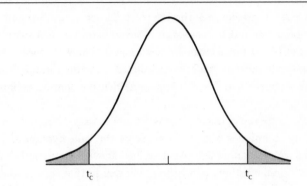

t_c' t_c

Levels of confidence		90%	95%	98%	99%
Area in two tails (*p*-value)		0.10	0.05	0.02	0.01
Critical values t_c	df				
	1	6.31	12.71	31.82	63.66
	2	2.92	4.30	6.97	9.93
	3	2.35	3.18	4.54	5.84
	4	2.13	2.78	3.75	4.60
	5	2.02	2.57	3.37	4.03
	6	1.94	2.45	3.14	3.71
	7	1.90	2.37	3.00	3.50
	8	1.86	2.31	2.90	3.36
	9	1.83	2.26	2.82	3.25
	10	1.81	2.23	2.76	3.17
	11	1.80	2.20	2.72	3.11
	12	1.78	2.18	2.68	3.06
	13	1.77	2.16	2.65	3.01
	14	1.76	2.15	2.62	2.98
	15	1.75	2.13	2.60	2.95
	16	1.75	2.12	2.58	2.92
	17	1.74	2.11	2.57	2.90
	18	1.73	2.10	2.55	2.88
	19	1.73	2.09	2.54	2.86
	20	1.73	2.09	2.53	2.85
	21	1.72	2.08	2.52	2.83
	22	1.72	2.07	2.51	2.82
	23	1.71	2.07	2.50	2.81
	24	1.71	2.06	2.49	2.80
	25	1.71	2.06	2.49	2.79
	30	1.70	2.04	2.46	2.75
	40	1.68	2.02	2.42	2.70
	60	1.67	2.00	2.39	2.66
	80	1.66	1.99	2.37	2.64
	100	1.66	1.98	2.36	2.63
	∞	1.64	1.96	2.33	2.58

Looking up t-tables (Table 28.2), the value of 2.73 is very close to the value 2.75 for $p = 0.01$ with 30 degrees of freedom. Hence $p = 0.01$ and the result is significant at the 5% level and almost at the 1% level. Similar results were found for the second stage of labour and so those who received pethidine had significantly longer first stages of labour (on average 4 hours longer). The 95% confidence interval for the difference in means can also be calculated using the formula from Appendix 28.1, giving an interval of 1 to 7 hours. Note that the confidence interval excludes the value zero.

Strictly speaking, this study was set up to assess differences in outcome between pushing techniques and this represents the null hypothesis to be tested. The secondary exploratory analysis described above is not strictly a test of a pethidine 'effect' and the authors rightly point out that further studies would be necessary to establish whether such a relationship does exist (Thomson & Hillier, 1994).

Comparison of two independent proportions

Consider the example of a study of quality of assessment visits in community nursing (Kerkstra & Beemster, 1994). A 2 × 2 table can be constructed concerning the collection of dietary information (Table 28.3). The table shows that the criterion for assessment of diet during assessment visits was 50% overall, but nursing auxiliaries (67%) collected data for this criterion more often than community nurses (48%). This poses the question 'Is this difference a chance finding or does it represent a real difference?'.

Table 28.3 Extent to which nurses have been collecting data concerning the physical condition of patients during assessment visits (Kerkstra & Beemster, 1994).

	Community nurses	Nursing auxiliaries	
Diet data collected	183 (48%)	35 (67%)	218 (50.3%)
No diet data collected	198 (52%)	17 (33%)	215 (49.7%)
	381	52	433

In order to compare two independent proportions, the chi-squared test is used. This is based on the chi-squared (χ^2) probability distribution which is continuous and approaches the Normal distribution for large degrees freedom. However, in comparing two proportions the χ^2 distribution with one degree of freedom is used, which is highly positively skewed.

In order to facilitate the test, the data are laid out in a 2 × 2 contingency table. The two rows in Table 28.4 represent the two samples, with the column totals being the total number in each sample, and the first row, divided by the column totals, representing the two proportions which are to be compared. The test compares the two proportions $p_1 = a/s_1$ and $p_2 = c/s_2$. If the proportions in the two populations

Table 28.4 General form of 2×2 contingency table.

Sample 1	a	b	r_1
Sample 2	c	d	r_2
	s_1	s_2	n

are the same, then a/b and c/d should be similar and so $|ad-bc|$ should be small. (The symbols $||$ simply mean that the result of the arithmetic between the vertical bars is given a positive sign.) The table can be rearranged so that the columns become the rows if this is more convenient. The test is one of association between the two dimensions which make up the table.

The null hypothesis is that $p_1 - p_2 = 0$ and the test statistic is given by

$$X^2 = \frac{(ad - bc)^2(n - 1)}{r_1 r_2 s_1 s_2}$$

(X^2 is the sample value which is then compared to the χ^2 distribution.) The value of this calculation is then compared to the theoretical value from chi-squared tables (Table 28.5) with one degree of freedom and if it is larger the result is significant at that level. A formal test of this difference involves the calculation of the X^2 statistic as described above. The test statistic X^2 is calculated as follows from the data in Table 28.3:

$$X^2 = \frac{(183 \times 17 - 35 \times 198)^2 432}{381 \times 52 \times 218 \times 215}$$
$$= 6.78 \text{ with one degree of freedom}$$

Table 28.5 Critical values of the chi-squared distribution with one degree of freedom (df).

Significance level (p-value)	0.10	0.05	0.02	0.01
Critical value χ_1^2	2.71	3.84	5.41	6.64

This is statistically significant as this value is above the 1% value in tables (6.64) and hence the difference is not a chance finding but represents a real difference between the rates of data collection. This can be written as $p < 0.01$. To further describe the results a confidence interval for the difference between the percentages, which is 19%, would be calculated. Using the formula in the Appendix the 95% confidence interval for the difference in proportions is 5% to 33%.

More than two groups

So far, I have only considered one variable and a comparison of this measure in two groups (or samples). There are extensions of the methods described for comparing more than two groups: for example, one way analysis of variance for comparison of more than two means. Lack of space prevents their description here; for details of these methods see Armitage & Berry (1994) or Altman (1990).

Correlation

The next step is to consider relationships between two quantitative variables. As an initial step, a scatterplot, as described in Chapter 27, will display this relationship. A summary statistic of the relationship between two quantitative variables is the Pearson correlation coefficient. Table 28.6 shows some of the correlations from a study of work environment scales (WES) and psychological strain in a sample of hospital nurses (Fielding & Weaver, 1994). Note that these have been multiplied by 100 for ease of comparison. The correlations are all negative, indicating that high levels of one dimension (for example, Involvement) are associated with low levels of psychological strain (for example, emotional exhaustion). The p-values indicate that these correlations are not chance findings (i.e. they are significantly different from zero).

Table 28.6 Pearson correlations $\times$ 100 between work environment scales and psychological strain in a group of hospital nurses ($n = 67$).

Work environment scale	Depersonalization	Emotional exhaustion
Involvement	−29**	−32**
Support	−27*	−26*
Innovation	−25*	−22

* $p < 0.05$; ** $p < 0.02$

Linear regression

The correlation coefficient tells us the strength of the relationship between two quantitative variables. On the other hand, the method of regression tells us about the nature of the relationship between any two quantitative variables and precisely how they change numerically together. In regression, one is interested in by how much one variable increases for a given increase in the other. A linear relationship is assumed to model the data. In the study of pethidine use and duration of labour, a plot of the pH of venous cord blood showed an approximate linear relationship with duration of the second stage of labour in the control group (Fig. 28.4). One variable is considered as the outcome while the other is known as the predictor, although it is not always obvious which is the outcome. Even though the terms outcome and predictor are used, as with correlation, causality cannot be assumed.

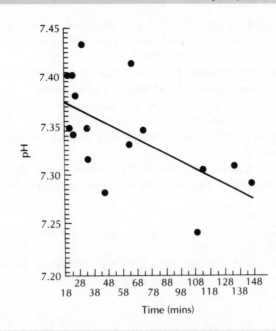

Fig. 28.4 Reduction in venous cord blood pH with duration of the second stage of labour in the control group (Thompson, 1993).

In reality, there will be many possible predictor variables. In the example of the study of the work environment scale and psychological strain, after the initial look at the correlations, the next step could be to assess whether the relationship between involvement and emotional exhaustion was still significant, allowing for differences in age, for example. The method of simple linear regression can be extended for this case and most computer packages (such as SPSS) contain programs which will carry out multiple regression. For an explanation of these methods, see Armitage & Berry (1994) or Altman (1990).

Summary

This chapter has introduced the powerful tool of statistical inference, in terms of estimation and hypothesis testing. These ideas are fundamental, and other more sophisticated methods, although not described in this chapter, also produce results which generally involve estimation of parameters, estimation of their confidence intervals, and the testing of hypotheses, followed by an interpretation of these procedures.

References

Altman, D.G. (1990) *Practical Statistics for Medical Research*. Chapman and Hall, London.
Armitage, P. & Berry, G. (1994) *Statistical Methods in Medical Research*. Blackwell Scientific Publications, Oxford.

Fielding, J. & Weaver, S.M. (1994) A comparison of hospital- and community-based mental health nurses: perceptions of their work environment and psychological health. *Journal of Advanced Nursing*, **19**, 1196–1204.

Gardiner, M.J. & Altman, D.G. (eds) (1989) *Statistics with Confidence: confidence intervals and statistical guidelines.* British Medical Journal, London.

Kerkstra, A. & Beemster, F. (1994) The quality of assessment visits in community nursing. *Journal of Advanced Nursing*, **19**, 1205–11.

Norusis, M.J. (1993) *Statistical Package for the Social Sciences (SPSS) Release 6.* SPSS Inc, Chicago, Il.

Ryan, B.F. & Joiner, B.L. (1994) *MINITAB Handbook.* Wadsworth, Boston.

Siegel, S. (1988) *Nonparametric statistics for the behavioural sciences.* McGraw-Hill, New York.

Sprent, P. (1981) *Quick Statistics.* Penguin, London.

Thomson, A.M. (1993) Pushing techniques in the second stage of labour. *Journal of Advanced Nursing*, **18**, 171–7.

Thomson, A.M. & Hillier, V.F. (1994) A re-evaluation of the effect of pethidine on the length of labour. *Journal of Advanced Nursing*, **19**, 448–56.

Appendix 28.1: Formulae for confidence intervals

Confidence interval for a sample mean

The standard error for a sample mean $\bar{x}$ is given by $s/\sqrt{n}$ where s is the sample standard deviation. The confidence interval for a sample mean is:

$$\bar{x} \pm t_{(n-1)} \times s/\sqrt{n}$$

where t is the appropriate value from the t-distribution with $(n-1)$ degrees of freedom.

Confidence interval for a proportion

The standard error for a sample proportion p is

$$\sqrt{p(p-1)/n}$$

The confidence interval for a sample proportion is

$$p \pm 1.96 \times \sqrt{p(p-1)/n}$$

assuming n is large.

Confidence interval for a difference between two means

The pooled standard deviation is given by

$$s_p = \sqrt{\frac{((n_1 - 1)s_1^2 + (n_2 - 1)s_2^2)}{n_1 + n_2 - 2}}$$

where n_1 and n_2 are the sizes of the two samples.

The standard error of the difference $(\bar{x}_1 - \bar{x}_2)$ is

$$\text{se} \, (\bar{x}_1 - \bar{x}_2) = s_p \sqrt{1/n_1 + 1/n_2}$$

and the 95% confidence interval is given by

$$(\bar{x}_1 - \bar{x}_2) \pm t_{(n_1+n_2-2)} \times s_p \sqrt{1/n_1 + 1/n_2}$$

where $t_{(n_1+n_2-2)}$ is the 5% point of the t-distribution with $n_1 + n_2 - 2$ degrees of freedom.

Confidence interval for a difference between two proportions

For proportions p_1 and p_2 the standard error for their difference $p_1 - p_2$ is

$$\text{se} \, (p_1 - p_2) = \sqrt{p_1(1 - p_1)/n_1 + p_2(1 - p_2)/n_2}$$

and the 95% confidence interval is given by

$$(p_1 - p_2) \pm 1.96 \times \text{se} \, (p_1 - p_2)$$

(If p is expressed as a percentage, use 100 instead of 1 in the formula for the standard error.)

Chapter 29

Qualitative Analysis

Sam Porter

What is qualitative analysis?

The uniqueness of qualitative analysis is that it is not primarily concerned with numerical techniques of organizing, describing and interpreting data. It will be remembered from Chapter 11 that the basic premise of qualitative research was that the social world we live in can only be understood through an understanding of the meanings and motives that guide the social actions and interactions of individuals. That sort of understanding cannot be fully gained through the use of quantitative methods.

Qualitative analysis is concerned with describing the actions and interactions of research subjects in a certain context, and with interpreting the motivations and understandings that lie behind those actions. This is, of course, a very broad remit, and requires further elucidation.

The problem with attempting to be specific about the nature of qualitative analysis is that it cannot be reduced to a single formulation. Because there is no one method of qualitative analysis, it is impossible to lay down hard and fast rules about the way it should be done. However, there are some general guidelines that can be elaborated.

The place of analysis in qualitative research

Data analysis does not form a discrete stage of the qualitative research process. It is part of the process all the way through from the selection of the research problem to the writing of the final report.

In this section, I will examine the role of analysis in each stage of the research process, illustrating my points with a practical example. Because of my familiarity with the processes that were involved in it, my own work on interaction between nurses and doctors will be used as a demonstration model. That research was conducted by means of participant observation in an intensive care unit.

Developing research problems

All research begins with the identification of an issue or problem that the researcher feels is worthy of study. This problem often arises out of the researcher's knowledge of previous studies and theories, although it can also derive from personal experience, or the discovery of interesting or surprising facts. It should be borne in mind that to be worth pursuing, research problems need to be both answerable and manageable.

The identification of research problems involves focusing upon specific aspects of the social group that it is proposed to examine. These problems are not like scientific hypotheses; they are not designed to be predictive statements that can be verified or refuted by evidence from the data. They are much looser than that – the purpose is to focus the researcher on a general area of enquiry, without compromising the openness of the research by implying answers to their own questions.

My research into interaction between doctors and nurses began with the identification of a research problem that emanated from two sources – the reading of sociological and nursing literature on the subject, and personal experience as a clinical nurse. This combination led me to identify inequalities in professional relationships as a problem that was worthy of research. Thus, the problem in my research was how power relations affected and were manifested in interactions between nurses and doctors (Porter, 1991).

After research problems have been identified, the next stage is to manipulate them into a form whereby they can be more easily studied in the field, which is usually done by taking a rather general problem and making it more specific.

On thinking about how I should go about observing power relations between nurses and doctors, I decided that this could be most easily done if I restricted my examination to the manifestation of power in decision-making processes. This sharpening of the focus of the research onto a clearly defined type of interaction meant that I could more easily identify, record and analyse pertinent data. However, the increase in clarity involved in this step was bought at the price of excluding other, less obvious instances of the exercise of power; instances that may have been extremely important in the constitution of occupational relations between nurses and doctors. It is well to remember that sharpening the focus of research may mean the researcher is less sensitive to other important aspects of the research problem. Prior to hardening up research problems, the researcher should think seriously about these alternative avenues, and whether or not they are sufficiently peripheral to be excluded from the research.

A word of warning here. Many qualitative researchers are wary of making up their minds about the social world they are going to examine before they actually get round to examining it. They are suspicious of the sort of hypothesis testing favoured by quantitative researchers because they believe that it encourages researchers to see the world in the image of their own preconceptions, rather than keeping an open mind about what it will be like when they examine it. While it is useful, indeed essential, to have some sort of research problem worked out before entering the field, these problems should not be cast in granite. Be prepared to alter or abandon them in the light of the evidence you subsequently gather.

The reason for the inappropriateness of definitive hypotheses lies in the subject matter of qualitative research. Because it focuses on the actions and interpretations of subjects, each social situation examined will have a distinctive character which cannot be totally covered by a general theory. Abandonment of that which is particular to a given situation entails unwarranted distortion. However, it is also the case that there are commonalities between different social situations, so the complete rejection of common conceptual formulations would also be inappropriate. A sensible compromise has been offered by Blumer (1954), who advocates using theories as general guides, rather than fixed prescriptions about what researchers should be addressing.

Perhaps the danger of definitive theories can be best illustrated by looking at another study of the relationship between nurses and doctors. Hughes (1988) criticises previous analysts for taking the concept of the 'doctor–nurse game' (Stein, 1967) as being definitive of the nature of interoccupational relations. Hughes argues that, to the extent that analysts have accepted a model of interaction which assumes that nurses will invariably be deferent to doctors, they 'may have been guilty of assuming a homogeneity in the division of labour that is simply not justified by empirical evidence' (Hughes, 1988). Hughes goes on to demonstrate that the degree to which nurses are subservient or otherwise depends upon the specific situation that they find themselves in. In doing to, he does not reject out of hand the concept of the doctor–nurse game. Rather, he argues that it is only applicable in certain circumstances.

Even though they are not definitive, the identification of research problems prior to the commencement of qualitative research will guide the collection of data. However, these pre-understandings should not be seen by the qualitative researcher as iron cages. Phenomena that researchers come across and think might be useful, but which fall outside the remit of their preconceptions, should not be ignored. Rest assured that the data will reveal behaviours and ideas that the researcher could not have conceived of prior to entering the field and collecting data.

Reviewing the literature

As can be seen from Hughes's (1988) comments, the degree to which previous work should mould research is a matter of contention within the qualitative research community. My own opinion is that sole dependence on data for the generation of theory, an approach known as induction, leads to a tendency for researchers to continually re-invent the wheel. Previous literature, both descriptive and theoretical, is there to be used. Researchers should make the most of it, without allowing it to predetermine the outcome of their research.

The importance of the literature review to the process of analysis lies in the grounding that it gives researchers in the subject area that they are proposing to examine. It narrows the field of enquiry by indicating which problems and which perspectives might be appropriate. Examination of the literature will enable the researcher to judge which areas have not been adequately researched, or, conversely, which conclusions it would be profitable to test in a different setting.

Thus, in my study (Porter, 1991), I used the previous literature on nurse–doctor interactions to further refine the research problem by extracting from the literature four possible ideal types of interaction in decision-making processes: the total subordination of nurses, the use of the doctor–nurse game, informal nursing assertiveness in decision-making and open and formally sanctioned involvement of nurses in the making of decisions. However, I went into the research consciously trying to avoid any presumption about which concept would be most accurate – the ideal types were simply adopted as frameworks to organize the data. Thus, I was using the literature to generate ideas rather than to help me decide, before empirical examination, what was actually going on. As it turned out, I found examples of all four ideal types of behaviour.

The cycle of data collection and analysis

The process of data collection and analysis in qualitative research is a cyclical one. The researcher arrives in the field with some conception of the nature of the behaviour and understandings of the people being researched. These theories are then tested out on the data, which themselves suggest refinements to the original theories, or even entirely new theories. These new or improved theories then in turn need to be tested on the data (Hammersley & Atkinson, 1983).

The cycle of alternating between data collection and analysis can be demonstrated diagrammatically, as shown in Fig. 29.1. It should be noted that Fig. 29.1 is simplified. It is highly unlikely that a single cycle will enable the qualitative researcher to identify patterns of behaviour and meaning, or to discover variations and limitations to those patterns. The terms used in Fig. 29.1 will be discussed in the rest of the chapter.

It is through the cycle of data collection and analysis that the research becomes ever more acutely focused on the problem at hand. On the basis of this analytical discrimination, the researcher is able to construct a theoretical model that can, at least partially, explain the research problem that has been addressed. This process of analytical focusing can be divided into five stages.

(1) The first stage involves the qualitative researcher becoming familiar with the situation under study. The researcher will initially be confronted with a mass of undifferentiated information. The process of making sense of this information entails the *identification of patterns* of behaviour or discourse.

(2) Once patterns have been identified, the research can move on to the second stage, which involves fleshing out the data by mapping out *variations, limitations and exceptions* to the patterns being examined.

(3) The third stage of the collection/analysis cycle is concerned with the *explanation of patterns* that have been identified and elaborated. In qualitative research, this explanation is usually framed around an understanding of the meanings and motives of the research subjects that lay behind their observed behaviour.

(4) Having reached the point where patterns have been clarified and explanations for them posited, the next stage of the observation/analysis cycle is the

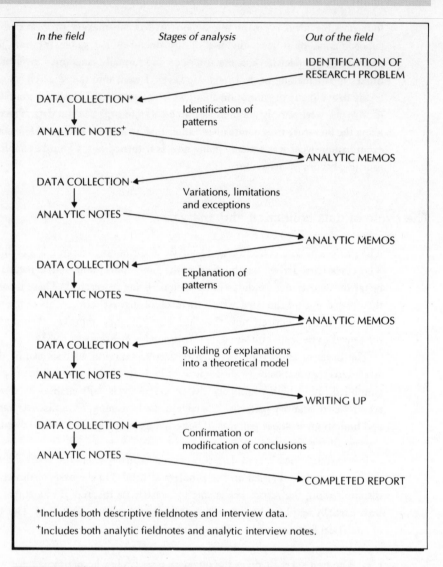

Fig. 29.1 The qualitative research cycle.

building of explanations into a theoretical model. This involves uncovering the relationship between patterns and tying together the various explanations that have emerged thus far.

(5) The final stage involves the *confirmation or modification of conclusions* that have emerged from the research. This is often accomplished by returning to the field towards the end of the research process.

To illustrate how this process works in practice, I will concentrate on a specific aspect of my participant observation of nurse–doctor relations, namely the influence of racism upon the dynamics of power (Porter, 1993).

Stage one

I entered the field with a theoretical concept that I had taken from Hughes's (1988) study of nurse–doctor relations. Hughes had noted that white nurses were considerably less deferential in their interactions with Asian doctors than they were with white doctors. Thus the concept that I arrived with was that, to some degree, racism would influence relationships between white health workers and those belonging to ethnic minorities. However, after several weeks in the field as a participant observer, one of the patterns of behaviour that I began to identify was that there was no appreciable difference in the power and status of black and Asian doctors in their interactions with white nurses, as compared to white doctors.

Stage two

Further examination of the behaviour of white nurses revealed that while they were deferent to black and Asian doctors in their open interactions with them, some nurses expressed racist views amongst themselves in private. Thus, I had identified a variation in the pattern of behaviour of nurses.

Stage three

Given the cycle of observation and analysis that I had thus far conducted, my task was now to explain the variable behaviour of some nurses, taking into account the concept that I had developed from Hughes's study. The explanation evolved around the understandings that nurses had of their occupational situation. I argued that nurses placed considerable faith in the ideology of professionalism. Part of this ideology involved the rejection of irrational judgements. This presented racist nurses with a problem in that racism, by definition, is irrational. Because of the significance of the ideology of professionalism, they were only able to express that racism using an apparently rational pretext. In Hughes's study, this was provided by the cultural unfamiliarity of the Asian doctors observed, which allowed nurses to cloak their racism under the rational veneer of criticism of the doctors' competence. Because the doctors in my study were familiar with the culture pertaining, this avenue of expressing racism was not available to those nurses who were racist.

Stage four

In my study of relations between nurses and doctors, I had noted that, in addition to racism, the quality of interaction was influenced by gender relations, and by economic structures. Thus, I had refined three separate theories to help explain the nature of the professional relationship that I was examining. I combined these discrete explanations into a theoretical framework which posited that the actions and understandings of nurses and doctors in their interactions with each other could not be solely understood through examination of factors internal to these occupations or the health care institutions within which they worked. Account also needed to be taken of the powerful influence of wider social structures upon the behaviour of health care professionals (Porter, 1996).

Stage five

In order to test the conclusions that I had come to, I returned to the field several times during the year that following the initial observation period of three months.

The point of this explanation is to underline the provisional nature of initial theoretical concepts, the requirement to identify the specificities of the social situation being examined and the need to frame qualitative explanations in terms of the understandings of the actors involved.

Having laid out this guide to the stages of qualitative analysis, I should remind readers that it is not a blueprint for every piece of qualitative research. For example, the research might concentrate on a single theme, rendering redundant the final stage of constructing a theoretical model. It is up to each researcher to decide which analytical procedures are appropriate for the research in hand. The only rule is that the researcher should be prepared both to describe and to justify the approach taken.

Triangulation

The key method of ensuring the validity of the processes of qualitative analysis is the use of triangulation. This can be done in two ways. The first method of triangulation involves comparing the outlooks of research subjects. By testing the validity of theories from the different perspectives of different subjects, the researcher can be more confident that the analysis is along the right track.

An example of the use of this sort of triangulation can be seen in research that I conducted into the degree to which the application of ideas emanating from the 'new nursing' has democratized relations between nurses and patients (Porter, 1994). A number of interviewed nurses, who supported the new nursing, claimed that relationships with patients had altered significantly. The danger of sole reliance on these accounts was that they might have led to over-optimistic conclusions about the effectiveness of the new nursing. However, by triangulating these opinions with the responses of subjects who disapproved of the new confidence enjoyed by some patients, but who nevertheless accepted that a degree of democratization had occurred, I was able to improve the validity of my research.

The second method of triangulation involves the collection of different forms of data from the same subjects. If the same sort of results are gained using two or more techniques, then the conclusions that can be drawn are all the stronger. Often triangulation involves the use of both qualitative and quantitative methods. Thus, for example, in an examination of how gender affects nurse–doctor power relations (Porter, 1992), I supplemented qualitative data that indicated that female doctors were more egalitarian in their dealings with nurses than their male colleagues, with some simple statistical analysis. Using the willingness of doctors to tidy up after performing clinical procedures as an indication of egalitarianism, I counted the number of times doctors were prepared to tidy up. I discovered there was a statistically significant association between a doctor's gender and the likelihood of them tidying up, female doctors being more likely to do so.

The practicalities of analysis during data collection

The practicalities of data analysis differ according to the method of qualitative research adopted. It will be remembered from Chapter 11 that I identified four major qualitative methods. Here I will concentrate on two – participant observation and in-depth interviews. Because similar techniques are used in in-depth interviews and oral histories, no specific discussion of analysis in the latter method is required. As far as conversation analysis is concerned, the complex technique of breaking down discourse is beyond the remit of this chapter. Interested readers should consult a specialist text, such as Atkinson & Heritage (1984), if they are interested in pursuing this line of research.

Participant observation

The first thing to note about analysis of material collected during participant observation is that it is dependent upon the quality of *data collection*. For this reason, the content of the researcher's written descriptions of the situation under study (known as descriptive fieldnotes) should be as full as possible. The recording of speech should be as close to verbatim as the researcher can manage, while non-verbal behaviour needs to be recorded in detail. The context of interactions, in terms of where and when they took place and who was involved, should also be clearly drawn.

Fieldnotes should not simply be descriptive, they should also constitute the first stage of analysis in the data collection/analysis cycle. Any ideas or comments that researchers have about the situation at the time of observation should be included. These comments are termed *analytical notes*. Because they will be subsequently examined and elaborated upon, analytical notes do not have to be fully worked out, or even consistent. Some will prove to be deadends, but some will supply promising lines of enquiry.

An example of the construction of descriptive and analytical fieldnotes can be taken from qualitative data of the interaction between doctors of different sexes and nurses during aseptic procedures, gathered during my examination into the effects of gender upon occupational relations (Porter, 1992). The first two fieldnotes describe two different social interactions that I observed. In the analytical note that was added to descriptive fieldnote 2, I compare the two interactions and attempt to come to terms with their social significance. The notes remain in the informal language that they were originally written in, although descriptive fieldnote 2 is abbreviated.

Descriptive fieldnote 1 (12/7/89)
'Male SHO and female SN inserting an intercostal drain. Sister has informed staff nurse to prepare. Nurse arrives at bed with trolley, and explains to patient what is going on. Doctor arrives, says nothing to either nurse or patient. Starts procedure. Doctor says nothing at all during procedure except to demand

"Gloves!". When he is finished he leaves the bedside without a word, leaving the nurse to clear up his debris.'

Descriptive fieldnote 2 (13/7/89)
'Female SHO and female SN performing intravenous insertion. SHO greets staff nurse and asks if she is free to do it. Both engage in smalltalk ... Both nurse and doctor talk to the patient about what is going on, along with smalltalk ... Doctor very polite to nurse ... SHO "Sorry, would you mind opening these gloves for me ... Thanks." ... On finishing, the doctor tidies away all her waste and thanks nurse.'

Analytical fieldnote (13/7/89)
'Stark comparison between female SHO's actions and those of male SHO yesterday. Two things: (1) She is far more polite, treating nurse and patient with respect. (2) She tidied up after herself and he didn't. Is this an example of gender differences? I could test this by counting whether female doctors tidy up more often than men.'

The main point to be made in relation to fieldnotes is that the participant observer is never *only* involved in the collection of data. The process of analysis, albeit at a rather crude and spontaneous level, is going on all the time the researcher is in the field.

The next level of analysis is the construction of *analytical memos*. In these, the researcher reviews the research to date, examining the relationship between the data collected and the theories that have been developed. These memos often take the form of short essays, which can be revised, extended or combined as the analytical cycle progresses. In the construction of memos, the researcher calls upon both descriptive and analytical fieldnotes, along with the literature reviewed and analytical memos from previous cycles of analysis. Analytical memos, while involving more reflection than analytical notes, are still provisional pieces of work. However, as the research develops, they will become increasingly sophisticated.

The final analytical stage of *writing up* allows researchers to step back, clarify their thinking and organize their ideas more elegantly. Almost invariably, new connections emerge at this stage that were not considered during the period of data collection. For this reason, if possible, it is wise to keep access to the field open, so that these new ideas can be subjected to some empirical testing. As can be seen, the data gathering/analysis cycle persists to the very end of the process of research.

As analytical categories are developed, the researcher will need to code the data collected according to those categories. Coding entails constructing a system whereby all instances of data pertinent to each category can be retrieved. There are a number of methods of going about this. In a grading of technological sophistication, these include the use of card indexes, cutting and pasting on a word processor and the application of dedicated software. The use of computers in qualitative analysis is discussed in Chapter 30.

Interview data

The process of analysis of in-depth interviews is very similar to that of participation observation data. Data collection takes the form of the interviews themselves, while analytical notes can be added immediately after the interviews, while the encounter with the subject is still fresh, or during the process of transcription. Interviews should be transcribed as soon as possible after they take place. The ideal is to transcribe the same day as the interview. This enables the researcher to remember the subtleties of interaction, and perhaps recall unclear pieces of recorded speech. The researcher should listen carefully to the tone and the emphasis of respondents, which can often tell a lot.

The same cycle of gathering data and analysing should be adhered to when the data come from interviews. For this reason, researchers should not arrange to conduct all their interviews in a condensed period of time. Spacing out interviews gives researchers the opportunity to use subsequent interviews to retest theories developed both in analytical memos and the writing up stage.

Reporting qualitative analysis

The variability of qualitative analytical techniques makes the recounting of methods in research reports a lot more cumbersome than it is in much quantitative research. Because of the differences of method between different qualitative studies, it is important that researchers clearly, honestly and comprehensively report the nature of the analytical methods that they use.

An example of good practice can be found in Sherblom *et al.*'s (1993) examination of nurses' ethical decision-making, where they clearly explain their use of the responsive reader method of analysis. This method of analysing interview transcripts was designed to emphasize the multiple voices of subjects, and indeed researchers, instead of narrowly focusing upon specific issues that the researcher had already decided were important. In Sherblom *et al.*'s research, the responsive reader method is used to analyse data gained from interviews with nurses in order to show how the concepts of justice and care animate their decisions. Sherblom *et al.* explain that each interview transcript was subjected to a number of readings. The aim of the first reading was to become attuned with the point of view of the subject. The second reading entailed searching for themes associated with the concept of justice. This process was repeated to identify themes related to caring. A fourth reading highlighted those concerns that did not fit into either the care or justice perspectives. Moreover, in presenting their analysis, Sherblom *et al.* grounded it in numerous quotations from the nurses interviewed, thus allowing the reader to conduct their own readings of the expressions of the participants.

The painstaking explanation provided by Sherblom *et al.* means that a reader of that research, who may not have been previously aware of the responsive reader method of analysis, is able to understand clearly the aim and process of the research, and to judge its accuracy and utility accordingly.

Conclusion

The reader will now be aware that the process of qualitative analysis is far from being simple or straightforward. The qualitative researcher is largely bereft of the sort of clear guidelines that their quantitative colleagues enjoy. To a considerable extent, success depends upon the curiosity, imagination and erudition of the researcher, not to mention the all-important factor of serendipity. This is another good reason for qualitative researchers to include in their written reports a clear description of their analytical procedures. It is only by doing so that they can demonstrate to readers that the path they took was a valid one.

One of the consequences of the uncertain nature of qualitative analysis is that it is impossible for textbooks such as this to provide a *cookbook recipe* for the prosecution of qualitative research. For this reason, anyone considering carrying out a piece of qualitative research for the first time is strongly advised to ensure that they have close supervision from an experienced qualitative researcher, who will be able to guide them through the unexpected pitfalls and opportunities that will inevitably arise.

That said, qualitative analysis, because it involves such close contact with people, is an extremely satisfying way of conducting research work. As such, it has much to commend it to nursing researchers.

References

Atkinson, J.M. & Heritage, J. (1984) *Structures of Social Action: Studies in Conversational Analysis.* Cambridge University Press, Cambridge.

Blumer, H. (1954) What is wrong with social theory? *American Sociological Review*, 19, 3–10.

Hammersley, M. & Atkinson, P. (1983) *Ethnography: Principles in Practice.* Tavistock, London.

Hughes, D. (1988) When nurse knows best: some aspects of nurse/doctor interaction in a casualty department. *Sociology of Health and Illness*, 10, 1–22.

Porter, S. (1991) A participant observation study of power relations between nurses and doctors in a general hospital. *Journal of Advanced Nursing*, 16, 728–35.

Porter, S. (1992) Women in a women's job: the gendered experience of nurses. *Sociology of Health and Illness*, 14, 510–27.

Porter, S. (1993) Critical realist ethnography: the case of racism and professionalism in a medical setting. *Sociology*, 27, 591–609.

Porter, S. (1994) New nursing: the road to freedom? *Journal of Advanced Nursing*, 20, 269–74.

Porter, S. (1996) *Nursing's Relationship with Medicine.* Avebury, Aldershot.

Sherblom, S., Shipps, T. & Sherblom, J. (1993) Justice, care, and integrated concerns in the ethical decision making of nurses. *Qualitative Health Research*, 3, 442–64.

Stein, L. (1967) The doctor–nurse game. *Archives of General Psychiatry*, 16, 699–703.

Chapter 30

Computer Assisted Data Analysis

David C. Benton

Computer technology continues to advance at a phenomenal rate. It is not that long ago that the only researchers with access to computers were those working for academic institutions or large corporations. However, in the last 5–10 years, many households now have their own computer and most health care establishments have a range of equipment available.

The purpose of this chapter is not to describe in detail the technology, hardware and software behind computer based data analysis, but to look at some of the practicalities. Accordingly, general principles rather than specific details will be explored.

Qualitative and quantitative data analysis

Throughout this text we have considered both qualitative and quantitative research methods. Today's computer technology can assist us in the analysis of data generated by either approach. Whilst computers have been used for many years for assisting researchers in the analysis of quantitative data, their use in analysing and exploring qualitative data is a relatively new phenomenon. It is not the intention to replicate the contents of Chapters 27 to 29 and therefore the detail of the analytical procedures being used will only be reproduced in this chapter if this adds clarity to the understanding of how computer analysis can be undertaken. Furthermore, reference is made to a number of computer programs throughout this text. In the case of qualitative software a list of contact points for further information is given in Appendix 30.1.

Computerized quantitative data analysis

Quantitative data can be analysed using a wide range of software packages. Some of these packages are specifically designed to conduct statistical analysis, whereas others often offer a limited set of statistical procedures as a feature of a broader specialized program. Programs such as spreadsheets, databases and graphics packages can all offer facilities that will enable statistical analysis to take place.

Spreadsheets, databases and graphics packages

A spreadsheet can best be thought of as an electronic data sheet made up of a series of rows and columns. Each row and column is labelled so individual squares can be cross-referenced. Statistical analysis can be undertaken either by writing specific formulae involving the contents of the various rows and columns or by using predefined procedures. For example, a column of numbers can first be added then divided by the total number of data elements. This would give the mean. Conversely the function MEAN, available on most spreadsheet programs, may be used to perform the same operation.

Databases can contain both textual and numerical information. Databases are in widescale use within health service settings. It is often possible for researchers to gain access to data that have already been recorded and stored as part of the patient information system. Researchers can then either formulate queries based on the various information stored within the database and/or take advantage of the wide range of specialized functions offered by the package. Like spreadsheets, databases commonly offer functions such as MEAN, standard deviation and other basic descriptive statistics. Graphics packages that can display information in bar, line or pie chart format frequently offer a range of basic descriptive statistical functions that can be applied to the data which generate the graphical output.

In summary, spreadsheets, databases and graphics packages can provide researchers with a restricted range of statistical procedures. On the whole, these non-specialist packages can calculate basic descriptive statistics. However, if more advanced techniques, in particular inferential statistical analysis, are to be conducted then a specialized package is required.

Specialized quantitative computer analysis programs

There are a number of statistics packages available on the market. This chapter will use, for illustrative purposes, one of the most widely used and comprehensive packages available. SPSS® which stands for Statistical Package for the Social Sciences has been developed over the past 20 or so years from a programme originally used on mainframe computers to one that is now available on standard desk top personal computers.

A sophisticated program such as SPSS® offers a wide range of statistical procedures. Not all of these come as standard and the package consists of a number of modules which can be purchased to meet the specific needs of the researcher. Having said this, it is important to recognize that even the base package is sufficiently comprehensive to meet the needs of most researchers unless highly specific and advanced tests are required (Frude, 1987; Norusis, 1990; Norusis, 1993).

Whilst it is not the intention to give a detailed review of the analytical tools available within the package or the syntax of how the analysis is conducted, a review of some of the basic features is now given. Since personal computers are available to many researchers, rather than examine the mainframe based version, discussion will be focused around SPSS Version 4 for MS DOS. This is the fourth generation of the package which runs under the MS DOS operating system. A version which runs under Windows, another type of computer operating system, is also available. The Windows version is perhaps even easier to use but does not give the researcher the same level of access to the underlying principles. For those researchers who are less confident with computers, then the Windows version certainly requires fewer computing skills.

Starting SPSS

SPSS is a large and sophisticated program. It can undertake both descriptive and inferential statistical analyses, present information in tabular or graphical form, import information from existing data sources such as a database or spreadsheet and produce output that is ready for inclusion in final reports. In addition to these functions, SPSS can also provide facilities that enable the researcher to create or reproduce on screen questionnaire structures which then can be used for entering data and preparing them for analysis.

Whether using SPSS for DOS or Windows, on starting the system the researcher is faced with a series of menu options. By highlighting one of these options, further related choices can be made. Figure 30.1 illustrates the top level options available, when using SPSS Version 4 for DOS, followed by the sub-menu that is offered once, for example, analysed data have been highlighted followed again by the statistical analysis that can be conducted once descriptive statistics have been highlighted. This process of selection from menus continues until the various commands required are reached. These can then be cut and pasted into an area that enables commands to be built. These commands can then be processed to undertake the required analysis.

Preparing data for analysis

It has already been illustrated in Chapter 26 that data can be stored in a variety of formats. SPSS enables data to be entered either directly into a template which resembles the original questionnaire, in a spreadsheet format or as a data list. Figures 30.2, 30.3 and 30.4 illustrate how these would look if such approaches were used. For illustrative purposes, a very simple questionnaire structure is used. Figure 30.2 illustrates a single set of answers relating to one subject or case. Figures 30.3 and 30.4 illustrate the same case as entered in Fig. 30.2 (case 1) along with the subsequent five cases. A case is the terminology used for the responses made by a single research subject.

Uncategorized data

The examples used in Figs 30.2, 30.3 and 30.4 are all data that reduce to numerical values. That is, the data are either a continuous variable, such as age, or capable of being categorized and coded, for example yes = 1, no = 2. SPSS can however handle uncategorized data. For example the open-ended question 'what did you

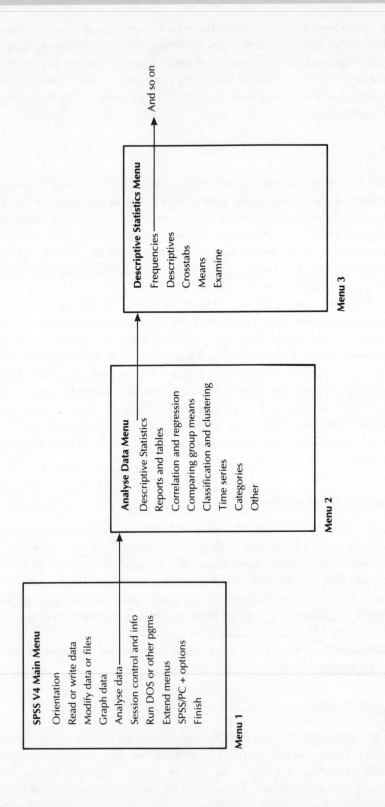

SPSS V4 Main Menu

Orientation
Read or write data
Modify data or files
Graph data
Analyse data
Session control and info
Run DOS or other pgms
Extend menus
SPSS/PC + options
Finish

Menu 1

Analyse Data Menu

Descriptive Statistics
Reports and tables
Correlation and regression
Comparing group means
Classification and clustering
Time series
Categories
Other

Menu 2

Descriptive Statistics Menu

Frequencies
Descriptives
Crosstabs
Means
Examine

Menu 3

And so on

Fig. 30.1 Menu selection in SPSS/PC+ version 4.

What is your age in years?

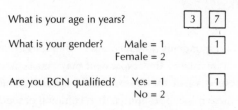

What is your gender?   Male = 1
                         Female = 2

Are you RGN qualified?   Yes = 1
                           No = 2

Fig. 30.2   Example of questionnaire entry screen [case 01].

Case No	Age	Gender	RGN
01	37	1	1
02	24	2	1
03	45	1	2
04	32	1	1
05	22	2	2
06	34	2	2

Fig. 30.3   Questionnaire data in spread sheet format.

```
Data List
/Case 1–2 Age 3–4 Gender 5 RGN 6.          Describes Location Of Variables
Variable Labels                            Within Data List
/Case "Subject Number"
/Age "Age of Respondent"                   Gives Labels to Variable Name
/Gender "Sex of Respondent"                which can be printed when
/RGN "Is Respondent RGN Qualified".        analysis is conducted
BEGIN DATA
013711
022421
034512
043211                                     Data [Case, Age, Gender, RGN]
052222
063422
END DATA
FINISH.
```

Fig. 30.4   Questionnaire data in data list format.

enjoy most about your RGN training?' could be stored within an SPSS data file. However, in this case it would be stored as a text string. SPSS would not allow any detailed analysis of this string to take place, but could print out all responses to this question so the researcher could then conduct some form of content analysis (see later in this chapter).

Missing data

Sometimes respondents do not complete all questions in a questionnaire. This may be simply a mistake or the respondent may choose not to answer particular questions. Irrespective of the reason, the researcher needs some systematic way of handling these missing responses. It is common practice to allocate a specific code to missing data. When missing data occurs, the code can therefore be entered. By examining the percentage of data missing in relation to any particular question, a researcher may gain valuable insights. For example, a lot of missing data relating to a particular question may indicate that the question is poorly structured and therefore respondents are unwilling or unsure as to how to offer a reply. On the other hand, it may indicate a question that respondents find particularly sensitive to answer. Such an example might include 'how much money do you earn?'. Missing data therefore may give additional valuable information.

Data entry and verification

As had been seen from Figs 30.2, 30.3 and 30.4, there are a variety of ways of entering data. Chapter 26 illustrated that it is sometimes necessary to code the subject's response into a numerical value. For example, a tick in a particular box might have to be given a numerical coded value. Obviously the more often this has to occur, the greater the chance of an error resulting. SPSS offers a number of ways of ensuring that errors in data entry do not occur. By displaying the information in the spreadsheet format, simple inspection of the layout may reveal errors in data entry. Alternatively the computer can ask you to re-enter perhaps 10% of all questionnaires, comparing the original entry with the subsequent attempt at verification. If a large number of discrepancies are flagged up, then clearly widescale verification is required.

Data cleaning

If the need for widescale verification is identified, then there are a number of ways of *cleaning* the data – removing errors. SPSS allows the researcher to set certain limits on the types of information that can be entered. For example, if the expected response to the question of gender is 1 for male and 2 for female, any other response such as 3, 4, 5 can be disallowed. This would prevent errors at the data entry stage occurring. It would of course not prevent a male respondent being classified as female.

Some conditional responses can also be pre-programmed. For example, if a respondent to a health questionnaire classified themselves as male, you would not expect any data to be entered in a section relating to menstruation. Data consistency can therefore be assured if such rules are entered and applied within individual cases.

Documentation

A piece of research can take anything from perhaps one month to several years to complete. The researcher may, after another few years, wish to return to the original data, possibly to compare it with updated information obtained, or to conduct further analysis. If the data are inadequately documented, then problems can arise. For example, did '1' mean male or female? It is essential that the manner by which data are coded is adequately documented. Some researchers refer to this process as creating a *data dictionary*. Each variable would therefore have information on the location within a data string, a label attached to the variable which explains in more detail what the information is about, a set of value labels which explain each and every coded response, for example 1 = male, 2 = female, and finally the code that is used for missing data. Only by carrying out such a detailed description can a researcher be assured that mistakes will not occur when they, or perhaps other researchers, explore the data set in the future.

Worked example

In this example, the researcher is trying to identify the barriers experienced by nurses in implementing research into their practice. The questionnaire consists of data from a number of sources: educationalists, community based nurses, health visitors and midwives. The respondents are asked to give their views on how significant a series of 29 statements are in inhibiting their ability to implement research based practice. Subjects are then asked to identify what they see as the top three barriers to implementation. Additional demographic information relating to gender, age and highest level of educational attainment is also recorded. Appendix 30.2 gives details of the structure of the data list file, and Appendix 30.3 an illustration of the data from the study.

The actual data file contained the responses of 424 respondents. A request to describe the staff group from which the various respondents were from resulted in the output detailed in Table 30.1. The analysis took less than five seconds to carry out.

Whilst the example given above only illustrates the use of a straightforward descriptive statistic, SPSS can perform a wide range of complex analytical proce-

Table 30.1 Frequency count of the staff groups of the respondents.

Value label	Value	Frequency	%	Valid %	Cumulative %
Educationalists	1	77	18.2	18.2	18.2
Community based nurses	2	159	37.5	37.5	55.7
Health visitors	3	71	16.7	16.7	72.4
Midwives	4	117	27.6	27.6	100.0
		Total 424	100.0	100.0	
Valid cases 424	Missing cases 0				

dures. For each analysis a well thought out layout which presents the results is available – the default format. These default formats, as can be seen from Table 30.1, are of a sufficiently high standard that they can be readily incorporated into the results section of a research report without the need for any modification.

Computerized qualitative research analysis

Several authors contend that computers can be used to assist the researcher in qualitative analysis (Baker, 1988; Norman, 1989; Fielding & Lee, 1991; Taft, 1994). As computer technology has become more readily available, qualitative researchers have had at their disposal a new means of supporting the conduct of analysis of interview transcripts, ethnographic field notes and other data sources. These new, high technology techniques are far more sophisticated than the scissors, copier and card indexes traditionally used.

Gerson (1984) has suggested that the computer can assist the qualitative researcher by doing anything that it is possible to do on paper but more quickly, easily and with greater efficiency and precision. Conrad & Reinharz (1984) have suggested that the ability of the computer to tirelessly search large volumes of material has enabled qualitative researchers to more easily identify key material embedded within lengthy transcripts. This in turn has made it easier for researchers to find deviant cases and to extract small but significant pieces of information which might otherwise go unnoted. Computer technology therefore provides the researcher with a dedicated assistant that can remove much of the tedium associated with qualitative analysis.

Software available for qualitative analysis

Computer programs for the analysis of qualitative data fall into two distinct types – off the shelf solutions and dedicated/specialist programs.

Researchers can make use of generally available software packages such as word processors or database management programs. Both these off the shelf solutions offer many of the facilities that can assist the qualitative researcher in analysing their data. In addition, however, there are available a number of specialist programs which have been developed for a qualitative researcher. These fall into three main types: chunking and coding programs, qualitative modelling programs and expert systems. Both off the shelf and specialist package styles are now described.

Off the shelf programs

Off the shelf programs such as word processors and database management systems can both be used for qualitative data analysis.

Word processors

It has been suggested by both Norman (1989) and Baker (1988) that standard word processing packages can be used for the analysis of qualitative data sets. In short, they are ideally suited to identifying words or individual blocks of text. With the advent of more sophisticated packages such as Microsoft Word® version 6, several files can be searched at once. This could mean, for example, that an interview with an individual subject may be recorded in a single file. By searching all the files, all interviews could be searched for the occurrence of certain word groups or phrases. In addition, such packages can automatically generate an index detailing the frequency of occurrence and location of the various phrases being searched for.

Database management systems

Relational databases are becoming increasingly sophisticated. Initially they were thought of simply as a means of holding numerical data. However, as each generation of program has been developed, increased sophistication in text management has become a significant feature. Again, like word processors, they can store large quantities of text, search for information and index this for further use.

Specialist packages

Whilst off the shelf packages can offer a range of basic analytical tools, for more sophisticated techniques specialist programs are required. Many of these programs have been developed by qualitative researchers who wished to take advantage of the computer's ability to manipulate large quantities of data in a flexible and efficient manner.

Chunking and coding programs

Chunking and coding programs have been specially developed to meet the needs of qualitative researchers and are especially useful in analysing field notes and transcripts. The field notes and transcripts are inspected and codes are then assigned to various segments which are of interest to the researcher. The computer program can then be asked to abstract these various *chunks* of *coded* material and display them together with the text with which they are associated. In short, these programs offer little more than the more sophisticated word processing packages that are now currently available. Programs such as ETHNOGRAPH were developed in the early to middle 1980s when word processing packages were generally not as sophisticated as the current generation.

Qualitative 'modelling' programs

Qualitative modelling programs try and expose the underlying connections and structures of the data being analysed. According to Heise (1991) many qualitative researchers are wary of these systems since they contend that there is a danger that a mechanical approach to the generation of qualitative theory may result in 'mechanical' solutions. However, if researchers do not blindly accept the connections being suggested but critically consider the material, then the researcher stays in control thereby choosing to either accept or reject the structures being suggested by such programs. ETHNO is an example of such a package.

Expert systems

With the increased sophistication of computer technology, expert systems are being developed which can sift through vast quantities of data in such a way as to distil out phrases, their associated linkages and thereby the developing categories and theory. Gerson (1984) has suggested that the further development of expert systems could be considered analogous to the computer turning from dedicated clerk to supervised research assistant.

Teaching

Irrespective of the program being used, an added advantage that computerized analysis programs offer is the ability to enable qualitative analysis to be more readily taught. Generally speaking, the principles of qualitative analysis are given to student researchers, but it is not until they actually conduct a piece of research that they use the techniques live. With the advent of computer technology, lecturers can offer students the opportunity to analyse existing data sets with the assistance of the various programs available. Since it is the researcher who is controlling the process, this does not mean that all students would necessarily come up with the same or similar analytical solutions, but would at least in a reasonable time frame have had experience of analysing the same data. Accordingly, not only do students gain insight into using the various computer packages on offer, but also via discussion with their peers gain a more comprehensive insight into qualitative analysis (Fielding & Lee, 1991).

Software analytical capabilities

Whilst there are significant differences between various qualitative analytical approaches (see Chapters 11, 12 and 29) there are certain commonalities which do exist. These commonalities include:

- Locating individual words and phrases.
- Creating alphabetic word lists which include the frequency of occurrence of the various words.
- Creating indexes (locating the various words within the overall data source).
- Attaching key words to segments of text.

- Attaching codes or categories to segments of text, linking codes to identify and align relationships.
- Connecting codes.

Locating individual words and phrases

As already noted, there is no need to buy sophisticated and specialized qualitative analysis packages to enable the researcher to locate individual codes or phrases. The FIND command available in both word processors and database management packages is perfectly adequate for this purpose. In most cases a dialogue box (the way the user requests access to a specific command) is used. Various constraints can be placed on the 'search', for example forwards, backwards, finding whole words only or using a phonetic search to find words that sound like the word being searched for. The computer will then search through the file for all occurrences of the word or phrase being sought. This will then be highlighted and the researcher can view on the screen the various locations. As an illustrative example, Fig. 30.5 displays the output of a search for the word 'research' in a short piece of interview text. Only exact matches, that is, research as opposed to researcher, were sought. Figure 30.5 does not illustrate the use of any particular software program since the syntax varies one from another and therefore it is only the principles that are illustrated here.

FIND: **research**

LIMITS OF SEARCH:- WHOLE WORDS ONLY, WHOLE DOCUMENT

While there might have been more lofty aims to do with integrating **research** into practice and all that sort of thing, it was much more about safeguarding nursing. It was about getting influence, I felt that nursing had lost influence when general management came in. Because of the kind of **research** that was put forward I got the feeling that general managers didn't value what was being done. To get any sort of credibility there was a need to take the initiative by getting it right. Playing the game by their rules. Researchers needed to be politically aware if nursing was to progress the **research** based agenda advocated by Briggs and others.

Fig. 30.5 FIND dialogue box and resultant search of an interview text.

Creating alphabetic word list and counting the frequency of occurrence of words

The ability to identify not only the words used by research subjects but their frequency often gives qualitative researchers valuable insights into the vocabulary of the research subjects. Such a tool often provides a basic starting point for content analysis. By comparing the words and their frequency across a number of interview subjects, commonalities can be found. There are a variety of programs that enable this to happen, for example TEXT COLLECTOR, CONCORDANCE and ZYINDEX. These programmes allow the researcher to indicate common words such as 'the', 'and', 'he', 'it' which are in effect background noise which can then be discounted. This reduces the total extensive list to a manageable list of words which may provide real insight into the content of the transcript.

Creating indexes

Whilst comparing the vocabulary of one subject to another, or indeed one part of a transcript to another originated by the same subject, it is the ability to locate the occurrences of words within the totality of the document that is important. The production of an index can provide information on several levels. It can identify the source document, the chapter or segment in which the word is located, the page and perhaps even more importantly for qualitative researchers the paragraph and line numbers. By comparing the relative location of the occurrences of such words an understanding of the context can be obtained. The key word under consideration can then be placed in the context of the data sources. It may then be possible to identify, for example, that the word 'research' has been mentioned by every respondent and that it typically occurs within the first three paragraphs of the interview conducted. Whilst standard word processing packages are becoming far more sophisticated in offering such facilities, specialized qualitative research analysis packages do provide a more comprehensive range of options. TEXT BASE ALPHA, a relatively cheap program, excels in this task in that it not only provides all the necessary indexing information but also prints the 30 succeeding and the 30 preceding characters associated with the word being indexed. This obviously gives the researcher significant contextual information upon which to base a more sophisticated analysis rather than simply that which can be derived from location and frequency of occurrence.

Attaching key words to segments of text

It is not always the case that we mention a specific key word when trying to communicate a concept or idea. In Chapter 12, when illustrating memo writing, the category of empowerment was identified. Figure 30.6 illustrates how the key word of empowerment is attached to the various segments of text which convey and verbalize this idea.

Attaching codes to segments of text

It is important to note that there is a difference between key words and codes. In short, key words can be considered as one word summaries of the content of a text segment whereas codes are the abbreviations of category names. Codes can be attached to various chunks of text which then produce or convey a particular category of meaning. Coded text can be overlapping or indeed codes can be nested within existing segments. A search using one of the codes will therefore result in the

While there might have been more lofty aims to do with integrating research into practice and all that sort of thing, it was much more about safeguarding nursing. **It was about getting influence**, I felt that nursing had lost influence when general management came in. Because of the kind of research that was put forward I got the feeling that general managers didn't value what was being done. **To get any sort of credibility** there was **a need to take the initiative** by getting it right. Playing the game by their rules. **Researchers needed to be politically aware** if nursing was to progress the research based agenda advocated by Briggs and others.	**Empowerment** **Empowerment** **Empowerment** **Empowerment**

Fig. 30.6 Illustrating the attachment of key words to segments of text.

reproduction of all segments to which that code is attached. Such a search will yield information regarding the location of the segment within the original text. All qualitative analysis programs offer such facilities and QUALPRO is one such program which enables the user to segment material, code it, then perform searches.

Connecting codes

If qualitative researchers are truly to understand the nature of the subject under investigation, then it is not simply sufficient to code material but they must gain an understanding of the underlying structures. The ability to link coded sections in a meaningful way provides such a facility. By undertaking this step it is possible then to develop propositional statements or to make assertions regarding the structure of the linkages so various concepts can be related, thereby enabling the researcher to discover the underlying principles. In short, this feature enables theory building to take place. Programs such as NUDIST and ATLAS provide the researcher with such facilities. By looking at the pattern of coded segments both within an individual interview and across interviews it is possible to discover underlying principles and theories. Similarly, by testing for the absence of linkages it is also possible to either confirm or refute the hypothesis being developed.

Conclusion

This chapter has not attempted to provide in-depth critique of how the various computer programs can be used in both quantitative and qualitative analysis. It has, however, identified some of the basic principles and provided some direction as to how the researcher can take the subject of computer based analysis further. Extensive texts have been written on this subject, but the selection of these will be dependent on both the hardware and software resources available to you. Many researchers with links into academia will have ready access to many of the programs described in this chapter. Hence before pursuing the specifics any further, early contact should be made with local research experts and/or computer specialists. A failure to do so may result in much wasted time.

It is important to note that computer technology does not replace the thinking and decision-making required by researchers to intelligently analyse and interpret their data. Computer science only removes the tedium of repetitive calculation and data organization. The time freed from such activities can therefore be applied to data interpretation, hopefully adding to the quality of the research undertaken.

References

Baker, C.A. (1988) Computer applications in qualitative research. *Computers in Nursing*, 6(5), 211–14.

Conrad, P. & Reinharz, S. (1984) Computers and qualitative data. *Qualitative Sociology*, 7(1), 3–15.

Fielding, N.G. & Lee, R.M. (1991) *Using Computers in Qualitative Research*. Sage Publications, London.

Frude, N. (1987) *A Guide to SPSS/PC+*. Macmillan Education, London.

Gerson, E. (1984) Qualitative research and the computer. *Qualitative Sociology*, 7(1), 61–74.

Heise, D.R. (1991) Event structure analysis: a qualitative model of quantitative research. *Using Computers in Qualitative Research*, (eds N.G. Fielding & R.M. Lee). Sage Publications, London.

Norman, E.M. (1989) How to use word processing software to conduct content analysis. *Computers in Nursing*, 7(3), 127–8.

Norusis, M.J. (1990) *SPSS/PC+ 4.0, Base Manual*. SPSS Inc, Chicago, Il.

Norusis, M.J. (1993) *SPSS for Windows, Base System User's Guide Release 6.0*. SPSS Inc, Chicago, Il.

Taft, L.B. (1994) Computer assisted qualitative research. *Research in Nursing and Health*, 16(10), 379–83.

Acknowledgements

SPSS is the registered trademark of SPSS Inc, 444 North Michigan Avenue, Chicago, IL60611, USA.

Microsoft Word is the registered trademark for Microsoft Ltd, Microsoft Place, Warfdale Road, Winnersh Triangle, Wokingham, Berks RG11 5TP.

Appendix 30.1: Qualitative software programs

ATLAS IFP ATLAS Sekr Hab 6 Hardenbergerstr 28, D-1000, Berlin 12, Germany.

CONCORDANCE Dataflight Software, 10573 West Pico Blvd. Los Angeles, CA90064.

ETHNO The National Collegic Software Clearing House, Duke University Press, 6697 College Station, Durham NC27708.

ETHNOGRAPHP Qualitative Research Management, 73425 Hilltop Road, Desert Hot Springs, California CA92240.

NUDIST La Trobe University, Bundoora, Victoria 3083, Australia.

QUALPRO Qualitative Research Management, 73425 Hilltop Road, Desert Hot Springs, California CA92240.

TEXT BASE ALPHA Qualitative Research Management, 73425 Hilltop Road, Desert Hot Springs, California CA92240.

TEXT COLLECTOR O'Neill Software, PO Box 2611, San Francisco, CA94126.

ZYINDEX ZyLab Corporation, 233 Erie Street, Chicago IL60611.

Appendix 30.2: List of variable definitions, variable labels and value labels for research barrier questionnaire

data list file = "dcb.dat"
/source 1 id 2–4 q1 to q29 5–33 great 34–35 second 36–37 third 38–39 sex 40
age 41 educ 42
variable labels source "Staff Group"
/ID "Questionnaire Number"
/q1 "Reports Availability"
/q2 "Practice Implications"
/q3 "Stats Understandable"
/q4 "Practice relevance"
/q5 "Nurse awareness"
/q6 "Implement facilities"
/q7 "Time to read"
/q8 "Research replication"
/q9 "Benefits minimal"
/q10 "Results believable"
/q11 "Methods inadequate"
/q12 "Literature compiled"
/q13 "Authority to change"
/q14 "Not Generalizable"
/q15 "Nurse Isolation"
/q16 "Little self benefit"
/q17 "Reports old"
/q18 "Dr's non-cooperation"
/q19 "Admin non-cooperation"

/q20 "Research value"
/q21 "No stimulus for change"
/q22 "Conclusions not justified"
/q23 "Literature conflicting"
/q24 "Research unreadable"
/q25 "Staff Not Supportive"
/q26 "Unwilling to change"
q27 "Too much information"
/q28 "Not able to critique"
/q29 "Insufficient time"
/great "Greatest Barrier"
/Second "Second Gt Barrier"
/third "Third Gt Barrier"
/sex "Gender of Subject"
/Age "Age of Subject"
/educ "Highest Educational Level"
Value Labels source 1 "Educationalists" 2 "Community Based Nurses"
3 "Health Visitors" 4 "Midwives"
/q1 to q29 "To no extent" 2 "To a little extent" 3 "To a moderate extent"
4 "To a great Extent" 5 "No opinion"
/sex 1 "Male" 2 "Female"
/Age 1 "Under 25" 2 "25 to 34" 3 "35 to 44" 4 "45 to 54" 5 "55 and Over"
/educ 1 "O grade/level" 2 "A level/H grade" 3 "Diploma" 4 "Basic Degree"
5 "Advanced Diploma" 6 "Taught Masters" 7 "M. Phil" 8 "Doctorate" 0 "None"
missing values q1 to q 29 sex to educ (9)
/great to third (99).

Appendix 30.3: Sample of data list from barriers to research questionnaire

```
10772424324551314343231232125533429071  5146
10763332432232333343233332234334928250  5126
10753342344425244544354211234334431252  8232
10744333443334344443444243434444433303  2135
10733334434233344343444335234214415121  8134
10721442322434444433333322233334931323  3135
10713341432442233344155344235333221051  5134
10702232431143243245152445224314905150  1224
10694322333322142321231211122213429120  1244
```

.

.

.

Continues to end of data file.

Chapter 31

Data Presentation

Desmond F.S. Cormack and David C. Benton

The dissemination of research has long been, and continues to be, recognized as being crucial to the development of nursing's research base (Horsley *et al.*, 1983; Philips, 1986; Department of Health, 1993). However, not only have there been difficulties in gaining access to much of the material produced, but there have also been problems in comprehending some of the material. Data presentation, or to define it more explicitly, getting your results across and understood by your readers, is a critical element of any study.

By examination of the definition given, it is evident that it is not adequate to simply display results, since they must also be understood. Unless results are comprehended by your audience, there is no opportunity to receive feedback or for readers to consider and reflect on their own practice in the light of new information. It is essential that data are presented in a manner that is clearly understood via an appropriate medium, using an appropriate format, so as to facilitate both individual and our profession's development.

Data can be presented in many ways. The book that you are currently reading is a data source; it has a wealth of information about the research process. Hopefully, the information will be read, reflected upon, integrated into your personal knowledge base and used at some point in the future.

As you can see from this text, in addition to the written word you can also find numerical, graphical and pictorial data, all of which have particular strengths and weaknesses. Before dealing with each of these specific approaches, a number of general issues relating to data presentation are examined.

Data presentation techniques – general issues

The method chosen to present data is obviously dependent on a number of factors such as the type of data, the target readership and the overall design of your study. In today's technological world, there is an ever increasing number of aids which can be used to assist in the presentation of our material. If communication of results is to be effective, the appropriate use of technological aids must be made.

Whether these aids are used to prepare a scientific paper, a journal article, a book chapter or an overhead transparency, there are a number of fundamental principles which must be considered.

Computer technology has given the researcher, via the word processor and desk top publishing system, access to a wide variety of means of emphasizing data (Powell, 1989). Figure 31.1 lists a number of commonly available means of gaining readers' attention.

- Highlighting
- Capitals
- Size of print
- Markers and pointers
- Colour or variations of shading
- Change of colour
- Different fonts
- Indenting – sub-sections

Fig. 31.1   Approaches to gaining your readers' attention.

There are several means of *highlighting* data so as to enable them to stand out and attract attention. **Bold** and <u>underlining</u> can easily yet effectively help focus attention on a particular point. Another simple yet effective way of drawing attention to a point is to use CAPITALS. This can be particularly effective when the rest of the data are presented in lower case.

The ready availability of word processors and desk top publishing systems have given easy access to a number of techniques which were in the past only generally available to printers, graphic artists and designers. With new technological assistance, it is easy to produce **print in a variety of sizes**. This feature is particularly useful if you are using overhead transparencies or a poster presentation format. Unless data are presented in large bold characters, an audience will have great difficulty in seeing and hence interpreting the value of your work.

Markers or pointers in their simplest form may only simply be an asterisk, and are commonly used as a means of highlighting statistically significant associations (see Table 31.1). However with the introduction of new technology, much more sophisticated characters can be used. For example,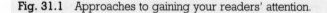

With high technology printers, it is possible to use either colour or variations in shade as a means of enhancing the clarity of data presentation. Colour laser pho-

Table 31.1   Correlation Table demonstrating pointers.

	Variable 1	Variable 2	Variable 3	Variable 4
Variable 1	1.000	0.857**	−0.486	−0.403
Variable 2		1.000	−0.771**	−0.692*
Variable 3			1.000	0.820**
Variable 4				1.000

$N=17$

1 tailed significance level $*P = 0.01$ $**P = 0.001$

tocopiers can produce material (at a cost) such as photographs or other figures which can add significantly to the quality of a presentation. Consider how effective it is to show a photograph of a wound rather than trying to accurately and succinctly describe it. However, great care must be taken when colour print is used on colour background. If an inappropriate choice is made the colours may clash or worse still, due to poor contrast, be illegible. As an example the colour combinations indicated in Fig. 31.2 are acceptable and easy to read.

Text colour	Appropriate background colour
White	Red, blue, black
Yellow	Blue, black
Cyan	Black
Green	Black
Red	White, yellow
Blue	White, yellow, cyan
Black	White, yellow, cyan

Fig. 31.2 Legible text and background colour combinations.

Even the most basic word processing systems offer the researcher the use of at least two *different fonts*. A font is the term given to a particular typeface in a particular size of print. Commonly a font such as italics is readily available in addition to a basic style. Italics is particularly useful for reporting quoted subject material. By incorporating both italics and *indenting*, verbal quotes from subjects can be effectively and efficiently identified from the main text. For example:

> *'We think new technology offers the researcher a great number of useful and easy to use means of improving the clarity and quality of data presentation'*

Unfortunately, new technology can be seductive and there is a danger that it will be over used. The net result is that instead of enhancing clarity, the effect is one of confusion resulting in poor data presentation. A good guide is to try and keep the number of techniques you use in any one table, text or figure, to a minimum. Use highlighting techniques to help get your message across, not just as a means of showing that you have the facility available.

Presenting data as text, numbers, graphs and pictures

Text

The written word is a useful and powerful means of getting views and results across, and is particularly efficient when an individual is attempting to describe a situation or event that is charged with emotion. It also has a potential ability to convey large amounts of data and considerable detail in a relatively compact form.

There are times, however, when such an approach is less than ideal. For example when reporting the results of a survey, it is common to see material presented in the following form:

'A total of 257 questionnaires were distributed of which 204 were returned. Of these, 87, 47, 39 and 31 were received from the Acute, Mental Health, Learning Disabilities and Community Services Units respectively.'

Data presented in this form, despite being accurate and factual, are unattractive from the visual and literary view point. More worrying is the point that such a presentation lacks clarity, for it requires considerable concentration and re-reading to ensure that the correct numbers are associated with the correct unit. Furthermore, the use of text to present numerical data gives the reader little visual assistance in relation to identifying trends or differences between groups.

It is not always possible to present data in descriptive formats; equally, it might be extremely difficult to do so. Consider how difficult it would be to describe the layout of your ward or office compared to the relative ease of drawing a plan.

Numbers, graphs and pictures

By using numbers, graphs and pictures as an alternative form of data presentation, you can take advantage of the reader's ability to interpret more visually stimulating material. How often have you flicked through a journal, stopping momentarily to examine an article which catches your eye, usually as the result of an interesting heading, graph, picture or table.

Visually dynamic data does not only attract an audience, but it can also be an efficient method of summarizing large quantities of information in such a way as to illuminate underlying trends. It is not always the case that the researcher takes an either/or decision and quite often will use both textual and graphical data presentation. The use of two approaches can help clarify the data and also emphasize their importance.

Tabular data presentation

Certain types of data do not lend themselves to textual presentation. Survey data often require the researcher to summarize findings in tabular form. For example, the skill mix of staff working in a hospital can be effectively and clearly displayed by use of a table (Table 31.2).

Presenting data in tabular form is perhaps one of the most common means of summarizing large quantities of numerical data. Despite the popularity of this approach, it is common for writers to produce tables which are poorly laid out and confusing to the reader. Common mistakes are inadequately descriptive titles, misaligned columns, use of abbreviations or units within data columns, omission of totals, totals that do not add up correctly and omissions of the number of respondents upon which the data are based, detracting from the quality and clarity of the presentation.

Table 31.2   Skill mix of nursing staff, by grade, in a medical unit.

Grade	Number of staff (N=47)	Percentage of staff in each grade
G	3	6
F	6	13
E	16	34
D	6	13
C	4	8
A	12	26
Totals	47	100

All percentages are rounded.

With the aid of new technology, many of these mistakes can be avoided and many of the basic problems of layout can be dealt with automatically. For example, the statistical package for the social sciences (SPSS) is now available on microcomputer and can present data in tables in an adequate and accurate manner, avoiding all the above flaws.

Tables are extremely useful and relatively easy to construct, but care is needed not to overload them with information. Always remember that the primary objective is to ensure that your reader gets the correct, accurate and clear information intended. It is far better to use two or more tables that are effective than one that leads to confusion.

Graphic presentation formats

There are several different ways of presenting data in a graphic form. In the past it has been necessary for writers who wish to present their data graphically to draw the figures by hand and then to physically 'stick' them into their report at the appropriate point. Thankfully, for those with access to new technology, all these steps can be automated. Data can be exported from statistical analysis packages into graphics packages and then electronically 'pasted' into the final report.

There are many programs available which will enable you to perform such activity. The specific program you may decide to use will be a personal choice which will inevitably be constrained by the type of computer you have access to and the amount of money you have to spend on the software. In view of the cost of some of these packages, it is recommended that you should attempt to negotiate access to such a facility through your employer. Most Health Authorities or Boards and Trusts will have these resources and people skilled in their use who can advise. Generally, the types of package that can be particularly useful when presenting data are integrated software packages. These packages incorporate word processors, spreadsheets, databases and graphics. In addition, desk top publishing systems that enable you to paste together the output from other programs such as stand alone word processing, statistical analysis or graphics packages are also available.

For those who cannot gain access to new technology, do not despair: all the graphical presentation formats that follow can be produced by hand. The end product can be just as effective, although it does take a little longer.

There are several types of graphs that can be used for data presentation. Examples of graphs that can be used include those of line and bar which may or may not be stacked. Furthermore it is possible to use either two or three dimensions when plotting data, thus further adding to the repertoire of actions available.

Whichever option is selected to present data, it is important that the scales on both axes are chosen appropriately. In most cases it is usual, as in Fig. 31.3, to plot the independent variable, in this case, 'months' along the x (horizontal) axis and the dependent variable, here, 'shifts lost due to sickness' along the y (vertical) axis. The scale for the dependent variable is extremely important since the scale can over- or underemphasize any trends present. A small gradual increase in sickness rate can be made to look extremely dramatic if the scale is so sensitive that a single day's sickness is represented by a visually dramatic rise. Great care and common sense are obviously required when selecting the scale.

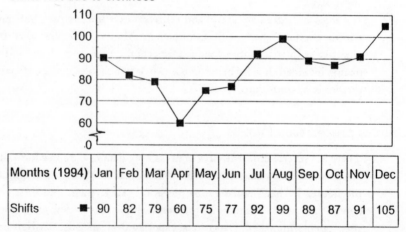

Months (1994)	Jan	Feb	Mar	Apr	May	Jun	Jul	Aug	Sep	Oct	Nov	Dec
Shifts	90	82	79	60	75	77	92	99	89	87	91	105

Fig. 31.3 Shifts lost due to sickness during 1994.

With the advent of new technology, some graphics packages will automatically scale the data for you and will attempt to emphasize differences of trends – trends are the tendency for a set of observations to increase, decrease or remain static in relation to time or some other variable. However, because of this feature sometimes these differences of trends are overemphasized. Under such conditions it may be necessary to over-ride the automatic scaling. The omission of the source of the data is also a frequent error and prevents the interested reader from checking it.

Certain issues are specific to the construction of various types of graph and these are dealt with in the following paragraphs.

Line graphs

Line graphs are particularly useful for displaying changes and are ideal for showing recurring patterns over time; it is important, however, to ensure that the timings along the horizontal axis are equal. A common error seen in graphical data presentation in line graph format is the omission of any discontinuities in the scale. That is, if the first scale point is, for example, '60' then the discontinuity between 0 and 60 should be indicated as in Fig. 31.3 (⪝).

There is no real limit as to the number of points that can be shown on a line graph; indeed, the greater the number, the more accurate any interpretation between points. However, for clarity, it is advisable to limit the number of lines (variables displayed) on any one graph to five or six, particularly if the lines frequently cross.

Bar graphs

This type of graph is one of the most commonly used in the presentation of data. The bar graph is particularly useful when trying to convey the concept of *leader* or where there are pre-set targets, since such an approach clearly demonstrates those who are meeting the goals and those who are not (see Fig. 31.4). Unlike line graphs, it is unusual to have discontinuities in the y axis since it is then necessary to show the discontinuity in each of the bars.

When drawing a bar graph, it is extremely important to keep the widths of the bars constant since it is in fact the area of the bar which conveys the information. Although Fig. 31.4 illustrates the presentation of variation along the x axis, it is more usual for the y axis to be used; that is variations in the height of the columns, rather than their length, convey the information.

Bar graphs are often *stacked* when the most important feature is to convey the

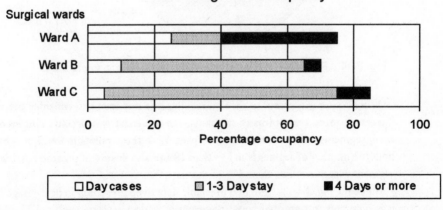

Fig. 31.4 Surgical unit bed occupancy for August 1994.

total magnitude of the dependent variable being measured. For example, there may be some interest in the breakdown of the component parts of the variable and it is then that the total magnitude can be shown as a sum of a number of elemental parts (see Fig. 31.4). It is important to note that, as in Fig. 31.4, it is necessary to illustrate the meaning of the elements by the inclusion of a legend.

Pie charts

Pie charts, as the name suggests, are circular in format. The overall circular structure is divided into segments which proportionally represent, by area, data to be presented. Many computer packages will generate the pie chart automatically, but if such a facility is unavailable, a pair of compasses for drawing the circle and a protractor for dividing it are required.

As an example, the data previously presented in Table 31.2 are displayed in the form of a pie chart in Fig. 31.5. The entire pie represents 100% of the data (47 members of staff). Since it is necessary to rotate compasses through an angle of 360° to fully describe the circumference of the circle, 1% of the data is represented by a segment with 360 ÷ 100° at the centre. Therefore every 1% of the data is multiplied by 3.6° to enable the segment to proportionally represent the percentage fraction of the data.

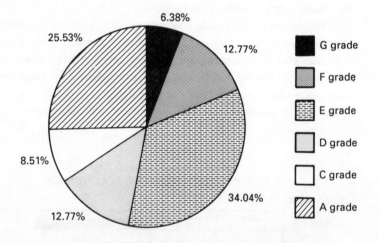

Fig. 31.5 Skill mix of 47 nursing staff by grade, in a medical ward.

When using pie charts to display results, it is important to consider the visual impact. If there are too many divisions, the pie chart will become cluttered and small segments will be difficult to interpret. With these points in mind, it is best to limit the number of segments to less than 10 and also ensure, if possible, that no one segment represents less then 5% of the data.

Since the pie chart is designed to enable data to be presented in percentage form, it is common to note that some researchers neglect to state the total number of subjects upon which the data are based.

Pie charts are labelled in several ways. First, it is possible to label each segment within the circumference, that is to superimpose the labelling upon the specific segments if both the segments and the pie chart are big enough. Second, it is common to see labelling attached to, or placed just outside, the circumference of the circle. Third, it is possible to use different types of shading and then use a suitable legend to define the various areas. Figure 31.5 uses two of these techniques: percentages are placed outside and adjacent to the various segments, but a legend is also used to define the meanings of the shades used.

Sociograms

Sociograms are particularly useful in the display of interactions between a number of individuals. Not only can they visually represent who talks to whom, but they can also be used to analyse the types and quantity of each member's contribution over a certain time period.

From the sociogram (Fig. 31.6), it is possible to identify those individuals who dominate group conversation (subject L), those who did not contribute (subject H), and those who form a sub-group (subjects E and F). A communication directed to the group as a whole is indicated by an arrow which goes to the centre of the figure.

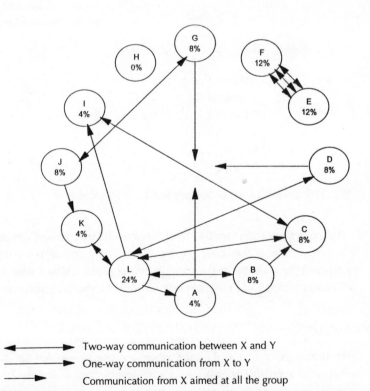

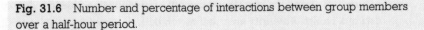

Fig. 31.6 Number and percentage of interactions between group members over a half-hour period.

Problems can arise with researchers who use too long a sampling time period, causing the sociogram to become cluttered and extremely difficult to interpret. Similarly, if the technique is being used by an observer to record the interactions of a very vocal group, it can be extremely challenging to ensure that all conversations occurring are noted.

Organizational chart

The purpose of an organizational chart is to demonstrate the (usually formal) managerial relationship and lines of responsibility between individuals or positions in various parts of an organization. Traditionally, health service provision is managed by means of a hierarchical management structure, although this has started to change significantly since the introduction of the NHS reforms. Figure 31.7 illustrates the use of the organizational chart as a means of succinctly representing the formal lines of communication within a functional unit of a health provider.

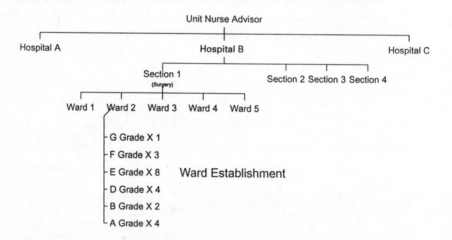

Fig. 31.7 Formal lines of communication in an acute unit.

Although these charts are frequently used to illustrate lines of communication, it is important to note that these are the 'official' or 'formally' recognized paths. In many cases these will not be the actual paths along which information flows and this can cause problems and mislead naive researchers who take things at face value.

Geographic mapping

This technique is frequently used when a researcher wishes to show the distribution of a variable in relation to a geographic area (Laborde *et al.* 1989). A geographic area can be an entire country, a county or even a postal code zone. Figure 31.8 shows the population density of individuals as identified from census data in a Health Authority area, and as can be seen increased population density is

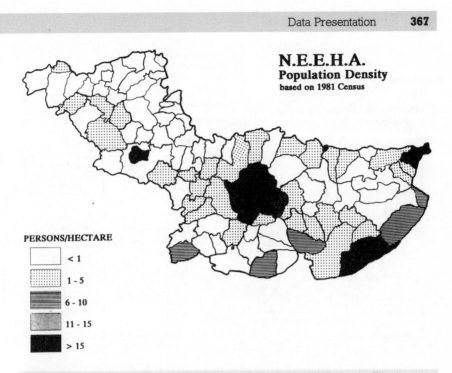

N.E.E.H.A.
Population Density
based on 1981 Census

PERSONS/HECTARE

☐	< 1
▦	1 - 5
▤	6 - 10
▨	11 - 15
■	> 15

Fig. 31.8 Population density for North East Essex Health Authority District based on 1981 census data (reproduced with permission from the North East Essex Health Authority).

represented by increasing depth of shading. Such a mapping as shown in Fig. 31.8 can be produced by hand, but with new technology it is possible to translate data directly from data files into the format by means of a suitable software package.

Flow charts

Originally, flow charts were used by systems analysts as a means of interpreting and representing the actions required to guide the development of computer software production. However, many researchers have recognized the utility of this approach for succinctly conveying to readers the relationship and sequential direction of ideas, concepts or propositions. Although it has a use which is, strictly speaking, often different from actual presentation of data, it remains a very useful and powerful tool for the researcher. The flow chart in Fig. 31.9 represents the phases in complaints handling.

Flow charts should have definite start and end points which are clearly defined, enabling readers to understand how the sequence of events is triggered and completed. The layout of flow charts is extremely important if clarity of information flow is to be ensured. The best and most easily understood charts should read from top to bottom, with feedback loops going in the reverse direction. Specific activities or processes should be included in rectangular boxes and decision points in diamond shapes.

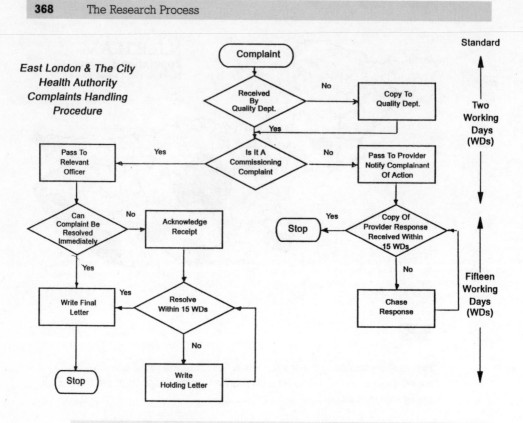

Fig. 31.9 Flow chart of complaints handling process.

Common errors seen in the production of flow charts include:

- The omission of decision conditions, that is, the requirements that have to be met before the particular path is followed.
- The omission of arrows to guide the reader through the chart.
- The cross-over of feedback paths over preceding sections of the chart.

Photographs

Both black and white and colour prints can be used as a means of presenting data which would be extremely difficult to show by other means. For example, photographs are an ideal medium to demonstrate pictorially 'before and after' views of some treatment such as the effects on posture of an intensive exercise programme on a child with multiple physical handicap.

Although the cost of producing the original photograph may be relatively inexpensive, the researcher, if planning to publish the material, should note that not all journals will accept photographic plates; equally, they may require a special size or type of negative. It is therefore essential, if considering submitting work for publication, that you should enquire about such points at an early stage. However, in recent years with the advent of sophisticated scanning equipment, it is now relatively straightforward for such material to be processed and integrated into reports and publications.

One positive point to bear in mind is the fact that most medical and nursing colleges may have a small illustrations department which may be quite willing to help with the production of photographic prints. These departments are usually both small and overworked so it is important to give sufficient warning if you require assistance. The production of monochrome or colour prints can be achieved by means of suitable photocopying machines, but although colour is perhaps more striking, it is also far more expensive. You should therefore assess the benefits versus the cost of using colour.

Blueprints – scale drawings

Blueprints or scale drawings are used to portray size, contents, position and spatial relationship of an item or area such as a hospital, ward or room. Figure 31.10 is an example of such a blueprint. If the blueprint needs to be drawn to scale, each of its parts must be carefully calculated, measured and drawn. While a scale drawing may be essential in some instances, it may not always be needed. The reader, however, must be informed whether or not it is a scale drawing.

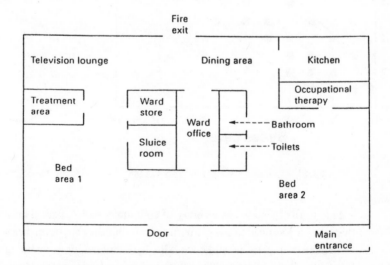

Fig. 31.10 Blueprint of ward 1 layout (not to scale).

Only items which are necessary should be included in the blueprint. If a major point of the presentation is to indicate the position of each of the rooms in the ward, it would obviously be inappropriate to include individual beds, hand wash basins and windows.

Scatter diagrams

Before the development and ready availability of computers, researchers who wished to examine data for correlations used the initial technique of plotting a scatter diagram. By plotting the value of the independent variable against the dependent variable, it is possible to visually determine whether there is likely to be a statistically significant correlation between the two variables. The decision can then be taken as to whether a statistical calculation should be performed. Examination of the overall shape of the data distribution pattern can reveal such information as positive, negative or no correlation between the variables. The closer the data pattern resembles a straight line, the greater the degree of correlation between the variables. It is common practice to encompass the data points so as to highlight the overall data pattern (Fig. 31.11).

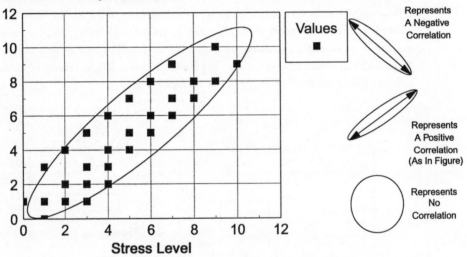

Fig. 31.11   Correlation between stress and days lost due to sickness.

Due to the increased availability of computers and statistical analysis packages, there is now less need to use scatter diagrams, but they are nevertheless a useful way of demonstrating to an audience who have limited understanding of statistical techniques the correlation between two variables under examination.

Contour plots

Perhaps the most readily recognized contour plot in the UK is that of the air pressure over the British Isles displayed by the weather forecasting service on television. In that plot, points of equal air pressure are connected, thus displaying a series of contour lines.

Contour plots are frequently used in diagnostic medical physics departments where the emission of radioactive isotopes are recorded as a means of identifying, for example, vascular lesions. However, researchers can put the technique to use for far less technologically based applications. For example, if you are interested in the effect of a new treatment on the granulation of a decubitus ulcer, it might be useful to plot the outline of the wound at specific time intervals. It would then be possible to calculate the rate of wound granulation for the patient. The technique would provide an objective, accurate, visual record, over time, of a healing process. Figure 31.12 illustrates the technique.

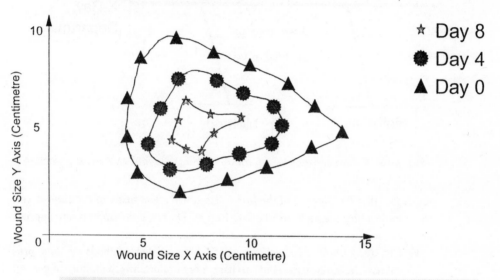

Fig. 31.12   Contour plot of outline of granulating wound.

Cause and effect diagrams

Cause and effect diagrams can be used to identify and illustrate the relationships between an effect or problem and possible causes or factors that contribute to it (McLaughlin & Kaluzny, 1994). Researchers can therefore use this tool to display results that are frequently conceptual or thematic. Cause and effect diagrams are sometimes called fishbone diagrams (see Fig. 31.13) and have been used in the field of quality improvement for many years and were originally developed by one of the great quality theorists Ishikawa in the early 1940s (McLaughlin & Kaluzny, 1994).

Conclusions

Many techniques are available for the presentation of data and if results are to have optimum impact, great care must be taken to ensure that the appropriate method is selected. Unless results are presented in a clear and visually dynamic format, readers may have difficulty in interpreting findings or, worse still, they may not be read. New technology offers a wide variety of aids which can enhance the standard of data presentation and reduce the time taken to prepare material. Nevertheless,

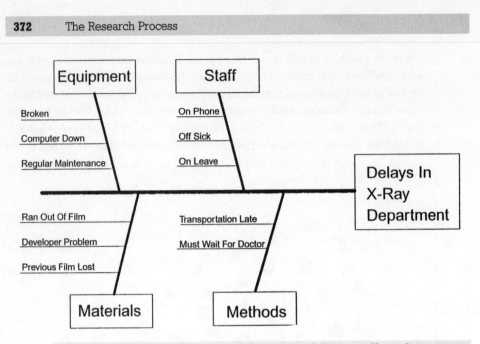

Fig. 3.13   Cause and effect diagram describing delays in an X-ray department.

remember that the purpose of the presentation will affect many of the choices you make in deciding the most appropriate format. Do not use inappropriate approaches just because they happen to be readily available to you.

Finally, throughout this chapter, specific specialized methods of data presentation have been illustrated but, perhaps more importantly, a number of general points have been emphasized. These points can be easily remembered by use of an acronym VACUME. That is, is the format Visually stimulating? Are the results Accurate, Clearly Understandable and Meaningful? Is the format chosen the most Efficient means of getting the message across? If the answer to all these questions is 'yes', then it is likely that you have made the correct choices.

References

Department of Health (1993) *Report of the Taskforce on the Strategy for Research in Nursing, Midwifery and Health Visiting.* Her Majesty's Stationery Office, London.

Horsley, J.H., Crane, J., Crabtree, M.K. & Wood, D.J. (1983) *Using Research to Improve Nursing Practice – A Guide. CURN Project.* Grune and Stratton, Orlando.

Laborde, J.M., Dando, W.A. & Hemmasi, M. (1989) Computer graphics – a tool for decision making in nursing. *Computers in Nursing,* 7(1), 15–20.

McLaughlin, C.P. and Kaluzny, A.D. (1994) *Continuous Quality Improvement In Health Care.* Aspen Publishers, Gaithersburg.

Philips, I.R.E. (1986) *A Clinician's Guide to the Critique and Utilisation of Nursing Research.* Appleton Century Crofts, Norwalk.

Powell, D. (1989) How to get your message across with maximum effect. *Business Graphics Review,* 1(1), 8, 10–11, 13.

Chapter 32

Reporting and Disseminating Research

Alison J. Tierney

The research process is not complete until a written report of the study which has been undertaken is prepared and disseminated. Through the activities of reporting and dissemination, the 'doer' of the research communicates with the potential 'users' and, of course, without this there is little point in having done the research in the first place.

This chapter looks at what is involved in writing a research report, preparing research papers for publication and, more generally, at research dissemination. The guidance given should be particularly useful for nurses who are writing up research for the first time. But, equally, the chapter may be helpful for others who are not doing research but who simply wish to learn about the research process. An understanding of how research reports and papers are structured helps one to read this kind of literature and, importantly, to evaluate it critically.

Writing a research report

Preparing a research report on completion of a study is a researcher's responsibility even when there is no obligation to do so. Usually there is this obligation. If the study has been supported financially, it is usual for the funding body to make the submission of a written research report one of the conditions of the grant contract. Many nursing research studies are not grant-supported but are carried out in an education context. In such circumstances the requirement would be in the form of a dissertation or thesis. However, even if there is no formal requirement to produce a written report – for example, in the case of a small, unfunded study carried out in the context of a nurse's work – there is still the need for some form of written research report. This need applies to small-scale studies as much as to large-scale research, and to studies which produce inconclusive findings as well as research which generates new insights and knowledge. It is from the written report that others can be made aware of the work, be able to critically appraise its relevance and, as appropriate, make use of its findings.

The format of a research report

Obviously, depending on the nature of the study and the circumstances, there are variations in the way research reports are written and in their length. A pilot study or small-scale project report may be quite short, containing only brief details of the background and method and with main findings succinctly presented. In contrast, a complex large-scale study is likely to merit a full report in order to provide a comprehensive account and discussion of all steps of the research process. If the research is being written up in the form of a thesis to be presented for a higher degree, there are specific requirements laid down by the education establishment concerned which govern the format and length of the report. In other cases, it may be that the grant-giving body specifies how the report is to be presented and in what amount of detail.

Although the style and length of presentation may vary, there is, in all cases, a basic format for a research report. This format is simply a logical reflection of the research process and, following the sequence of the steps, the report is usually structured into the following sections:

(1)   Introduction
(2)   Literature review
(3)   Method
(4)   Findings
(5)   Discussion
(6)   Conclusions and recommendations.

Some basic guidance is given below on each of these sections in turn. First, it may be helpful to suggest that much of the ground-work for the final report can be done long before the study itself is completed. As each stage of the research is completed, notes for the relevant section of the report can be made and even some first draft writing up attempted, for example, in the case of the literature review and method sections. By doing this, time will be saved (not to mention panic!) when work on the final report has to be got down to in earnest; the danger of forgetting details or mislaying vital information will be avoided; and, perhaps most important of all for the newcomer to this exercise, some valuable practice at writing will have been obtained.

Introduction

The very beginning of a research report needs to be especially clear and engaging if the reader is to be persuaded to venture further. First of all, there should be a clear statement of what the research was all about. It has been emphasized earlier in the book that the business of identifying and formulating the research question is a vital, but difficult, first stage of the research process (see Chapter 6). Assuming the task was accomplished properly, then it will not be difficult to provide a clear statement of the research aims in the introduction to the report.

It is also interesting, and often helpful, to outline the thinking which was involved in translating the original idea into the researchable question or hypothesis which the study was designed to explore, answer or test. It is useful, too, if the boundaries of the research are explained; in other words, what was *not* being studied as well as what *was* included. In explaining the focus and scope of the study, some background is often both interesting and informative; for example, the reader might be told what prompted the researcher's interest in the study, particularly if its origins lay in direct practice experiences or problems.

After reading the introductory section of the report, the reader should be clear about the precise nature of the research being reported and know something about its background and context.

Literature review

The tasks of searching and reviewing the literature have already been described (see Chapters 7 and 8) and, in the final report, an account of these early steps in the research process is given. This is not simply a case of listing a string of references which were consulted; nor is it an endless discourse on the literature. The aim is to present a distilled and critical analysis of the relevant literature, showing how the study being reported was based on previous research and existing knowledge, and how the new work was intended to take that forward. This is no easy task, even for experienced researchers. If a good job is made of it, however, the reader will benefit from the literature review in its own right as well as being able to judge the extent to which the present study was properly grounded. The reader is, of course, entitled to be informed about all relevant literature and all perspectives on the subject. This includes references to theories and studies which conflict with, as well as support, the perspective and approach adopted in the research.

Writing the literature review section of the report will be made easier if, as suggested earlier, some work has been done towards this already. It is, of course, imperative that references have been documented in full, and helpful if summaries and/or copies of material consulted were filed away carefully. At the stage of writing up, there will be little time available to hunt for lost references, check incomplete ones, or, even worse, scour the library for that crucial chapter in the book by Anderson (... or was it Henderson? ...), the one with the purple cover! Organization and diligence at the time of the original review of the literature will pay off when the final report has to be written up. All that remains to be done in terms of new reading is to cover more recently published work, noting any important new research which impinges on the present study.

When writing up the literature review section of the final report, a clear structure is needed; sub-headings facilitate this, even in a short review.

Method

Information about how the study was designed, planned and conducted is a vital part of a research report. A re-cap of the research problem/question(s) and a statement of the aims of the study should be given at the start of the method section. Thereafter, how this section is structured and presented needs to take account of the nature of the study and the method(s) employed.

With a more conventional research design, the description of the method is usually written up under a series of fairly standard sub-headings. After the research questions or hypothesis have been stated, the study setting is described and then the sample, this in terms of size, mode of selection, assignment to groups (if relevant), and consent procedure adopted. Any intervention must be detailed and data collection methods and instruments described, including any piloting and reliability testing undertaken. (Copies of instruments can be put in an Appendix to the report or offered as available on request.) Finally, methods of data analysis require to be described and statistical techniques explained.

In contrast, the method description of newer paradigm research (e.g. a qualitative study) may be less conventionally structured and is often more difficult to write up succinctly because the analytical processes are less linear and the distinctions between method and data analysis less clear-cut.

Whatever the approach, much of this information will be in written form already, in the research proposal. The proposal, however, will have been written in the future tense in terms of intentions, whereas, in the final report, the account is given in the past tense and is a description of how the study was carried out. Any significant changes made along the way should be explained, as should any major difficulties which were confronted. This information is important since it might suggest changes needed should the study be replicated and it also helps to bring the process of the research alive to the reader.

Findings

Unless described in the method section (under 'sample'), the characteristics of the sample are presented at the beginning of 'findings'. Specific characteristics such as age and sex, socio-economic status and health history, along with a description of the sample as a whole, provide background to the findings and their relevance. Response rates, for example to a questionnaire, are also reported at this stage.

Beyond that, how findings are presented really depends on their nature and the type of analysis undertaken. But, in all cases, this section of the report needs to be well organized so that the reader is taken through what was found in relation to the questions which the study set out to explore or answer.

In a qualitative study, findings are usually presented in terms of themes which emerged from the data and, by the way of substantiation and illustration, examples of raw data will be given (i.e. direct quotes from an interview transcription or accounts of observation). In contrast, quantitative analysis produces findings of a numerical type and much of the presentation will be in the form of tables (See Chapter 31). Each table must be numbered, given a legend and referenced in the text with explanation of statistical tests employed. The reader should not be expected to work out what all these tables show and what relationships were found. Such explanation is the responsibility of the reporter, as is comment on any inconclusive or contradictory findings or on results which were incidental (but interesting) or different from those which reasonably could have been expected.

Discussion

While some discussion may have been entered into in the course of presenting the various findings, the final discussion should provide a broader and deeper interpretation of the results of the study. This section of the report can be thought of as attempting to answer the question 'So what?'. The aim is to draw together the findings of the study and to discuss these in the light of what the research set out to do and in the context of previous research and the current state of knowledge of the subject.

For the reader, the results of this task should be illuminating and so should it be for the researcher. Preparing the discussion involves more thinking than any other part of the research process except perhaps the very beginning stage of teasing out the research idea in the first place. What is being provided by the discussion is an explanation of the meaning of the research findings – their inherent limitations as well as their value.

Conclusions and recommendations

From the discussion, the conclusions should follow fairly obviously and these require to be stated clearly and succinctly. On the basis of the conclusions, recommendations can be made concerning the implications of the study for practice, education, management and future research. By doing this, the researcher will stimulate and assist the readers to consider the relevance of the recommendations in relation to their own circumstances as well as appreciating the more general relevance of the study to nursing knowledge. This, after all, is the point of reporting research.

Publishing research

In the course of describing how a research report is written, numerous references were made to 'the reader' because, obviously, the only reason for producing a written research report is for others to read it. As such, however, research reports seldom have a wide readership. Reports in the form of a thesis or dissertation will be stored in a university or college library and borrowed only by students and the occasional outsider who finds out about the work and has a particular interest in it. Research reports submitted to a grant-giving body or steering committee, or clinical colleagues, will be scrutinized with interest by those groups but are unlikely to be disseminated more widely. Thus, for the most part, written research reports are not made widely accessible and, indeed, may be too detailed in that form for the needs of a wider readership. If the researcher is to make the work known more widely and available for public access, then the research needs to be published.

There are many reasons why publication of research is especially important in the case of nursing. Research is still a relatively recent development in nursing and much of the work is still in the form of small-scale, one-off studies. Further research will be all the more useful if it builds on studies previously undertaken and, for this to be done, there needs to be access to earlier work in published form. It is not only intending researchers who need access to this material. Students and teachers need it too if research is to be incorporated into nurse education. And, clearly, for nursing practice to be developed and changed on the basis of research, then those members of the profession who are in a position to bring this about – the practitioners and the managers – must also be kept informed through publication of the findings of recent research. The potential readership of nursing research is both large and varied and not confined only to members of the nursing profession.

Preparing research for publication

A number of decisions must be taken before any actual work begins on the reformulation of the research report into a form suitable for publication. The researcher has to decide what would be most useful to have published; how many publications are merited; who each of these is intended for; where publication would be most suitable in order to reach the targeted readership; and the form of presentation which would be most appropriate.

If it seems that the written research report or thesis merits publication more or less in full, then length dictates that this will be in the form of a book or monograph. Usually publishers are only interested in a research publication of this type if it is of sufficiently wide interest to be commercially viable. There are a few publishers, however, with an interest in publishing nursing research monographs.

Publishing research material in the form of journal articles is much more common and, indeed, has a number of advantages over publication in book form. An article is usually in print much more quickly than a book, an important consideration when the subject is research. Journal articles are also much more likely to be read by many more nurses than a research monograph and, depending upon the journal selected, an article can be targeted at a particular section of the profession. Journal articles differ from monographs in two main respects: they are shorter, and they are selective in the aspects of the research reported.

What the researcher should not do is write an article and then look around for a journal willing to publish it. This sounds rather obvious but it is something that is often done by inexperienced writers. Before putting pen to paper, there are various decisions to be made.

Deciding on the focus

From the outset, it must be clear what is to be covered in the article. If it is considered that general rather than detailed information about the study would be most useful, the article could take the form of a resumé of the total research study (really an abridged form of the written research report). In another case it might be the findings of the study which merit concentration, particularly if these appear to be potentially influential on nursing practice. Alternatively, the focus of an article might be the research method employed, or perhaps even more specifically, the particular data collection instruments used or developed in the study. Or it may be that the most useful type of publication is the literature review undertaken. Usually there is sufficient material of interest and importance in any one research study to merit several articles rather than just one.

Identifying the readership

Once the topic for the article is clarified, it is important to turn attention to another issue: who the publication is intended for. Being clear about this is vitally important. Every journal has a quite distinct readership and so identifying the intended readership is essentially synonymous with selecting the right journal.

If the article being planned is aimed at a large and varied readership then the researcher should seek publication in a nursing journal which has a large circulation among nurses representing various levels and branches of the profession – *Nursing Times* or *Nursing Standard* would be the likely choice in this case. If the article is of special relevance to nursing practice, a journal which caters especially for practising nurses may be most suitable: the *Journal of Clinical Nursing*, the *Journal of Gerontological Nursing*, or *Cancer Nursing*, to mention some examples. However, if the research is concerned with an aspect of nursing education, and the article planned is aimed at nurse educators, then *Nurse Education Today* would be a suitable choice. If the article is to be longer, and intended for readers with knowledge of research methods, the *Journal of Advanced Nursing* might be selected. For an article of interest to an international readership, the researcher might seek publication in the *International Journal of Nursing Studies*.

The journals named above are simply mentioned to illustrate the point that selection of the journal is dependent on having clearly identified the targeted readership. In some cases, the researcher may consider it appropriate to seek publication in a non-nursing journal or a multidisciplinary journal (for example, *Health and Social Care in the Community*) if the research has relevance for other health care professions or academic disciplines.

If the choice of journal does not immediately seem obvious, then a helpful step is to spend time in a library which is well stocked with a wide range of current periodicals. Browsing through many different journals, even quite quickly, is a good way of getting to know their various readerships and assessing likely interest in the research material you have available. The guidelines for contributors which each journal produces usually give a clear idea of the focus and scope of its content.

Structuring the paper

The decision about which journal to write for to a great extent predetermines the length, format and style of the article. Careful scrutiny of back issues of the selected journal will provide a good idea of how a scientific paper should be presented. Most journals have specific guidelines concerning length, format and style of presentation, including illustrations and style of references. If the journal does not carry notice of these, the editor will provide guidelines for prospective authors on request. It is vital that a manuscript is submitted in accordance with the guidelines. An article should not be submitted to more than one journal at a time.

With all this planning accomplished, there is only one job left to do – to sit down and write the article for publication!

Writing for publication

The actual prospect of writing for publication often seems daunting to those with no experience and, perhaps, a self-consciousness about writing. Nurses seem particularly prone to thinking that writing for publication is something which only the exceptionally talented can accomplish! Writing *well* is, of course, a very skilled activity and there is no simple formula to follow. There is no quick and easy way to write and it is perhaps reassuring for the rest of us to realize that people who do have a flair for self-expression and a good command of language and grammar are the exception rather than the rule. Mostly, writing is a slow, laborious and often frustrating business but, when done, it gives a great sense of satisfaction and accomplishment.

The key is to allow plenty of time for writing (and, even more important, for rewriting), and not to become discouraged by the slow progress or the seemingly disproportionate number of drafts consigned to the wastepaper basket! Some of the hints about writing for publication which are given below may be helpful. These, of course, are equally pertinent to the business of writing a research report.

Planning the writing

The drafting of an article for publication becomes instantly easier if sufficient time is spent on planning it out. This involves making an outline, which consists of headings and sub-headings, with brief notes of the main points to be included under each. This exercise helps to organize ideas and material logically and into a sequence. It also divides the writing task into manageable portions, so making it all less daunting. Most journals restrict the length of particular kinds of articles so, bearing this in mind, each section can be allocated an approximate number of words so that, from the start, there is a clear sense of how much detail can be afforded.

Drafting

Once a satisfactory outline has emerged, and thought has been given to the content, a first draft of the article can be attempted. It may be helpful to start at the beginning, but it is often encouraging to work first on the parts which seem the easiest to write. Knowing how important it is for the introduction to be clear and engaging, starting here can often result in getting quickly bogged down in pursuit of inspiration and perfection. Better just to get writing. The putting together of all the sections of the article, each linking logically with the next, is a job which can be done later.

Once an initial draft is done, the next step is to re-read it carefully and review it critically and objectively. Revision and rearrangement are usually needed. If you are using a word processor, this is a relatively easy and rather enjoyable job. If drafting with pen and paper, the same process of rearrangement can be done by 'cutting and pasting', with revisions marked up alongside. The goal at this stage is to produce a paper which is organized in a sensible way, which deals with the points to be covered in the various sections, and which, overall and in its parts, is balanced and approximately of the right length.

Finalizing the paper

Even when the paper is in final draft, however tedious, a final stage of work still remains. This involves one last, but detailed, check of the finished research paper. What is being looked for now is that each sentence conveys what was intended: every detail is correct (check especially the accuracy of data, quotations, references and cross-references); language and grammar are as good as possible; spelling and punctuation are correct; and the style is readable, even if not remarkable. Improving and refining writing takes a lifetime of practice, but many of the features of poor writing can be avoided if adequate time and concentration are invested on this final stage of the process.

A frequent criticism of research publications is that they are too full of technical language and jargon. Avoiding unnecessary terms greatly extends the readership but, if such terms need to be used, their meaning should be explained. Nursing, like other disciplines, runs the risk of becoming jargon-laden. The goal should be concise and natural language, and this is especially important if nursing research is to be read and appreciated by all members of the profession. Many journals now not only encourage, but require, 'reader-friendly' research writing. A scientific paper need not be boring!

Preparing tables, references, appendices

A research report or article normally involves a combination of text and visual forms of presentation of data. Tables, graphs and charts can be valuable for presenting complex information in a concise and ordered way. But, if poorly presented or too complicated, they can confuse the reader. Each table must be numbered, accompanied by an explicit legend, and placed in the report or article following the reference to it. Any necessary explanation of the table or figure should be provided in the text (see Chapter 31 for a full discussion of data presentation).

It is essential for one standard style of referencing to be used consistently throughout the report or article; in this book, the Harvard system is adopted. This particular style involves reference to the surname of the author(s) and year of publication in the text, with the full reference provided in the reference list at the end, ordered alphabetically by authors' surnames. Alternatively, a numbering system can be used: numbers are inserted in the text and then the references are detailed in a numbered list at the end of the paper. Whichever system is employed, details of references should be checked and double checked.

A written research report (although not usually a journal paper) is likely to contain appendices for the inclusion of material which is too lengthy or too detailed to include in the body of the report – for example, a copy of a questionnaire used. Appendices are placed at the end of the report and referred to at the appropriate point in the text.

The contents (i.e. chapter and/or section titles), appendices, tables and figures should be at the front of the report. The full range of items which may precede the text of the report are:

(1)   Title page
(2)   Contents page
(3)   List of tables and figures
(4)   Preface
(5)   Acknowledgements
(6)   Abstract.

In a research paper intended for publication in a journal, any acknowledgements would normally be inserted at the end. The inclusion of an abstract (at the beginning) is usually a requirement.

Preparing an abstract

An abstract (a concise summary) is a useful feature of a research report or article; it is usually a requirement in a thesis. It is also possible to have an abstract of a research report published in its own right. Abstracts of nursing studies are printed, for example, in *Nursing Research Abstracts* published by the Department of Health (see Chapter 7 for further details).

Titling the report or article

Although the title is the first thing a reader looks at, it is very often the last thing the author of a research report or article attends to. It is extremely important for a research publication to have a meaningful and unambiguous title. Nurse authors (and, dare it be said, editors of some nursing journals) still sometimes show a preference for titles which are intriguing and anecdotal, but which are not always informative and are sometimes downright misleading. It is the title which clarifies the topic of the research being described and gives the potential reader an indication of the content and scope of the report or article. More importantly, the title is reproduced in references, bibliographies, indexes and abstracts. As literature retrieval through on-line computer systems uses 'key words', it is vital for the title to contain the most relevant words. Nurse researchers should not be tempted to dream up clever but totally useless titles for their reports and publications – these can be reserved for that bestselling novel, yet to be written!

Preparing the manuscript for submission

A research report or article must be produced in typed form and in strict accordance with the guidelines on presentation which are laid down by the educational establishment (in the case of a thesis), publisher or journal in question. A writer who is not an experienced typist should have their manuscript retyped (or tidied up on disk) by a professional secretary.

Only one job – careful proofreading – remains to be done before the hard work is over and the report or article is at last ready to be submitted.

Disseminating research

The completion of a written report and the preparation of articles for publication are really only the starting point of research dissemination and not, as is sometimes assumed, the job completed. Making available the information in written form cannot automatically ensure that the research becomes known about and appreciated, or that appropriate use will be made of its findings.

As Florence Nightingale wrote in a margin note on her draft of the Report of the Sanitary Commission on the Health of the Army (July 1857) 'Reports are not self-executive'. Serious attention to the matter of disseminating research, however, has only very recently come to the fore. The nursing profession is not alone in its neglect of this matter. Dissemination has been equally neglected in health services research and, indeed, in industry there has been longstanding concern that science does not adequately impact on new technology and work practice.

Strategic developments

In 1990, the UK Department of Health published a document called *Taking Research Seriously* (HMSO, 1990), the aim being to improve research dissemination and use through a strategic approach at policy level and greater activity on the part of researchers themselves.

Building on this, the *Research and Development Strategy for the National Health Service* (HMSO, 1991) addressed the need for strategic initiatives in the area of dissemination, and facilities for central review and widespread distribution of research findings have since been established. Integrating nursing research in this information systems strategy is one of the key objectives of the *Report of the Taskforce on the Strategy for Research in Nursing, Midwifery and Health Visiting* which was published in 1993 (DoH, 1993) and which is steering nursing research development in the UK through the 1990s.

Responsibilities of researchers

In *Taking Research Seriously* (HMSO, 1990), it is made clear that researchers must assume *principal* responsibility for dissemination, this specified in terms of the following:

- Write time for dissemination into research plans and proposals.
- Complete reports and publications on time.
- Target publications to specific audiences.
- Prepare attractive and accessible material.
- Produce and distribute summaries of the research.
- Disseminate research imaginatively and widely.

Picking up on these recommendations, the Annex on dissemination and implementation of research findings to the publication by DoH (1993) draws particular attention to the value of *speaking* about research as well as writing.

Nurse researchers can accept and seek opportunities to talk about their research at anything from large conferences and international meetings to small-scale study days and in-service education sessions. Giving talks is a particularly effective way for the researcher to communicate research findings to others. In particular, talks can be targeted at practising nurses who may well be in the best position to consider the implications of research for nursing practice.

For the researcher, a talk is not only a means of information giving, but also of stimulating questioning and discussion. However, preparing and giving talks and engaging in face-to-face discussion is a time-consuming business and allowance of time needs to be made for researchers to concentrate solely on this dissemination phase. Increasingly, nurse researchers are making more use of modern audio–visual technology to disseminate research findings in an appealing way to a wider audience. There are signs, too, that radio and television and the national press are beginning to be seen as vehicles for publicising the profession's science more widely.

Thus, there are signs that the government, the researchers and the profession are beginning to attach a higher priority to research dissemination. This, at last, is a step in the right direction towards ensuring that research which has been undertaken and adequately reported has the best possible chance of being put to good use.

References

DoH (1993) *Report of the Taskforce on the Strategy for Research in Nursing, Midwifery and Health Visiting*. Department of Health: Research and Development Division (RD3), Quarry House, Quarry Hill, Leeds LS2 7UE, UK, with annexes published by the Royal College of Nursing, London.

HMSO (1990) *Taking Research Seriously: Means of Improving and Assessing the Use and Dissemination of Research*. Her Majesty's Stationery Office, London.

HMSO (1991) *Research for Health: A Research and Development Strategy for the National Health Service*. Department of Health, HMSO, London.

Further reading

Cormack, D.F.S. (1994) *Writing for Health Care Professions*. Blackwell Scientific, Oxford.

Tornquist, E.M. (1987) *From Proposal to Publication: An Informal Guide to Writing about Nursing Research*, 2nd edn. Addison-Wesley, California.

Watson, G. (1987) *Writing a Thesis: A Guide to Long Essays and Dissertations*. Longman, Harlow.

Part III

The Use of Research Nursing

The main reason for undertaking research is that it be used by practitioners, educators and managers. The three chapters in the final part of this book will be of use to those who make use of, and facilitate, nursing research in nursing practice (see Chapter 33), nursing education (see Chapter 34) and nursing management (see Chapter 35). These chapters also apply to potential researchers in these areas who are considering a possible focus for their own research. Although each of these topics is dealt with individually, it is recognized that considerable overlap and similarity exists.

The ability to make use of completed studies, and to initiate or facilitate new ones, depends on a firm understanding of the research process generally. For this reason, this section, dealing with the use of nursing research, is placed at the end of this text.

Chapter 33

Research in Nursing Practice

Alison J. Tierney

'Applying research findings in nursing practice is perhaps the biggest challenge facing nursing research' (Sheehan, 1986). This remains true.

The preceding chapter stressed the importance of effective dissemination of research findings. Dissemination which is targeted at those who are in position to use research in practice, and in a form which encourages its use, is especially important if research is to make its proper impact on patient care. The *raison d'etre* of research in nursing is, after all, to improve the quality of patient care and to increase the effectiveness and efficiency of the nursing service. The mere existence of research cannot in itself alter nursing practice; research has to be *used*.

Using research is a complex task; this is true for all applied disciplines, not just nursing. In nursing, however, we have been slow to appreciate the complexities of 'research utilization'. It tends to have been assumed that use of research in practice would somehow 'just happen' if only researchers reported their findings and practising nurses read their reports.

The apparent lack of research use in nursing practice is discussed in the first part of this chapter. The need to understand the notion of 'research utilization' is then addressed. Finally, the challenge of improving research utilization in nursing practice is explored. This chapter does not provide simple guidelines for the use of research in nursing practice. Rather, it seeks to stimulate readers into thinking more deeply about an issue which tends to have been oversimplified and neglected but which now, in the context of a fast-changing health service in which the crucial importance of research and development are better recognized (HMSO, 1991), is an issue which can no longer be ignored.

Research use

As the amount of research in nursing continued to expand through the 1970s and 1980s, so too did concern about what was seen to be its apparent lack of impact on, and use in, practice. In a hard-hitting analysis of clinical nursing, Walsh & Ford (1989) drew attention to numerous examples of regular practice which appeared to ignore research evidence. They argued that much of nursing practice remained rooted in myth and traditional ritual, with nurses acting in these ways because 'this is the way it has always been done'. They asked questions about why, for example, nurses spent time drying out a pressure sore with piped oxygen when research had shown that the best environment for wound healing is a moist one; about why patients continued to be subjected to unnecessarily long pre-operative fasting times in the face of all the evidence of its adverse effects; about why pre-operative skin preparation had failed to change in the light of all the research; and so on. Perhaps the most catching of their examples is 'the myth of the salt bath'. Walsh & Ford (1989) referred to studies which suggest, on the one hand, that there is no evidence to support the notion of the salt bath as therapeutic for infected wounds and, on the other hand, surveys which indicated regular continuation of this practice. While it may not be dangerous, it is at the very least a waste of nurses' time ... not to mention the good salt! Were Walsh and Ford to look again now for examples of nursing practices which fly in the face of research evidence, no doubt they would still find plenty to write about.

Why isn't research used?

'Why don't we use the findings?' was the question asked by Hunt (1984) in an early article on the issue of lack of use of research in nursing practice. Hunt suggested several reasons. Some of these are what could be regarded as deficiencies in nurses themselves: for example, their lack of knowledge of research and disinclination to 'believe' the findings. Other reasons given reflect deficiencies in the system; for example, the lack of encouragement and incentive for nurses to use research in practice. Greenwood (1984) concurred with this analysis but, in explaining why 'the impact of research findings on the clinical nurse and her work is minimal', he ventured to suggest that:

'Clinical nurses do not perceive research findings as relevant to their practice because frequently they are *not* relevant ...' (emphasis added).

It is certainly true that practising nurses have expressed criticism of nursing research as an essentially academic exercise which can seem remote from, and largely irrelevant to, their practice. This was a common criticism in the early years of research development in nursing in the UK. Even then there were examples of research findings which were very obviously relevant to practice but, even so, appeared not to being used: for example, research relating to the prevention and management of pressure sores. Much of that research had very directly relevant implications for practice and yet, as Gould (1986) discussed, the findings were not being applied.

What can be concluded from all of this? Does the problem lie with researchers failing to effectively disseminate research findings? Or is it that practising nurses and nurse managers do not keep up-to-date with research or, if they do, are simply failing to appreciate its relevance for practice? Or do they possess this knowledge and appreciation but, for whatever reason, find themselves unable to make use of it in practice? The answer is that we really do not know because there has been so little investigation of research utilization in nursing.

Studies of research use

The few studies which have been undertaken on use of research in nursing are, therefore, interesting. In the USA, Ketefian (1975) investigated nurses' use of research findings related to temperature taking. She chose this topic because it represented a commonplace nursing activity and, further, because the research findings had been published widely, and had been available for some time and, importantly, had been reported with the implications for practice clearly stated. Despite this, Ketefian found that only one of the 87 registered nurses studied knew the correct way to take oral temperature and, indeed, many used this site while believing it to be less accurate than rectal temperature assessment. She concluded that 'the practitioner was either totally unaware of the research literature ... or, if she was aware of it, was unable to relate to it or utilize it.'

A rather more optimistic picture emerged from a later study by Brett (1987). She identified 14 nursing research findings and, from data collected from 216 practising nurses in hospitals of varying size, assessed their awareness of, persuasion about and use of the findings. The majority reported awareness of most of the findings and, for seven of the innovations, felt persuaded about use in practice. Actual use of various findings varied greatly but at least one (relating to closed sterile urinary drainage) was in routine use. Brett concluded that 'at least for the group of nurses and innovations studied and reported here, the findings suggested that research dissemination and use is occurring'.

Lacey's (1994) study of research utilization among nurses in two general hospitals in the UK also found some positive evidence of use of research in practice, for example in the form of research-based protocols for wound care. But, again, this was a small-scale investigation with methods being piloted and so its results are not widely generalizable.

If little is known about the extent of research utilization in nursing, even less is understood about what effects or inhibits it. An attempt to explore this was made by Champion & Leach (1989) in relation to the variables of:

(1)   Support from the work environment.
(2)   Availability of research findings.
(3)   Nurses' attitudes.

From data on self-reported use of research findings in practice from a sample of 59 nurses, both perceived availability of research findings and a positive attitude towards research were strongly related to research utilization.

In an overview of reported obstacles and solutions to the integration of research in nursing practice, Bassett (1992) categorizes the constraints as:

(1)   Educational.
(2)   Communicational.
(3)   Organizational.

It is clear that, in broad terms, study to date of research use in nursing serves to reinforce the importance of a positive attitude towards research being encouraged in the process of nurse education as well as the need for effective dissemination of research findings to practising nurses.

But even if nurses were to feel positive towards research and be informed about research, the use of research in practice would not automatically follow. Closs & Cheater (1994) argue that widespread improvements are needed to achieve the type of culture, level of interest and extent of support which are required for active utilization of nursing research to succeed. There is also the need for nurses to understand the *nature* of research utilization and how to act on this knowledge.

Understanding research utilization

Fawcett (1984) pointed out:

> 'In the past, many nurses expected all nursing research to have immediate applicability for practice. This expectation probably was based on a mis-understanding of knowledge utilization ...'

Research rarely produces new knowledge which is instantly usable. Certainly, any single nursing study is unlikely to result in a straightforward and immediate pre-scription for practice. To expect this is to misunderstand the processes of knowledge building and utilization of knowledge and, as a result, to devalue research.

In nursing especially, where much of the research to date has been small-scale and both exploratory and descriptive in nature, it is inappropriate to expect results which are immediately applicable. The production of explanatory and predictive knowledge for practice can only be obtained through larger-scale and longer-term cumulative investigation and, importantly, with the replication of studies to test applicability and generalizability of findings.

But even if research studies do not have any obvious or legitimate direct application to nursing practice, it is seldom the case that there is no potential for utilization. Appreciating that 'utilization of research' and 'implementation of research findings' are not synonymous is a helpful starting point in thinking through this argument. It is also useful to distinguish between 'direct' and 'indirect' uses of research.

Direct uses of research

Horsley (1985) highlights a helpful but rarely made distinction between using the *products* of research (i.e. the findings), and using the *methods*.

Using research findings

The most obvious direct use of research is when findings do have potential for application in practice. Here, we *are* talking about 'implementation of findings'. Findings from research which justify implementation (albeit with need for on-going review as new knowledge becomes available) are now available in relation to many nursing practices and across the range of patient/client groups with which nurses work (for an overview see, for example, Macleod Clark & Hockey, 1989, or Smith, 1994). In a few areas there is now a well-developed research-based body of knowledge to underpin nursing practice. Perhaps the outstanding example is patient teaching: Wilson-Barnett (1989) describes this as one of the few aspects of nursing care which have been subjected to rigorous analysis through original and replicated research. Reflecting on 25 years of patient education research in nursing, Redman (1993) concluded that 'the research base ... show(s) patient education to be an effective intervention'. A set of 'generalizations' which provide clear guide-lines for the use of the accumulated research in practice is provided by Lindeman (1988) on the basis of her comprehensive and critical review of the patient education literature.

The increasing availability of research reviews and meta-analyses in the nursing literature should greatly assist practising nurses with the challenge of *using* research findings in practice. Many of the nursing journals now publish research reviews regularly; and the *Taskforce on the Strategy for Research in Nursing, Midwifery and Health Visiting* (DoH, 1993) has recommended that the Review Commissioning Facility set up under the auspices of the overall *Research and Development Strategy for the NHS* (HMSO, 1991) should build a nursing and midwifery dimension into their programme and be commissioned to undertake and publish regular critical overviews of research in specific fields.

Using research methods

Although the findings of a particular research study (or even a set of studies) may not be sufficiently robust for legitimate use in nursing practice, the *methods* employed may well be directly useful in practice (Horsley, 1985). Increasingly, nursing research studies are using (or validating) measurement instruments and many of these have potential for use in nursing practice for purposes of patient assessment and/or evaluation of the outcomes of nursing intervention. From nursing research on the topic of patients' pain and its management, for example, methods for assessing pain can be found: these range from detailed questionnaires to simple rating scales. Kitson (1994) provides a short description of the main types of instruments available and, although each has limitations, such instruments can be useful in practice. Indeed, with the increasing emphasis throughout the health service on 'outcomes' and 'effectiveness' and 'quality' of care, there is an urgent need for reliable methods of outcome measurement and quality assessment. The transfer of research methods and instruments into nursing practice is, therefore, an increasingly important area of direct research utilization.

Indirect uses of research

Seeing the usefulness of research only in terms of its potential for direct use, however, is to ignore its contribution to 'enlightenment'. The concept of 'an enlightenment model' of social research is contrasted with 'the technological approach' of natural science in Robinson's (1987) discussion of the relationship of knowledge to action.

A similar idea was conveyed by Stetler & Marram (1976) in their use of the term 'cognitive applications' of research. Stetler & DiMaggio (1991) use the term 'conceptual' (as distinct from 'instrumental'). By this they mean using research findings to enhance one's understanding of a situation. Almost by definition, all research and certainly all descriptive studies, encourage reflection and extend understanding of nursing practice. Many examples from the nursing research literature come to mind in support of this suggestion.

Thinking back to some of the earliest research, one obvious example is the work which Stockwell (1972) published under the title *The Unpopular Patient*. That study set out to establish whether there were some patients who nursing staff enjoyed caring for more than others and, if so, why were some patients more or less 'popular' and did the 'unpopular' patients receive 'less good' nursing care? While a great deal was 'found out' by this study, it did not really produce findings with potential for direct use. Nevertheless, it was enlightening. Surely that study could not have failed to stimulate nurses who read it to reflect on their own relationships with patients and, thereafter, to be more sensitive to factors and circumstances which might influence how they regarded and treated different patients.

Enlightenment of this kind is to be found particularly in nursing studies which have explored little researched areas of practice through qualitative/phenomen-ological methods. For example, although there can be few community nurses who do not appreciate the significance for parents of caring for a chronically ill child, their 'lived experience' is brought alive in a remarkably enlightening way by Whyte's (1994) detailed study of four families caring for a child with cystic fibrosis and Jerrett's (1994) account of the experiences of parents of ten children with juvenile arthritis. Neither study produced 'results' which could be 'implemented' in practice but each provides invaluable insights into the complexity of parents' experiences and, for community nurses, these could not fail to be 'useful' by influencing, albeit indirectly, their commitment to providing support for families in which there is a chronically sick or handicapped child.

Perhaps, if the indirect value of research was more explicitly recognized, and particularly so among practising nurses, then research in general would become more appreciated. The personal benefit to be gained from reading research reports would also become more obvious. For individual nurses, the feeling of being powerless to implement research findings in practice would then be offset by the knowledge that at least their own thinking had been extended, and become more enlightened.

Improving research utilization

Improving nurses' knowledge of research and their understanding of the com-plexities of research utilization is crucial, but not, in themselves, sufficient to ensure that research will be better used in nursing practice. The potential for research use in practice needs to be more clearly articulated by researchers and more systematically assessed by practitioners and managers. And once the potential for the use of research is recognized, the process of research utilization can begin. This requires planning, management and conditions which are conducive for change; and, of course, all of that requires resources – both human and material.

Identifying potentially useful research

The first step, then, towards improving research use in practice is for *potential* use to be better recognized. Researchers in general tend to be hesitant about pointing out how their research might be used. Quite reasonably, academic researchers may have no real interest or necessary concern with 'what gets done' with their research. Their primary concern is to contribute to the generation of knowledge and to stimulate further research. And so, reasonably, they concentrate on reporting the theoretical and methodological aspects of a research study and discuss the findings in that context.

There are good reasons why nurse-researchers should go beyond that, attempting to delineate the consequences of their work in terms of its potential for application in practice. Tornquist *et al.* (1989), in an article on writing research reports for clinical audiences, make just that point. What practising nurses need, they argue, is a readable research report which provides adequate information about the study method, and a clear presentation of the findings; but, most of all, they need a full and helpful discussion of the relevance and potential usefulness of the research for nursing practice.

Given that, practising nurses are more likely to see the potential for use of research in practice. The researcher's recommendations should not be unconditionally accepted, of course. The importance of critical appraisal of research has been emphasized elsewhere in this book (see Chapter 8) and the ability to assess the validity and relevance of newly published findings becomes ever more crucial as the amount of nursing research increases.

In judging the relevance of research to practice, whatever the field, a number of issues need to be considered. According to Robinson (1987) these are:

(1) The relevance of the research findings to actual day-to-day work.
(2) The quality, objectivity and cogency of the study itself.
(3) The plausibility of the research given prior knowledge, values, and experience.
(4) The explicit guidance which is given for the feasible implementation of the research.
(5) The challenge presented to existing assumptions, practice, and arrangements.

Many factors are involved, therefore, in decision-making about research utilization in practice. The potential user is not only challenging the robustness of the research, but is also being challenged by its findings. Even if the findings are judged to be relevant, the feasibility of their application cannot be taken for granted. There is a need to assess the readiness and receptiveness of the practice setting for the changes which will have to be made if the findings are to be implemented.

Viewing research utilization as organizational change

While it is certainly within the powers of an individual nurse to identify the *potential* for use of research findings in practice, it is rarely possible for one individual alone to act on that, except in the most limited of circumstances where personal control can be exercised. Indeed, Hunt (1987), on the basis of experience gained in the course of an innovative project concerned with the process of translating research findings into nursing practice, concluded that the task of research utilization is 'generally beyond the capacity of any one individual'. She also concluded that it has been simplistic to hope that if individual nurses could be educated to read research, they could then be enabled to change their practice.

Whose responsibility is it, then, to tackle research utilization in practice? Fawcett (1980) described nurse administrators as the 'key to making research an integral part of nursing practice', and suggested:

'They alone hold the power and authority to effect the requisite changes and to provide the necessary incentives and rewards.'

While this view of research utilization as requiring organizational change and management support is now well established in North America, it has been slow to develop in the UK, even though individuals have highlighted the need for managers to become more responsible in this regard. For example, Melia (1984) bravely challenged managers to 'grasp the real nettle of research'. Objecting to their idea that researchers should be responsible for getting research used, Melia bluntly suggested that while 'researchers make the bullets, it is up to the managers to fire them'.

The argument for research utilization being accepted as an aspect of the management of change within organizations is put forward forcibly by MacGuire (1990). Her paper begins as follows:

'The problem of utilization of research findings in nursing is usually characterized in terms of why nurses in clinical areas do not modify their practice in response to the new knowledge that has been generated . . . I feel that the position has been oversimplified in much of the writing on this subject.'

She takes up the whole question of research utilization as an aspect of the management of change, and comments that:

'The process of *intentional* change in large-scale organisations is complex and involves a great deal more than bringing about modifications in attitudes and behaviours of individual people.'

In concluding, she says:

'What is clear (is) that the whole process is . . . more difficult that any of us imagine when we blithely talk about a wholescale change to research-based practice.'

Research utilization has to come to be viewed, then, as an organizational process, and resources need to be directed towards finding ways of understanding that process and translating it into practice. There are clear indications now that this is beginning to happen. *The Research and Development Strategy for the National Health Service* (HMSO, 1991) acknowledges the need for an infrastructure which supports and resources the systematic utilization of relevant research findings and, indeed, the need for research to be undertaken to establish the best ways and means of securing the uptake of tried and tested developments throughout the health service. In *The Strategy for Research in Nursing, Midwifery and Health Visiting* (DoH, 1993) it is suggested that the field testing of promising research results should be concentrated in selected centres and it is acknowledged that time will be needed to dissolve the barriers which have isolated researchers and practitioners 'in their separate worlds'. Hopefully, advantage will be taken of knowledge and ideas already generated by innovative attempts at improving research utilization in nursing.

Examples of research utilization initiatives

The first major research utilization initiative in nursing was launched in the USA in the 1970s. Called the 'WICHE programme', this was a regional programme for nursing research development run by the Western Inter-State Commission for Higher Education (hence, WICHE). It provided workshops for clinical nurses to develop skills for research utilization and, as such, it was essentially an educational programme.

The need to view research utilization as an organizational process rather than an individual endeavour was recognized by Horsley *et al.* (1983) in the development of a later project in the USA, the CURN project (i.e. conduct and utilization of research in nursing) and this is now recognized as the flagship of North American efforts in this field. It took the form of a major collaborative study conducted with the purpose of developing and testing a model to facilitate the use of scientific nursing knowledge in clinical practice settings. Research findings relating to selected nursing practices were synthesized, translated into clinical protocols, implemented and evaluated.

Although there has been no comparable initiative in the UK, individual nurse researchers have been active in tackling the challenge of research utilization in practice. An innovative approach described by Wilson-Barnett *et al.* (1990) involved the introduction of individuals with a researcher-teacher role to work alongside practitioners. Two studies (one relating to nursing care of patients with a tracheal stoma, the other concerned with nurses' knowledge and attitudes to cancer), were used to demonstrate how a researcher can work with practising nurses to improve patient care on the basis of research. In this 'experiment', both the researchers and the nurses appeared to be persuaded of the benefits of this type of ward-based research and teaching by the researcher.

Other examples of initiatives aimed at closing the so-called 'gap' between research and practice include Tierney & Taylor's (1991) successful researcher-practitioner collaboration on a project in a breast cancer unit which led to subsequent utilization of the research findings in practice; and Titchen & Binnie's (1993) collaborative action research initiative designed to assist the move in two wards from traditional methods of care delivery to primary nursing.

Conclusion

Clearly, this is an era in which such innovative approaches to improving research use in nursing practice are needed. For its survival, and certainly to justify its growth, nursing research will have to begin to be able to demonstrate that it does make a difference in terms of positively influencing nursing care. It may well be that its apparent lack of impact has resulted more from a lack of understanding of the complexities of research utilization – and misplacement of responsibility on individual nurses – than from a lack of desire to see research used in practice. Whatever the reasons, the time has come for us to stop thinking that use of research in practice will somehow 'just happen'. We need to make it happen and all of us – researchers, managers, educators, and practitioners – have a part to play in that. And, at least in the UK, we now have the benefit of a framework in which to do so, in the form of *The Strategy for Research in Nursing, Midwifery and Health Visiting* (DoH, 1993) and *Research for Health: A Research and Development Strategy for The National Health Service* (HMSO, 1991) which, together, are designed to strengthen the commitment to knowledge-led practice in nursing and throughout the health service.

References

Bassett, C. (1992) The integration of research in the clinical setting: obstacles and solutions. A review of the literature. *Nursing Practice*, **6**(1), 4–8.

Brett, J.L. (1987) Use of nursing practice research findings. *Nursing Research*, **36**(6), 344–9.

Champion, V.L. & Leach, A. (1989) Variables related to research utilization in nursing. *Journal of Advanced Nursing*, **14**, 705–10.

Closs, S.J. & Cheater, F.M. (1994) Utilization of nursing research: culture, interest and support. *Journal of Advanced Nursing*, **19**, 762–73.

DoH (1993) *Report of the Taskforce on the Strategy for Research in Nursing, Midwifery and Health Visiting*. Department of Health, Leeds.

Fawcett, J. (1980) A declaration of nursing independence; the relation of theory and research to practice. *Journal of Nursing Administration*, **10**, 36–9.

Fawcett, J. (1984) Hallmarks of success in nursing research. *Advances in Nursing Science*, **7**(1), 1–11.

Gould, D. (1986) Pressure sore prevention and treatment: an example of nurses' failure to implement research findings. *Journal of Advanced Nursing*, **11**, 388–94.

Greenwood, J. (1984) Nursing research: a position paper. *Journal of Advanced Nursing*, **9**, 77–82.

HMSO (1991) *Research for Health: A Research and Development Strategy for the NHS.* Department of Health, Her Majesty's Stationery Office, London.

Horsley, J. (1985) Using research in practice: the current context. *Western Journal of Nursing Research*, **7**(1), 135–9.

Horsley, J., Crane, J., Crabtree, M.K. & Wood, D.J. (1983) *Using Research to Improve Nursing Practice: A Guide.* (Conduct and Utilization of Research in Nursing Practice: CURN). Grune & Stratton, New York.

Hunt, J. (1984) Why don't we use these findings? *Nursing Mirror*, **158**,(8), 29.

Hunt, M. (1987) The process of translating research findings into nursing practice. *Journal of Advanced Nursing*, **12**, 101–10.

Jerrett, M.D. (1994) Parents' experience of coming to know the care of a chronically ill child. *Journal of Advanced Nursing*, **19**, 1050–56.

Ketefian, S. (1975) Application of selected nursing research findings into nursing practice: a pilot study. *Nursing Research*, **24**(2), 89–92.

Kitson, A. (1994) Post-operative pain management: a literature review. *Journal of Clinical Nursing*, **3**, 7–18.

Lacey, E.A. (1994) Research utilization in nursing practice – a pilot study. *Journal of Advanced Nursing*, **19**, 987–95.

Lindeman, C.A. (1988) Patient education. *Reviews of Nursing Research*, **6**, 29–60.

MacGuire, J.M. (1990) Putting research findings into practice: research utilization as an aspect of the management of change. *Journal of Advanced Nursing*, **15**, 614–20.

Macleod Clark, J. & Hockey, L. (eds) (1989) *Further Research for Nursing.* Scutari Press, London.

Melia, K. (1984) Using research (letter). *Nursing Times*, **80**(49), 14.

Redman, B. (1993) Patient education at 25 years: where we have been and where we are going. *Journal of Advanced Nursing*, **18**, 725–30.

Robinson, J. (1987) The relevance of research to the ward sister. *Journal of Advanced Nursing*, **12**, 421–9.

Sheehan, J. (1986) Nursing research in Britain: the state of the art. *Nurse Education Today*, **6**, 3–10.

Smith, J.P. (ed.) (1994) *Research and its Application.* (The Advanced Nursing Series.) Blackwell Scientific Publications, Oxford.

Stetler, C.B. & DiMaggio, G. (1991) Research utilization among clinical nurse specialists. *Clinical Nurse Specialist*, **5**, 151–5.

Stetler, C. & Marram, G. (1976) Evaluating research findings for applicability in practice. *Nursing Outlook*, **124**, 559–63.

Stockwell, F. (1972) *The Unpopular Patient.* The Study of Nursing Care, Series 1 No 2. Royal College of Nursing and National Council of Nurses of the UK, London.

Tierney, A.J. & Taylor, J. (1991) Research in practice: 'an experiment' in researcher-practitioner collaboration. *Journal of Advanced Nursing*, **16**, 506–10.

Titchen, A. & Binnie, A. (1993) Research partnerships: collaborative action research in nursing. *Journal of Advanced Nursing*, **18**, 858–65.

Tornquist, E.M., Funk, S.G. & Champagne, M.T. (1989) Writing research reports for clinical audiences. *Western Journal of Nursing Research*, **11**(5), 576–82.

Walsh, M. & Ford, P. (1989) Rituals in nursing: 'We always do it this way'. *Nursing Times*, **85**(41), 26–35.

Whyte, D.A. (1994) *Family Nursing: The Case of Cystic Fibrosis.* Avebury, Aldershot.

Wilson-Barnett, J. (1989) Patient teaching. In *Further Research for Nursing*, (eds J. Macleod

Clark & L. Hockey), Chapter 12. Scutari Press, London.

Wilson-Barnett, J., Corner, J. & DeCarle, B. (1990) Integrating research and practice – the role of researcher as teacher. *Journal of Advanced Nursing*, 15, 621–5.

Chapter 34

Research in Nursing Education

Patricia Osborne

He who teaches and does not do research is like a man who drinks from a stagnant pool. He who teaches and does research is like a man who drinks from a flowing stream.

Chinese proverb

The function of research in nursing education

Nurse education had been in a state of flux for some years. The cause of this is complex, but the underlying reason has to do with nursing's desire to be identified as a profession in its own right. The main stumbling block to this had been the lack of a solid research based foundation upon which to build and strengthen the professional identity of nursing. It has long been asserted that research is essential to the survival of nursing. Simpson (1981) considered that the aim of research was to maximize the contribution of nursing to health care.

Without research the unique knowledge base of nursing is stunted and cannot grow. Nursing has been accused, rightly, of borrowing theory from other disciplines (Akinsanya, 1994). Clearly the need for distinctive theoretical development is increasingly important if nursing's uniqueness is to be recognized and the dilution effect of the borrowed theories can be stemmed.

It is common sense that if the profession is addressing the issues of the day from a research perspective then nurse educators and nurse education must adopt the same stance. This will ensure that all concerned are in accord, and that nurse educators are able to anticipate the needs of the profession and can respond appropriately.

The wholesale move of nurse education into higher education in the UK and elsewhere has not only presented a more 'academic front', but has also facilitated the development of nursing research being undertaken by nurse educationalists. This they are doing in several ways: undertaking degrees and higher degrees with a strong research component, as well as entering the world of academic research. This has high academic status and involves grant applications and full-time study and may culminate in research directorships and the establishment of departments whose specific term of reference is the development of quality research for the nurse educational establishment as a whole.

In a study of the career patterns of nurse educators, Clifford (1992) identified that research did not feature as a major reason for nurses to enter nurse education, nor did lack of time for research feature as a cause of dissatisfaction. Clifford suggests that this indicates lack of awareness regarding the potential importance of research as part of the nurse-educator's role. Bassett (1994), in his phenomenological study of nurse-teachers' attitudes to research, observed a general awareness of the requirement in higher educational arenas to undertake research and publish academic works. Reaction to this was mixed, with some nurse-teachers expressing positive feelings towards this opportunity whilst others expressed anxiety and doubt about the benefits of this for them.

Now that the arena in which nurse education has entered is larger, more complex and open to scrutiny by colleagues of neighbouring departments in higher education establishments, the opportunities for nurse education research have greatly increased. The chance to guide and influence the future of nursing has never been better. The consequences of not doing so could result in decisions and plans for the future being taken out of our hands.

Recent developments in nursing education research

In reviews of recent British literature, a wide range of issues have been identified. Some of these are the maturation of previously identified research, reflecting the process approach to nursing education. Others are completely innovative, providing opportunity for new growth and dynamism within nurse education.

Curriculum development

If the arrival of Project 2000 (United Kingdom Central Council for Nursing, Midwifery and Health Visiting, 1986) did anything, it created an unprecedented flurry of activity on a nationwide scale. Curricula which had not been addressed proactively for many years were dusted down and reconsidered, and curriculum planning groups evolved. The intention was that nurse education, with its new roots now in academic settings, should focus more rigorously on academic, research-based learning. The subsequent challenge for nurse educators, highlighted by MacDonald (1992) has been the ability to respond to change in curriculum intention and an increase in student–teacher contact time. Conceptual frameworks have been identified and built up to form course models which had to reflect the way in which nursing operates in the broadest framework of skill, knowledge and experience (Frost, 1990).

Central to the curriculum development process must be the philosophy of the nursing faculty, and this should be congruent with the philosophy of the larger, educational establishment to which the nursing faculty belongs. This facilities opportunities within a broader institutional network, to influence curriculum development and the whole educational process.

The relationship between educational philosophy and educational practice, has been addressed by Gates (1990). His ethnographic study highlighted that the process of striving to remain true to the original ideology and philosophy was problematic. This was due to the complexities of functioning within the larger organization, along with the range of ideologies that exist within nurse education, and he concluded that these difficulties may negate the utility of stating an educational philosophy.

Nursing curricula have been undergoing evolutionary changes since the late 1980s in terms of the content, process and structure of students' learning experience. Much current thinking has been influenced by critical social theory and feminist epistemology. There has been criticism of the emphasis on empirical knowledge, traditional scientific research methodologies, behaviourist models of teaching and evaluation and of the hierarchical organization of educational institutions (Diekelmann, 1988; Bevis & Murray, 1990).

Of central concern within this curriculum revolution has been the social responsibility of nursing to challenge the patriarchal value of dominance and control, which pervade current health care systems. Caring has been reclaimed as a core value (Tanner, 1990) and the teacher–student relationship is claimed as a means of role modelling caring. Nurse education emphasizes the process of education where critique, discussion and the development of critical reflective skills are considered the core elements to learning and developing the skills of clinical practice. Such processes encourage a shared, egalitarian responsibility for learning between the student and teacher (Spence, 1994).

It would appear from literature that nursing colleges have collectively adopted a change of strategy regarding curriculum development. A comprehensive study undertaken by Crotty (1993a) reveals this to be a change towards the process approach, with the adoption of less rigid models, all of which reflect a humanistic ethos. This represents a major conceptual shift in nurse education where the aims of Project 2000 are being addressed in earnest along with the realization of a critical, analytical practitioner.

Evaluation of the curriculum

When considering research developments in nurse education, it is appropriate that the curriculum should take precedence. With the curriculum as the main artery of nurse education, most recent education research has been as a consequence of the transformation described above. Without curriculum development, much research would go unchallenged, and without research the curriculum would become sterile. In order to accommodate the requirements of these changes in curricular intention, there needs to be an integrated approach to evaluation of the teaching of curriculum content.

In the past, many evaluation models have over-emphasized either the process or product of education, and have not addressed adequately both of these components of professional learning. Evaluation of curricula has taken various forms, the most commonly used being the accreditation model, which makes use of quantitative analysis to assess results. Hogg (1990) comments that traditionally the nursing curriculum had been a complex entity, difficult to evaluate, and which left many nurse-educators struggling with inappropriate and time-consuming procedures, yielding little reward. The theoretical framework proposed by MacDonald (1992) for curriculum evaluation is action research which, as a form of social enquiry, allows participants to reflect on their own practices (see Chapter 15).

Sconce & Howard (1994) state that the introduction of the internal market to the Health Service in the UK requires colleges of nursing to adopt a customer-led approach to education and this should be reflected in evaluation. They consider that a suitable model for curriculum evaluation is that which concentrates on the decision-making processes involved in design and delivery of a curriculum, such as that proposed by Stufflebeam (1968). This model allocates these decision-making processes to one of four categories: context-input-process-product (CIPP).

Other approaches to curriculum evaluation include the use of repertory grids, although this can be time-consuming and complex (McSweeney *et al.*, 1991). Odro (1992) proposes a more innovative, pictorial approach to curriculum evaluation. He states that embracing humanistic principles and philosophy in nurse education requires more than adoption of a flexible and facilitative style in course content delivery. Atkinson (1993) is also a proponent of aesthetic evaluation through the use of music, stating that it evokes memory, thoughts, feelings and intuition. Both these approaches encompass the belief that course evaluation should allow for manifestations of the many humanistic learning processes to be properly identified and evaluated.

The teacher experience: the role of the nurse-teacher

Teacher preparation

There have been several reports of the changing role of the nurse-teacher as a consequence of the advent of Project 2000 diploma courses, in conjunction with the wholesale move into the higher education system. (English National Board for Nursing, Midwifery and Health Visiting, 1990; Webster, 1990; Crotty & Butterworth, 1992). The research undertaken by Crotty (1993a) addressed the preparation teachers received, in relation to undertaking perceived new activities relating to new diploma programmes. She noted that teachers felt they had not been adequately prepared for their changing role, commenting that teacher preparation was generally informal and self directed, and there appeared to be an urgent need to review the preparation of teachers and their continuing education and development. She identifies the main source of preparation as Certificate of Education courses and expresses concern about this, due to the known dissatisfaction with these (English National Board for Nursing, Midwifery and Health Visiting, 1990). Experience was valued particularly highly as a means of preparation, past experience as a nurse or a manager being of particular importance. Similar findings were also reported by Clifford (1992), who suggested a cross-cultural study of the impact of teachers' role in centres where nurse-educators do not undergo specific preparation for their role.

With the development of academe in nurse education, the role of the nurse-educator in the clinical area remains under consideration. Practitioners are being encouraged to become more educationally aware, whilst at the same time many of the institutions which influence the path of British nursing expect teachers to be more clinically aware.

There has been great debate over what is meant by clinical credibility or competence (Webster, 1990; Osborne, 1991; Acton *et al.*, 1992). Crotty's (1993b) study noted that teachers perceived their role as updating theoretical knowledge and basic skills, rather than being expert practitioners, and demonstrated a commitment to clinical liaison to support clinical staff. There are currently two main approaches used to bring teachers closer to practice.

The lecturer practitioner

Burke (1993) defines this role as

'the nurse who is employed by both the clinical area and the college and has responsibility for teaching and direct patient care.'

Several authors have described how the lecturer practitioner role successfully integrates theory to practice (Simons, 1984; King Edward's Hospital Fund for London, 1984) and more recently Lathlean (1992) has evaluated the contribution of lecturer-practitioners to theory and practice. Lecturer-practitioners, however, are few and far between and this role may only suit a minority of educationalists. Nevertheless, as Cave (1994) points out, there is a danger of recreating the divide that previously existed between clinical teachers and nurse tutors in the past.

The link teacher

The most common approach to maintaining clinical credibility is that of the link teacher. Kershaw (1990) states that this role has so far not been adopted effectively, due to lack of funding preventing teachers from having sufficient time to pursue this function. Teachers often have several links, but a study by Payne *et al.* (1991) has demonstrated that only half a day each week was spent in this role. A study by Jeffree (1991) suggests that clinical teaching is given low priority by teachers because they feel inadequately equipped to work in the clinical areas, as it may be some time since they worked there. Elsewhere it has been suggested that nurses move into education out of a sense of disillusionment with clinical practice, which makes them reluctant to return (Osborne, 1991). Neary (1993) further suggests that preparation for nurse teachers does not emphasize teaching in clinical settings adequately and that the role is ill defined. At the time of writing the Department of Health in the UK has commissioned research into this issue. Clearly this is one major arena that has not yet been resolved.

The student experience

Mentorship

The concept of mentorship has originated from North America over the last decade. It has become a key element of clinical support and is perceived to be necessary to the quality of the clinical experience for student nurses. Various authors have drawn attention to the ambiguities in the way the term is used, and of the notion itself (Burnard & Chapman, 1990; Donovan, 1990; Hart, 1990), yet there appears to be a paucity of empirical evidence for the apparent successes of mentorship schemes.

'Despite apparent consensus that mentorship is an important aspect of learning in the practice continuum, there has been no real critical appraisal of the literature for its research base.'

Maggs (1994)

Past studies have concluded that mentoring should be available throughout the training programme and that mentees should be able to change mentors at any time and dictate the amount of time spent together. Currently, these recommendations have largely been adopted by colleges of nursing, although there is still some uncertainty as to the true effectiveness of mentorship schemes.

Leonard & Jowett (1990), in their report on the six pilot schemes of Project 2000 in England, drew attention to the lack of clarity in the meaning and utilization of mentorship. An examination of current student nurse issues by Wood (1992) identified stress and the clinical environment and in particular the presence or absence of mentorship as major issues for student nurses. Currently, the National Foundation for Educational Research is undertaking research with learners and mentors to evaluate the mentoring process.

Assessing clinical competence

When continuous practical assessments for registration programmes began to be introduced in the UK in the late 1970s, they were generally hailed to be more valid, reliable and realistic methods of assessment (Girot, 1993). Now, however, with increasing pressures on the role of the ward manager, supernumerary status for students and shorter clinical placements, there is a danger that skills assessment may decline altogether. As part of research into the implementation of Project 2000, Elkan & Robinson (1991) identified that the gap between theory and practice was still very much in evidence, and that students were very much left to reconcile these differences themselves. At the heart of this was the difference in approach between tutorial and clinical staff to equipping students with practical skills during the Common Foundation Programme of Project 2000 diploma courses.

Students who reported feeling awkward and ill at ease during some of their ward placements ascribed these feelings to a lack of practical competence, feeling that too little emphasis has been placed on acquiring practical skills. According to Smith

(1994), most Project 2000 diploma students consider themselves to be less competent in practical skills than they believe traditionally trained students nurses to be at an equivalent stage in training.

In response to this and the radical changes in delivery of care as a whole, with increased emphasis on community care, day care and outpatient teaching with the concomitant increase in dependency and throughput of inpatients, Studdy *et al.* (1994) report on a joint initiative to develop a clinical skills learning facility. The aim of this skills facility is to provide a focus for the learning and assessment of clinical and communication skills in a multi-disciplinary environment. Clifford (1994) warns that dilemmas relating to the assessment of clinical skills hinge upon several factors: the development of new educational programmes, who should assess clinical skills, clinical expertise of teachers, and the design and location of the assessment system. Coates & Chambers (1992) state that suitable assessment instruments are difficult to locate and design. Their evaluation of 11 clinical assessment tools revealed that, in the majority of cases, use of a systematic research process to guide them was not evident. They conclude that there is a need for more rigorously designed and tested instruments of clinical assessment, particularly in light of the plethora of new courses being developed and implemented. They caution that it is vital that those involved in instrument development must have suitable skills to undertake this task, and that thorough testing must be done.

Learning strategies

Reflective practice

Ever since the popularization of Schon's (1983) seminal book, reflective practice has been a constant theme among professional groups. Reflective practice has been adopted as a concept within nursing, as a way of dealing with the relationship between theory and practice.

'... To reflect in action, is the core of professional artistry. Professionals reflect in the midst of action without interruption; their thinking shapes what they are doing whilst they are doing it. The goal of reflection in action is to change indetermined situations into determined ones, and the key to successfully completing this problem-setting activity is to bring past experience to bear on current action.'

Cervero 1988 p.44.

Nursing literature in relation to reflection is relatively new, even though it has been endorsed as an important concept for some years. Most of this literature is deliberative, and it is clear that there is still some debate over what constitutes reflection as a concept. James & Clarke (1994) endorse the need to critically examine the notion of reflective practice. They examine the attraction of models of reflection and argue their appeal is because they ground practice in established theory which offers practitioners and educators a framework in which to operate.

One such model of reflection is the clinical learning spiral developed by Stockhausen (1994). It draws upon other models of experiential learning and action research, and was developed to emphasize the importance of reflective practice to the professional growth of the nurse. It is suggested that this spiral adds structure and focus to the process of reflection on action and provides an avenue for the student and teacher in the clinical area to set mutual goals of action to trial for future experiences. This process allows the teacher to be an integral component of success to the students' learning in the clinical context.

Self and peer assessment

The assumption implicit in the traditional approach of student assessment is that the assessor, by virtue of her knowledge and experience, is the best person to make judgements of the students' performance. It has been argued, however, that the process of reflection should be examined from the perspective of both students *and* teachers, and that a range of assessment tools need to be developed and tested, in keeping with new forms of student participation in the assessment process (Runciman, 1990). This collaborative approach to the process of assessing students' work is perceived to be an important learning opportunity for participants and is welcomed as a fairly recent contribution to nurse education research.

In a study by Costello (1988) students identified their colleagues as their main teachers of practical skills, suggesting that the role of the nurse-teacher in peer teaching and learning requires further investigation. Proponents of self and peer assessment argue that if this process is adopted widely, it can become an integral part of group life. It is a personal activity yet maintains a sense of objectivity, and encourages openness of expression and support.

An exploratory study conducted by Wondrak & Goble (1992) identified that students, peers and tutors found themselves in agreement, at statistically significant levels, about the merits of their written work. They note that in fact students tended to award themselves lowest marks, dispelling the myth that students left to assess themselves will simply award themselves passes.

Future directions of nursing education research

Throughout this chapter, discussion has related to the influence of research in nursing education. It is extremely encouraging to note the advances that have been made in response to the range of developments and initiatives within nursing and the UK health service as a whole.

One of the most important developments that has occurred is that of curriculum design. It is no coincidence that this should be so. The needs of diploma courses as a result of Project 2000 have required that innovative strategies and models be adopted when considering curricula. This will continue well into the millennium with the implementation of post registration education and practice (PREP) (United Kingdom Central Council for Nursing, Midwifery and Health Visiting,

1990) and the need to cater for nurses' educational needs at all levels of under-graduate, postgraduate and continuing professional development.

In tandem with this has been the uptake of curriculum evaluation in nurse education. This is a very positive move and demonstrates a commitment to ensuring that the delivery of nurse education remains dynamic and relevant to current needs. The introduction of the internal market requires a customer led approach to education and it is their views that are important in ensuring fitness for purpose. Evaluation is a meaningful way of achieving this end. Further research needs to be undertaken to develop models and instruments for evaluation of the curriculum to accommodate the range of courses available. Perhaps it is most appropriate that the evaluation tool is developed simultaneously with the curri-culum design, thus ensuring that the ethos and philosophy of the course are adequately addressed.

It is apparent that the role of the nurse-teacher in relation to clinical practice is far from resolved. The debate continues as to what constitutes clinical credibility and how to maintain this. Much more research needs to be undertaken regarding the best role for nurse-educators in clinical practice. The role of the lecturer-practitioner needs to be evaluated in depth. If this is the way forward then should they exist in every clinical area or just as specialists in chosen fields? Is the concern expressed by Cave (1994), that the divide between clinical teachers and nurse-teachers will re-emerge, real or imagined? How do clients fare in areas where this role exists? The results of the research commissioned by the Department of Health on the role of teachers in the clinical area will be greeted with great interest. The role of the link tutor is one which remains ill-defined and open to wide inter-pretation and yet there is tremendous pressure upon nurse-educators to undertake such a role. It is manifest that the whole issue of clinical credibility for nurse educators will remain on the agenda for the foreseeable future.

In conjunction with the issue of clinical involvement, the challenge to nurse-teachers is also to find systems of assessing practice in nursing that will fully utilize their professional expertise in the assessment process. The assessment of practice is the mechanism by which the ability of student nurses to deliver care in a practice setting is determined. However the means by which this practice is assessed is far from clear and it is important that these matters be addressed.

Mentorship has been adopted wholesale by colleges of nursing as a way of providing support in the clinical field for student nurses. However it is evident that this is a complex issue, and the lack of understanding regarding this notion is a matter of great concern. As Maggs (1994) suggests, further research is required to clarify the nature and role of mentorship and indeed whether the educational system is enriched by the mentorship system.

Modularization of courses for the purposes of the credit accumulation and transfer schemes (CATS) is topical within nurse education and is in keeping within a higher education continuum. Modules can be versatile and the net result is the increase of courses available for nurses to undertake. Accessibility of courses has been enhanced by the adoption of accredited prior learning schemes (APL), and for the first time the possibility of awarding credits for achievement of clinical competencies. APL offers significant educational and service advantages, notably to meet the increased need in the face of limited resources, and the challenges implicit within PREP. It is apparent that APL as an individual strategy (perhaps with the use of portfolios), and as a corporate strategy, to ensure uniformity of interpretation, is very much in a developmental phase and this is set to continue.

Conclusion

In an editorial, Walker (1992) talks about a 'paradigm shift' in nursing over the last two decades. Nursing is no longer largely a matter of custom and practice closely following developments in medicine. Students are now educated in a culture of research and critical thinking and post-graduate opportunities for research are better than ever.

It is clear that this new paradigm is exciting, innovative and set to continue. Over the last few years there appears to have been an awakening within nurse education of the importance of research for the maintenance and indeed survival of the profession. Opportunities for undertaking research have increased and as nurse education becomes settled within a higher education framework, these openings will continue. The consequences of returning to a status where educational research was not integral to it would be the return of a profession with a fragmented, discordant voice, losing sight of its aims and losing its influence on health care settings and client care.

References

Acton, L., Gough, P. & McCormack, B. (1992) The clinical nurse tutor debate. *Nursing Times*, **88**(32), 38–41.

Akinsanya, J.A. (1994) Making research useful to the practising nurse. *Journal of Advanced Nursing*, **19**(1), 174–9.

Atkinson, A. (1993) The use of music in curriculum evaluation. *Nurse Education Today*, **12**(2), 133–8.

Bassett, C. (1994) Nurse teachers' attitudes to research: a phenomenological study. *Journal of Advanced Nursing*, **19**(3), 585–92.

Bevis, E. & Murray, O. (1990) The essence of the curriculum revolution: emancipatory teaching. *Journal of Nursing Education*, **29**(7), 326–31.

Burke, L.M. (1993) The future of the specialist nurse teacher: two different models explored. *Nurse Education Today*, **13**(1), 40–6.

Burnard, P. & Chapman, C. (1990) *Nurse Education: The way forward*. Scutari Press, London.

Cave, I. (1994) Nurse teachers in higher education – without clinical competence, do they have a future? *Nurse Education Today*, **14**(5) 394–9.

Cervero, R. (1988) *Effective Continuing Education for Professionals*. Jossey Bass, San Francisco.

Clifford, C. (1992) The role of the nurse teacher. *Nurse Education Today*, **12**(5), 340–9.

Clifford, C. (1994) Assessment of clinical practice and the role of the nurse teacher. *Nurse Education Today*, **14**(4), 272–9.

Coates, V. & Chambers, M. (1992) Evaluation of tools to assess clinical competence. *Nurse Education Today*, **12**(2), 122–9.

Costello, J. (1988) Peer and self assessment. *Nursing Times*, **183**(33), 62–4.

Crotty, M. (1993a) Curriculum issues related to the newly developed nursing diploma courses. *Nurse Education Today* **13**(4), 264–9.

Crotty, M. (1993b) The emerging role of the nurse teacher in Project 2000 programmes: a Delphi survey. *Journal of Advanced Nursing*, **18**(1), 150–7.

Crotty, M. & Butterworth, A. (1992) The emerging role of the nurse teacher in Project 2000 programmes – a literature review. *Journal of Advanced Nursing*, **17**(11), 1377–87.

Diekelmann, N. (1988) Curriculum revolution: a theoretical and philosophical mandate for change. In *Curriculum Revolution Mandate for Change*. National League for Nursing, New York.

Donovan, J. (1990) The concept and role of mentor. *Nurse Education Today*, **10**(4), 294–8.

Elkan, R. & Robinson, J. (1991) *The implementation of Project 2000 in a district health authority: the effect on the nursing service. An interim report*. Department of Nursing studies, University of Nottingham.

English National Board for Nursing, Midwifery and Health Visiting (1990) *Teacher Preparation Project*. ENB, London.

Frost, S. (1990) From Project 2000 to diploma of higher education curriculum and course development. *Nurse Education Today*, **10**(5), 384–90.

Gates, R.J. (1990) From educational philosophy to educational practice: fidelity and the curriculum in context. *Nurse Education Today*, **10**(6), 420–7.

Girot, E. (1993) Assessment of competence in clinical practice – a review of the literature. *Nurse Education Today*, **13**(2), 83–90.

Hart, K. (1990) *Mentorship in midwifery*. Unpublished MEd dissertation, University of Nottingham.

Hogg, S.A. (1990) The problem-solving curriculum evaluation and development model. *Nurse Education Today*, **10**(2), 104–10.

James, C. & Clarke, B. (1994) Reflective practice in nursing: issues and implications for nurse education. *Nurse Education Today*, **14**(2), 82–90.

Jeffree, C.A. (1991) A broken line in the chain. *Senior Nurse*, **11**(3), 4–6.

Kershaw, B. (1990) Clinical credibility and nurse teachers. *Nursing Standard*, **4**(51), 46–7.

King Edward's Hospital Fund for London (1984) *Joint Clinical Appointments in Nursing*. King's Fund, London.

Lathlean, J. (1992) The contribution of lecturer practitioners to theory and practice in nursing. *Journal of Clinical Nursing*, **1**(5), 237–42.

Leonard, A. & Jowett, S. (1990) *Charting the Course: A Study Of the Six ENB Pilot Schemes in Pre-registration Nurse Education*. National Foundation for Educational Research, Slough.

MacDonald, J. (1992) Project 2000 curriculum evaluation: the case for teacher evaluation. *Nurse Education Today*, **12**(2), 101–7.

Maggs, C. (1994) Mentorship in nursing and midwifery education: issues for research. *Nurse Education Today*, **14**(1), 22–9.

McSweeney, P., Fisher, B. & Russell, T. (1991) Course evaluation. *Senior Nurse*, **11**(6), 43–7.

Neary, M. (1993) Teacher preparation into the 21st century. *Senior Nurse*, **13**(3), 32–9.

Odro, A.B. (1992) A pictorial approach to course evaluation. *Nurse Education Today*, **12**(1), 57–60.

Osborne, P. (1991) Nurse teaching and ward based learning. *Senior Nurse*, **11**(4), 28–9.

Payne S., Jowett, S. & Walton, I. (1991) *Nurse Teachers in Project 2000: The Experience of Planning and Initial Implementation*. National Foundation For Educational Research in England and Wales, Slough.

Runciman, P. (1990) *Competence Based Education and Assessment and Accreditation of Work Based Learning in the Context of Project 2000 Programmes of Nurse Education. A Literature Review*. Scottish National Board for Nursing, Midwifery and Health Visiting, Edinburgh.

Schon, P. (1983) *The Reflective Practitioner. How Professionals Think in Action*. Basic Books, New York.

Sconce, C. & Howard, J. (1994). Curriculum evaluation – a new approach. *Nurse Education Today*, **14**(4), 280–6.

Simons, W. (1984) Towards integration. *Senior Nurse*, **1**(28), 14–16.

Simpson, H.M. (1981) Issues in nursing research. In *Current Issues in Nursing*, (ed. L. Hockey) Churchill Livinstone, Edinburgh.

Smith, J. (1994) Project 2000 assessed: is nursing education a means or an end? *Journal of Advanced Nursing*, **19**(2), 411.

Spence, D.G. (1994) The curriculum revolution: can educational reform take place without a revolution in practice? *Journal of Advanced Nursing*, **19**(1), 187–93.

Stockhausen, L. (1994) The clinical learning spiral: a model to develop reflective practitioners. *Nurse Education Today*, **14**(5), 363–71.

Studdy, S., Nicol, M. & Fox-Hiley, A. (1994) Teaching and learning clinical skills Part 1 – Development of a multidisciplinary skills centre. *Nurse Education Today* **14**(3), 177–85.

Stufflebeam, D.L. (1968) *Evaluation as Enlightenment for Decision Making*. Columbus Evaluation Centre, Ohio State University.

Tanner, C.A. (1990) Caring as a core value in nursing education. *Nursing Outlook*, **38**, 70–2.

United Kingdom Central Council for Nursing, Midwifery and Health Visiting (1986) Project 2000: a new preparation for practice. UKCC, London.

United Kingdom Central Council for Nursing, Midwifery and Health Visiting (1990) *The Report of the Post Registration Education and Practice Project*. UKCC, London.

Walker, J. (1992) The development of nursing research – a paradigm shift in nursing. *Nurse Education Today* **12**(3), 161–2.

Webster, R. (1990) The role of the nurse teacher. *Senior Nurse*, **10**(8), 16–18.

Wondrak, R. & Goble, J. (1992) An investigation into self, peer and tutor assessments of student psychiatric nurses' written assignments. *Nurse Education Today*, **12**(1), 61–4.

Wood, V. (1992) An examination of selected current student nurse issues. *Nurse Education Today*, **12**(6), 403–8.

Chapter 35

Research in Nursing Management

James Connechen

Any review of research in nursing management should begin by raising awareness of the problems of definition. The first difficulty is in defining who are nursing managers and what is nursing management. The organizational changes which have arisen as a consequence of the National Health Service (NHS) reforms resulted in a proliferation of different structures and management roles. The Audit Commission (1991) noted that nursing management varied in structure, style and operational matters from one hospital to another. Increasing development of responsibilities and flat organizational structures have meant that ward sisters and charge nurses are often the main operational level of management in many health care organizations. Harrison & Pollitt (1994) note that the days when non-medical professionals were able to construct management hierarchies exclusive to themselves are gone. The development of clinical directorates has meant that professionals can be managed (at least) by clinical persons outside the particular professions. It is likely, as Batehup (1992) has suggested, that the directorate structure has the potential to produce a supportive environment to promote highly successful nursing practice. However, the new and diverse organizational arrangements need to be properly evaluated, not against ideological or policy considerations but against their impact on the outcomes of nursing care.

The National Health Service Management Executive (1991) has noted that over 70% of those exercising managerial functions are in nursing and midwifery grades, and that over 60% of managers are female and concentrated in the lower levels of management. The Audit Commission (1994) has reported that hospitals vary by up to 50% in their clinical productivity and that much of this variation is a result of the way staff are organized. This has inevitably meant that a substantial proportion of the research into nursing management has been on the preparation and role of the ward sister and charge nurse and the way that nursing care is organized and delivered at ward and department level.

It is well known that the largest item of expenditure on a hospital's budget will be the cost of nurses, accounting for about 50% of all NHS salaries. This also means that the nursing service attracts a great deal of interest in the research literature in terms of attempts to measure its efficiency and effectiveness. The rapid growth of activity in the managerial analysis of nursing skill mix and staffing levels can be seen to be driven by a primary concern for the economical and effective deployment of the most expensive resource in the NHS. A glance through *Nursing Research*

Abstracts illustrates this point by the number of research publications devoted to this area. Some authors, such as Clifford (1990), feel that the concern with measurement in research is a means by which managers can control health professionals and deny them autonomy. This notion presents a particular view about managers and the purpose of management. Nevertheless it beholds nurse managers to demonstrate, through their actions and behaviour, that their primary concern is not about planning staffing levels, but about developing effective nursing care.

The demands of a 'managed' market and the need to develop more patient-led services will mean that hospital and community units will find it necessary to make the transition from bureaucracies with sometimes diffused and confused accountability, to more streamlined and open organizations. Responsibilities for decision-making and performance of the nursing service are being delegated to levels closer to the patient. At the same time, there are demands for health care organizations to achieve substantial improvements in cost and quality while increasing their productivity. The ability to envisage new ways of organizing and delivering services, in order to achieve these sometimes conflicting objectives, will place many demands upon nurse managers. Many, however, are unsure of how best to manage the change in order to develop flexible, more patient-centred organizations. Research into nursing management practice and education must be seen as a tool to help managers understand the most effective ways to bring about change in their own practice, as well as enabling the delivery of effective nursing care. It is clear that in order to achieve these changes, different professional and managerial agendas need to be brought closer together. East & Robinson (1994) have pointed out that much of the nursing research is inward looking and rarely placed in a wider context, as if nothing happens beyond the ward door or even the individual patient's bedside. They also argue, however, that much of management research ignores nursing and by doing so ignores what goes on '... at the very heart of care delivery'. These differences must be made more explicit and addressed in order to explore the common ground throughout the development of research networks and local research strategies.

The second issue concerning problems of definition is about what constitutes nursing management research. Smith (1994), in an analysis of the nursing literature in three nursing journals, noted that it was possible to place much of the research she reviewed into different categories. An example is given in a research paper on skill mix and effectiveness in nursing. The paper could have been categorized as clinical as it was hospital based, or as management, because patient outcome measures were used. As it was also concerned with the measurement of care it could have been classified under research on nurses. The paper was in fact classified under research methods, as its primary concern was the measure of outcome which was nursing specific. Despite the problems of definition and difficulties in implementing research, there is, none-the-less, a welcome and discernible increase in interest in nursing management research. The arrival of the new *Journal of Nursing Management* in the UK market reflects this interest and provides further opportunities, as well as a forum for debate for nurse managers to establish themselves as key players in the development of patient care.

Role of the manager in nursing management research

Lorentzon (1993), in her review of the management of nursing research, suggests that nurse managers often receive criticism as blockers of innovative research. Their role is often that of 'whipping boy' for practitioners, researchers and educationalists alike. She goes on to explore possible reasons for the 'ambivalence and occasionally frank hostility' between researchers and managers. She postulates that the possible differences in educational background between the two groups may be a contributory factor, as well as the perceived inability of nurse managers to use nursing research to promote innovative nursing practice.

Nurse managers, in common with most other managers, are not a particularly reflective or introspective group. Mintzberg (1975) found that managers worked at an unrelenting pace and their job is characterized by discontinuity, brevity and variety. This action orientation was also described by Stewart (1967) in describing the manager's day as typically fragmented, with constant switches in attention caused by endless interruptions. Thus, Lorentzon (1993) notes that 'the most commonly stated reason for nurse managers' lack of interest and involvement in research is pressure from other commitments'.

Rolfe (1994), however, is one of many writers on the subject of research application to argue that it is nursing research that has lost its way. He feels that there is a widening gap between nursing theorists and practitioners. This means that the results from much research are never translated into practical nursing interventions. He recognizes, however, that the relationship between theory and practice is complex. He goes on to argue for a new model of research which is planned in terms of outcome in which strategies for change are built into the model itself. Hunter (1994) feels that if changes in clinical behaviour are to occur as a result of research into health care effectiveness, then appropriate support, training and development work with clinicians is required and that this will take time.

The lack of awareness of research findings, and difficulty in implementing research amongst health care staff, is widely recognized. The Scottish Office Home and Health Department (1993) *Research and Development Strategy for the NHS in Scotland* states that 'There will be work to develop methodologies to facilitate the communication of new research findings of those who work in the NHS.' It goes on to say that it will be necessary to encourage the wide adoption of an 'evaluative spirit' among staff, managers and clinicians so that a 'more critical attitude' is generated in assessing the costs as well as the benefits of service developments. The report, in providing a strategic framework and focus for the development of research in Scotland, emphasizes the need for close collaboration between all those concerned. Research will not flourish then solely on the 'push' from research nurses, but will also require the 'pull' from managers and practitioners. In achieving this, nurse managers must be involved from the outset in determining research priorities within the context of the overall policies for the NHS in promoting good health, improving treatment and health care and service quality. If research is matched more closely to the health and social needs of people, then it becomes a more relevant and powerful force for change.

Facilitator, gatekeeper and user

Nursing managers can make a valuable contribution by developing the links with clinical and educational based researchers. This enabling role can be further enlarged by agreeing some key objectives for research and development. Burroughs (1993) wrote of the role of managers as identified in a locally developed research strategy as:

- Ensuring that nursing practice was based upon up-to-date research findings.
- Providing nurses with adequate support and guidance when carrying out the research programme.
- Disseminating information about research.
- Using educational programmes to promote research awareness.

To enable this to happen managers, having determined their research priorities, need to ensure that adequate resources in terms of money, time and equipment are allocated for nursing research. This must involve the development of a climate where existing nursing practice can be questioned and discussed, and where nurses can have easy access to research information. The existence of wider research networks and the presence of local research and development managers will greatly enhance the support available to practitioners and managers. Effective management is also about ensuring that managers' behaviour reflects the values and intentions of the service for which they have a responsibility. Managers should, in effect, do as they say. If nurses are being encouraged to develop research based practice, then their managers must lead by example and subject their own practice to critical scrutiny.

Bradbury (1992) supports the view that the role of the nurse manager is to enable the nurses they manage to deliver a high standard of nursing care. This can be best achieved by managers evaluating the quality of their own work. Bradbury (1992) goes on to describe a project developed by her region to assist nurse managers achieve their organizational goals by developing a set of management standards.

Applications of nursing management research

Much of the research into nursing is often driven by the need of managers to develop cost effective solutions to health problems, and to establish better value for money. The Scottish Office Home and Health Department (1993) highlights the principles underlying the introduction of a national research strategy. That report includes the notion that research and development should be used as an agent of change when introduced to health care practice, and to allow ineffective clinical practices to be stopped.

The Audit Commission (1991) recognized that nurses' skills must be deployed and managed as effectively as possible if quality of care is to be improved. Their review of nursing services also found that, in many places, standards, once set, were rarely monitored and that it was also rare to find a systematic review of ward nurse establishments. They also noted the large difference in staffing levels of wards on a day-to-day basis which did not reflect workload. There were also variations in the length of shift overlap periods and in the time nurses spent on non-nursing duties. The Audit Commission (1991) estimate that reduction of the shift overlap to a maximum of one hour throughout the country would result in a saving of many millions of pounds.

Much of the recent nursing management research, therefore, touches upon issues of ward staffing, organizational structures and processes, care delivery processes and outcomes. Differences between the intentions of nurses and their practice are also investigated, as is the difference between nursing theory and practice. The following examples are drawn from available research literature and are not intended to be comprehensive. They do, however, illustrate some of the directions of the available research, the methodologies used and the key questions and issues raised concerning nursing management.

Research into skill mix

Arthur & James (1994) reviewed the literature on determining nursing staffing levels and examined the strengths and weaknesses of different approaches. Most studies involved some attempt at nursing workload measurement and they discovered that 29 systems are currently available in the UK market. They recognized three broad categories of systems: consensus approaches (intuitive and consultative), top-down approaches (staffing norms and staffing formulae) and bottom-up approaches (nursing intervention and patient dependency). It was concluded that a perfect tool for measuring nurses' work is unlikely to exist and that '... no system can ensure a perfect match between the demand for nursing and the supply of nursing staff'. Arthur & James (1994) highlight several main areas of difficulty in using nurse staffing level systems. The systems need to be suitable to the local situation as well as facilitating comparison across wards or units, hospitals or regions. No such system exists at present. Issues involving philosophy of care are also important; a criticism levelled at workload measurement systems is that they tend to be task orientated and fail to recognize the complexity of nursing.

Few systems have the capability to address local ward situations and be useful for comparison purposes across wards. Hunt's (1990) analysis, for example, recognizes that nursing is a complex and subtle process that involves multi-functioning which is not always recognized by task measurement systems. Arthur & James (1994) recognize the importance of attempting to identify the appropriate number of nurses and skill mix at ward and hospital levels. However, managers must have realistic expectations of what can be achieved, and use such systems as facilitating tools rather than dictating staffing levels. Deciding on the appropriate overall skill mix of an individual ward is therefore a difficult task which depends upon many factors. These include the reasons behind introducing the exercise in the first place, the professional standards adopted, variations in workload that occur and the budget and staff available.

Rodrigues (1994) describes how a local initiative in a Community/Mental Health

Trust set out to address the skill mix issues through the establishment of a steering group, clear brief, outcome criteria against which to measure their pilot studies and the development of effective information systems. Membership of the steering group, while at senior/middle management level, was balanced by encouraging a bottom-up approach to the development of the studies. Successful outcomes included the development of a case load management framework customized to individual community nursing disciplines.

Job satisfaction studies

The relationships between organizational change, management style and staff satisfaction and morale have been known for some time. This area continues to attract considerable research interest, particularly in studies which attempt to evaluate the impact of these variables in nursing care.

East & Robinson (1994) embarked upon a two-year action research project to facilitate the management of change in a District General Hospital. Action research (See Chapter 15) is an effective way of bridging the gap between theory, research and practice, and is a way of empowering nurses through supportive collaboration between the researchers and researched. The main focus of East & Robinson's (1994) study was to support G grade ward sisters during the transition period from their traditional roles to a new 'standard setting, budget holding, ward manager'.

Early results from that study showed that the nurses felt alienated from many of the managerially derived initiatives such as the introduction of new information technology and the implementation of a quality strategy. There was little sense of ownership in the initiatives nor an 'enthusiasm or dynamism or excitement generated'. The authors felt that the initiatives were poorly understood and therefore a weak motor for change. It is important to note that nurses did not actually resist change as their senior managers appeared to suspect. When dealing with change arising from 'professional agendas' such as the introduction of team nursing or in areas where they try to update their practice, they were keen and enthusiastic. They were constrained in their efforts, however, in developing these initiatives by factors such as poor staffing levels or many staff being moved around wards. The senior nurses experienced high levels of stress and felt victims of organizational forces over which they had no control.

Mackenzie (1993) also looked at the effect of change on charge nurses during the development of clinical directorate structures in hospitals in one District Health Authority. Using convenience random sample methods (see Chapter 19) 93 ward sisters returned a questionnaire which utilized fixed/alternative questions. Eighty per cent of the respondents felt that their management responsibility had increased since the start of the NHS reforms, while 63% felt inadequately prepared to fulfil their new management obligations. Eighty per cent also felt that they would welcome the re-instatement of a purely nurse management structure above that of G grade in order to obtain better support. Mackenzie (1993) postulates different explanations for the findings, including that of the lack of preparation and support in fulfilling different role functions.

Gilloran *et al.* (1994) examined the experience of staff nurses in psychogeriatric wards and the relationship between job satisfaction and quality of care, using a specially designed self-completion questionnaire. Results showed that the staff nurses, as separate from other grades of nursing staff, felt that their potential was not being realized while working in these wards. They felt frustrated and inhibited and did not assess their charge nurses as exhibiting good leadership qualities.

Some studies attempt to relate job satisfaction with quality of patient care, although rarely against any empirical or outcome measures. Kivimaki *et al.* (1994) looked at 15 hospital wards in four medical departments. Two categories of ward emerged according to the level of satisfaction with management. These were called 'satisfied wards' and 'other wards'. The wards where high satisfaction levels were reported differed significantly in four respects from 'other wards'. There were: more opportunities to participate in decision-making, better communication, innovation experiences were higher and staff felt that they cared for their patients well. Nursing managers also related the quality of care in the 'satisfied' wards as higher. The authors concluded that further observation and sociometric research was needed in order to investigate leadership behaviour directly. The effects of low morale and low work satisfaction in nursing staff in terms of the cost implication of high turnover rates and high absenteeism will ensure that this area continues to attract funding and interest from researchers in the future.

Organizational and management characteristics and their effects on nursing practice

The development of the ward sister/charge nurse role into that of ward manager, the shorter length of stay in hospitals for patients and the shorter working week for nurses have had profound changes in the way care is organized at ward level. These have included the introduction of primary nursing and team nursing. Primary nurses have 24-hour responsibility and authority over all aspects of nursing care for a small group of patients. The ability of these systems to deliver effective personalized care is attracting considerable interest from researchers. The Audit Commission (1991) thought that there was no conclusive evidence that primary nursing improved clinical outcomes in ways that could be quantified. Jupp (1994) reviewed the different systems of organizing care in a hospital specializing in cancer treatment. Non-participant observation, patient and staff questionnaires and interviews were used. Results showed considerable differences between the system that nurses believed they were using and the reality of how care was being delivered. Primary nursing was criticized more by nurses for its lack of flexibility and many of the wards in the study were using a pragmatic mixture of the two systems. Patients rated the quality of care as being dependent on the individual nurse, whether primary nursing or team nursing was being practised.

Hendel & Bar-Tal (1994) conducted a large-scale study to evaluate the relationship between hospital and ward size and professional management and quality of nursing care in 119 medical and nursing wards. Their results showed that whatever the quality of management, ward size was the major determinant of the quality of nursing care. That is the more beds in a ward, the poorer the nursing care. Quality of ward management, however, was a significant factor in improving care in large hospitals. In small hospitals, the quality of top management was a more significant factor in improving care. The authors conclude that much more attention is needed to develop professional management at ward level.

Davis *et al.* (1994) set out to evaluate nursing process documentation, using an instrument constructed by them; a self-administered ward manager questionnaire was also used. The results showed some major differences between the stated purpose and intention of the nursing process documentation and effectiveness in practice. The authors recognized that the quality of documentation may not be an indication of the actual quality of care. Nevertheless, it was noted that individual care was not reflected in the documentation. There was also a considerable emphasis on biological and medical aspects of patient care. There was also little evidence of attempts to evaluate care. Results from the ward manager data suggested that some of the managers in the studies appeared to have little understanding of the principles and practice of the nursing process. The authors explored possible reasons which might explain the results, including lack of support from senior managers and shorter lengths of stay for many patients. The authors concluded by arguing for a more radical approach to the implementation of individual nursing care.

Future direction of nursing management research

The future direction of nursing research, including that of nursing management research, will be determined to a large extent by policy direction. The priorities and objectives set out in the Scottish and English national research strategies provide a framework in which purchasers and providers of health care are expected to develop a clear agenda where change priorities are needed. This agenda should determine hospital and community units' research and quality assurance programmes. The Scottish Office Home and Health Department (1993) *Research and Development Strategy* makes clear its view on the purpose of research in the statement

'...it is important that a demonstration of improving service delivery leading to better value for money should be part of the basis for decision making about investing in research and development.'

Guidance is also given for the introduction of local research and audit strategies, again with the emphasis on funding studies which are focused on achievements in health gain. Both national strategies and the guidance on the development of local strategies highlight the need for training in research methods for NHS career staff, not just academic researchers. It is clear that managers, educationalists and practitioners are all expected to have different, but complementary, parts to play in taking the initiative forward.

Outcome and effectiveness measures

It is not too difficult to see the areas where much of the research interest may lie. Hard pressed managers and clinicians will be keen for any reliable information that can help them in their day-to-day decision-making, as well as longer term policy formulation. Purchasers will be interested in placing contracts with those provider units that can develop better, validated outcome measures in the treatment of patients. Outcome measures in the field of health care, however, may lack the face validity claimed for them, by often excluding many relevant effects of care. It may also be possible that factors unrelated to health care systems will account for more of the outcome variance than do measures of health care input. Keppler (1990) further asserts that different criteria are meaningful to different users of information. Research would be needed, therefore, to validate specific indicators for particular client types in relation to various treatment outcome dimensions. Long (1994) argues that the research agenda must be influenced to ensure that appropriate criteria are used to address both user and clinical perspectives. Davis *et al.* (1994) point out that there is a need to involve the client as an active participant in an inter-disciplinary health service. It is clear that outcome measures which only include professional perspectives will be regarded as incomplete.

Hunter (1994) warns that the current claims of outcomes in research are excessive. He states that '... producing evidence on what is effective, when and for whom and at what cost is a mighty task ...'. This point is based on the understanding that effectiveness in the NHS is not a simple criterion. It is not simply a matter of cost efficiency or short-term performance improvements. In addition to satisfying the more overt measures of performance such as budgets or waiting list targets, there is a range of potentially incompatible expectations held by different groups. These expectations include value for money, a climate of long-term work satisfaction, customer focus, capacity for innovation and flexibility, public accountability and professional and technical excellence. It will be important when judging effectiveness of health care treatment to manage the balance between these demands and to develop clear operational definitions of outcomes in both quantitative and qualitative research. This will pose considerable challenges to nursing researchers since, at the moment, they have some difficulty in moving beyond structure and process issues. Another area that is increasingly attracting the attention of nurse managers and researchers is the move towards collaborative care amongst health care professionals.

Collaborative care

Greenhalgh (1994) illustrates the disadvantages of the uni-disciplinary approach to care in that patients' needs may be differently perceived and interpreted by different staff groups by virtue of their training. She claims that, under these circumstances, the real needs of the patient may not actually be addressed. Other disadvantages to the uni-disciplinary approach to care include the inability to prioritize the provision of total care for a particular patient. This is largely because only the activities within a professional staff group can be prioritized. This may result in the services of one profession being delivered when the services of another cannot be afforded. Greenhalgh (1994) describes new organizational models where care needs are identified by a multi-professional team (and the patient). A single (multi-disciplinary) care plan is produced and, although delivery is still uni-disciplinary, a care manager is appointed to assess and coordinate the provision of care. To maximize effectiveness, integrated clinical records would be developed, although resource constraints would probably mean that this would take some time to develop. Green (1993) describes the experience of how a psychiatric hospital used a multi-disciplinary approach and the development of specific outcomes to improve the care of old people. One key requirement was being able to challenge the relationship between the different models of practice adopted by each profession.

The collaborative approach to care is also seen as essential in 'patient focused' hospitals. These are defined by the Audit Commission (1994) as

'... an exercise in redesigning the basic processes by which health care is delivered so as to give the needs of patients priority over those of professionals.'

In effect this means that many of the routine tasks such as pathology and X-ray are performed by 'multi-skilled' staff at the patient's bedside. Nurse managers are in an ideal position to design or be involved in studies to validate the claims of increased efficiency and effectiveness in patient care in these 'redesigned processes'.

Competence and performance

If competence is what a person knows and can do under ideal circumstances, that is 'potential', then performance is actual behaviour, that is what is actually done in the real life situation. While (1994) recognizes that many variables affect the way we perform. These include how we feel, leadership style and patterns of communication. Experience tells us that apparently competent registered nurses do not always perform at an adequate level. Nurses frequently work in complicated and challenging situations where their performance will vary. More understanding is required about the variables that affect performance as well as tools which allow nurse managers to measure them more effectively.

Conclusion

The NHS is in a state of fundamental transition. In attempting to contain costs while improving services to patients, all health care organizations are looking to restructure their operations. The challenges facing nurse managers are formidable as they implement these major changes while maintaining morale. Personal transitions are also required as managers are required to learn new business and marketing concepts while retaining their professional values and identity. Increasingly, they will be expected to develop management styles which empower and encourage the acceptance of devolved responsibility and change by their staff. The important role that research will play in helping to develop more effective organization and management structures and processes in the NHS is recognized in the national research strategies and in the guidance for the development of local strategies.

Nurse managers must ensure that promoting, facilitating and participating in research is clearly established as part of their role. Time must be allocated for this and it should form part of their annual objective setting and performance management arrangements. To do this effectively they need to have access to research networks and information systems, and to develop working relationships with academic researchers and educationalists. Above all, they must be present at the levels where local research and development policy is being decided so that research into nursing practice and its management receives its fair share of resources.

References

Arthur, T. & James, N. (1994) Determining nurse staffing levels: a critical review of the literature. *Journal of Advanced Nursing*, **19**(3), 558–65.

Audit Commission (1991) *The Virtue of Patients. Making Best Use of Nursing Resources.* HMSO, London.

Audit Commission (1994) *Trusting in the Future. Towards an Audit Agenda for NHS Providers.* HMSO, London.

Batehup, L. (1992) Managing the nursing service in clinical directorates. *Senior Nurse*, **12**,(2), 10–12.

Bradbury, B. (1992) Standards for nursing management. *Senior Nurse*, **12**(6), 16–18.

Burroughs, J. (1993) Research based approach to nursing care. *Senior Nurse*, **13**(6), 46–7.

Clifford, B. (1990) Getting the job done properly. *Senior Nurse*, **10**(9), 16–18.

Davis, B.D., Billings, J.R. & Ryland, R.K. (1994) Evaluation of nursing process documentation. *Journal of Advanced Nursing* **19**(5). 960–8.

East, L. & Robinson, J. (1994) Changes in process. Bringing about change in health care through action research. *Journal of Clinical Nursing*, **3**, 57–61.

Gilloran, A., McKinley, A., McGlen, T., McKee, K. & Robertson, A. (1994) Staff nurses' work satisfaction in psychogeriatric wards. *Journal of Advanced Nursing*, **20**, 997–1003.

Green, S. (1993) Measured pace, *Nursing Times*, **89**(7), 46–8.

Greenhalgh, C. (1994) Programming professional boundaries, *Nursing Management*, **5**, 21–2.

Harrison, S. & Pollitt, C. (1994) *Controlling Health Professionals*. Open University Press, Buckingham.

Hendel, T. & Bar-Tal, Y. (1994) The moderating effects of structural characteristics of wards in general hospitals on the relationships between professional management and the quality of care. *Journal of Nursing Management*, **2**(12), 71–5.

Hunt, J. (1990) The activity balance. *Nursing Standard*, **4**(42), 47.

Hunter, D. (1994) Are we being effective? *Health Service Journal*, **104**,(5407), 23.

Jupp. M.R. (1994) Management review of nursing systems. *Journal of Nursing Management*, **2**(2), 57–64.

Keppler, S. (1990) Performance measurements for mental health programmes. *Community Mental Health Journal*, **16**, 217–34.

Kivimaki, M., Kalimo, R. & Lindsrom, K. (1994) Contributors to satisfaction with management in hospital wards. *Journal of Nursing Management*, 2(5), 229–34.

Long, A.F. (1994) Guidelines, protocols and outcomes. *International Journal of Healthcare and Quality Assurance*, 17(5), 4–7.

Lorentzon, M. (1993) Research for health. Managing the nursing input. *Journal of Nursing Management*, 1(11), 39–46.

Mackenzie, J. (1993) Effects of change on sisters/charge nurses. *Nursing Standard*, 7(36), 25–7.

Mintzberg, H. (1975) The manager's job: folklore and fact. *Harvard Business Review*, 53(4), 49–61.

National Health Service Management Executive (1991) *A Management Development Strategy for the NHS*. NHS Training Directorate, Bristol.

Rodrigues, L. (1994) Pick 'n' mix. *Health Service Journal*, 104(5412), 25.

Rolfe, G. (1994) Towards a model of nursing research. *Journal of Advanced Nursing*, 19, 969–75.

Scottish Office Home and Health Department (1993) *Research and Development Strategy for the NHS in Scotland*. HMSO, Edinburgh.

Smith, I. (1994) An analysis and reflection on the quality of nursing research in 1992. *Journal of Advanced Nursing*, 19, 385–93.

Stewart, R. (1967) *Managers and their Jobs*. Macmillan, London.

While, A.E. (1994) Competence versus performance. Which is more important? *Journal of Advanced Nursing*, 20, 525–31.

Epilogue

As nursing becomes a profession in the fullest meaning of the term, there can be no doubt that it is developing a firm research base. Without such a base, nursing would undoubtedly lack the support, academic and clinical credibility and professionalism which it deserves and requires. Although there continues to be a place for some intuition, opinion and untested theory in the art of nursing, this is being tempered with a much stronger research input than has been the case in the past. Although the change of emphasis which will result in a greater research mindedness is perceived by some as threatening, it need not be so. The nursing profession is not being criticized for the approaches to care which it has developed thus far; indeed it is to be applauded for the developments which have been achieved. Rather, it is embarking on a process of self-analysis and self-criticism which is making full use of a scientific tool not previously available to all its members – nursing research.

Now that the research process is becoming better understood by increasing numbers of nurses, the possibility of making it accessible to all professional nurses is becoming much more real. Thus far, the majority who have developed research skills have been based in academic establishments such as colleges and universities, a historical fact which is easy to understand in the context of research having a strong academic component. However, now that a number of academically based nurses have taken steps towards making nursing a research-based profession, the time is now right for introducing a greater degree of research mindedness into the thinking of all professional nurses.

Nursing is a clinically-based profession. It is composed largely of clinicians who are supported by a number of sub-groups such as managers and educators. As clinicians, the *raison d'etre* for all nurses and nurse groups, more fully understand and make use of the research process, nursing will become increasingly research-based. This book has been prepared with all nurses in mind, particularly those who are concerned with the delivery of direct patient care, and who wish to do so with a full appreciation of the value of *The Research Process in Nursing*.

Desmond F.S. Cormack

Index

2 × 2 contingency table, 325
3M scholarship, 27

abstract, 382
abstract, research, 68, 70–71, 80
abstracting journal, 28, 71
access, *see* research site, gaining access to
accountability 9, 31–3, 105
action research, 5, 44–5, 155–65
agreement–disagreement scales, 245
aims and objectives of research, 91–2, 374–5
analogue scale, 140
analytical memo, 338
analytical note, 337–8
anonymity, 35–6, 60, 107
  of institution, 35–6
  of organization, 35–6
  of subject, 35–6
appendices, 381–2
assessment, *see* measurement
Association of Medical Research Charities, 27
ATLAS, 353, 355
attitude
  measurement, 215–35
  scales, 216–22
    Guttman, 219–20
    Likert, 135, 182, 218–19, 245–6
    Semantic differential, 220–21, 246, 304
    Thurstone, 217–18
author index, library, 70
author, of research report, 80
average, *see* mean

bar chart, *see* bar graph
bar graph, 305, 342, 363–64
baseline conditions, 152

BASIC, 296
behaviour sampling, *see* sample, behaviour
bibliography, 68, 70–73, 382
biological sciences, 5
blind assessment, 149–51
blueprint, 369
boxplot, 313
British Lending Library, 65
British Society of Gerontology 25
budget, *see* finance

carry-over effect, 151
case control study, 185
categorical data, *see* qualitative data
categories, 127–30
  mutually exclusive, 139
category rating scale, 258
causal relationships, 17
cause and effect diagram, 371–2
CD-ROM, 28, 73, 75
central tendency, measurement of, 313
central value, 309
Charities Aid Foundation, 27
chart, 381
check-list, 139
chi-squared (χ^2) test, 324–5
chunking programme, 349
CINHAL, 73
citation index, 72
classification catalogue, library, 70
closed question, 292
COBOL, 296
coding, 338, 349
commissioned research, 37
comparative descriptive design, 184–5
comparison of groups, 303, 305
computer, 295–9, 341–56

data-base, 342, 349
  hardware, 296
  language, 296
  literature search, 27–8, 67, 69–70, 72–5
  main frame, 295–6
  personal, 296–8
  qualitative data analysis, 298, 348–54
  quantitative data analysis, 298–300, 341–8
  relational database, 70
  software, 296, 348, 350–53
concepts, *see* terms, research
conceptual definition, 180
conclusions, in research report, 81, 377
CONCORDANCE, 352, 355
conditions, constancy of, 141
confidence, 20, 319
  interval, 318–19, 325, 328
  level, 208–9, 323
confidentiality, 35–6, 60, 107
consent, 33–4, 107, 376
constant comparative method, 124, 129–30
constructs, 130
content analysis, 345
continuous measurement, 304–5
contour plot, 370–71
contract research, 30
control, 17, 140, 142–3
control group, *see* experimental group
conversation analysis, 120–21
Copeland–Chatterson (Cope–Chat) card,
    293–5
copyright law, 69
core categories, 128–9
correlation, 16, 326
correlation coefficient, 263
correlational research, 16, 140
critical incident technique, 266–74
critical science, 158–9
cross-over design, 150–51
cross-sectional design, 186–7
*Cumulative Index to Nursing and Allied
    Health Literature*, 71, 82
curriculum vitae, 98

Daphne Heald Unit, 24
data, 20, 333–6, 376
  analysis, 46, 81, 94–5
    computer assisted, 298–300
    descriptive, 302–15

inferential, 316–29
  qualitative, 46, 292–3, 303–5, 308, 330–
    41, 348–50
  quantitative, 94, 292–3, 302–15, 316–
    29, 341–8
cleaning, 346
collecting, 45, 81, 93–4, 333–6
collectors, nurses as, 32
entry, 346
handling, 45
interview, 339
missing, 346
numerical, 135, 139
presentation, 46, 357–72
recording, 125–6
storage, 45–6, 291–301
summary, 20
transcription, 126
uncategorized, 343
verification, 346
database management system, *see* computer
declarative research question, 53–4
deductive research, 5–7
degrees of freedom, 324
Delphi studies, 57
dependent variable, *see* variable
descriptive fieldnotes, 337–8
descriptive research, 16, 44–5, 138, 140,
    179–89
descriptive statistics, 46, 295, 306, 342, 347
Dewey Decimal Classification Scheme, 68
discussion, in research report, 81, 377
dissertation, 373, 377
disseminating research, 33, 47, 96, 373–85
distribution, 308, *see also* normal
    distribution
distribution, normal *see* normal distribution
distributional shape, 317

eclecticism, *see* methodological eclecticism
Economic and Social Research Council, 26–
    7
education for research, 22–3
electronic bulletin board, 67
epistemology, 114, 116
error
  sources of, 210
  types of, 321
ethical dilemmas, 31, 38, 263, 286

ethical problems, *see* ethical dilemmas
ethical responsibilities, 60
 of educator, 36–7
 of manager, 37–8
 of nurse, 31–2
 of researcher, 32–3
ethics, 30–39, 47, 81, 95–6
 committee, application to, 36, 60, 95, 105–6
 approval of, 36, 59
ETHNO, 350, 355
ETHNOGRAPH, 95, 349, 355
evaluating the literature, *see* reviewing the literature
evaluation research, 44, 190–201
Excerpta Medica, 71
experimental group, 141, 148, 305
experimental hypothesis, *see* hypothesis
experimental research, 5, 16–17, 44–5, 93, 140–41, 145–54, 179
exploratory descriptive design, 183
ex post facto design, *see* retrospective research

fieldnotes, 119, 337
field observation, 124
figure, 381
filter question, 228, 243
finance, 99–100
 assistance with, 26–7
 budget, 97–8
findings, 376
 inconclusive, 376
fixed alternative question. *see* closed question
Flanagan's critical incident technique, *see* critical incident technique
flow chart, 367–8
formative evaluation, 191–2
FORTRAN, 296
frequency count, 308, 347
frequency distribution, 309
funding body, application to, 99

Gaussian distribution, *see* normal distribution
generalization, 20–21, 136, 207–8, 391–2
geographic mapping, 366–7
grants, 373

graphics package, 305, 342
graphic rating scale, 258–9
graphics, 361–2, 381
grounded theory, 45, 123–34
Guttman scale, *see* attitude, scales

Harvard reference system, 85–6, 381
Hawthorne effect, 141
Health Promotion Research Trust, 27
Health Service Abstracts, 71
higher degree, 23, 69, 374
histogram, 305, 307–309, 317
historical research, 5, 166–78
Hospital Abstracts, 71
human subjects, *see* subject, research
hypothesis, 6, 16–17, 33, 80, 133, 179, 322, 331, 374, 376
 experimental, 147
 null, 319–20, 322, 324
 testing, 16–17, 319–21, 327

imprecision. *see* confidence
incidents, 129–30
inconclusive findings, 373
independent groups, comparison of, 138
independent proportions, comparison of, 145–6, 324–6
independent variable, *see* variable
index, 68, 70–71, 352, 382
indexing journal, 28
Index Medicus, 71
inductive research, 5–7
inductive theory, 123
inferential statistics, 46, 295, 316–29
information resources, 27–8
informed consent, *see* consent
Institute of Medical Ethics, 34
insurance, 107
integrity, 32–3
inter library loan, 69
International Confederation of Midwives, Ethical Guidelines, 31
International Council of Nurses, research guidelines, 8
International Nursing Index, 71–2, 82
inter-observer reliability, *see* reliability
interpretive research, 158
interpretive science, 157
inter-rater reliability *see* Reliability

interrogative research question, 53–4
interval data, 18
interval record, 260–61
interval scale, *see* interval data
interview, 44, 124, 126, 139–40, 181, 226–35
   ethnographic, 118
   closed end, 139
   in-depth, 118
   informal, 118
   open end, 139
   schedule, 139
   semi-structured, 118–19, 226, 292
   structured, 118, 139, 226, 232–3
   transcriptions, 292, 376
   unstructured, 118, 137, 232–3
interviewer training, 230–32
introduction, in research report, 80, 374–5
in-vitro measurement, *see* physiological
   measurement
in vivo measurements, *see* physiological
   measurement

journal clubs, 28

key words, 382

latency, 260
level of significance, *see* significance level
libraries, 27–8, *see also* searching the
   literature
   addresses, 76–7
   choosing, 67–9
Likert scale, *see* attitude, scales
linear regression, 326–7
line chart, *see* line graph
line graph, 305–6, 342, 363
literature review, 43, 78–88, 332–3, 375, *see*
   also reviewing the structure of a, 79–85;
   writing a, 82–3
literature search, *see* searching the literature
literature sources, 64–7
litigation, 107
logical positivism, 135–6
longitudinal design, 186

matrix questions, *see* checklist
Maws scholarship, 27
mean, 146, 311–14, 318, 342
measurement scales, 17–18

measure of spread, *see* standard deviation
median, 311–13
Medical Research Council, 26–7
MEDLINE, 73
memo, 129–32
methodological eclecticism, 161
methodology, 80, 114, 116–17
method, 17, 92, 114, 117–18, 375–6
microfiche, 69
microfilm, 69
MINITAB, 95, 313, 316
mode, 311, 313
monograph, research, 378
moral issues, *see* ethics
MSc, *see* higher degree

National Library of Medicine Classification
   Scheme, 68
needs assessment, 190–91
nominal data, 18, 303–4
nominal scale, *see* nominal data
non-parametric statistics, 317
non-participant observation, *see* observation,
   direct
non-response error, 210–11
no-treatment groups, 149
normal curve, 309
normal distribution, 208, 301–11, 313–14,
   317–18, 320, 324
normative beliefs, assessment of, 221–2
NUDIST, 95, 353, 355
null hypothesis, *see* hypothesis, null
numerical rating scale, 258
numerical referencing system, 86, 381
nursing
   education, 9, 378
   education research, 4, 6, 378, 401–12
   management research, 4, 6, 413–24
   practice research, 6, 378, 389–400
Nursing Bibliography, 71
Nursing Citation Index, 72
Nursing Research Abstracts, 66, 71, 382

objectives of research *see* aims and objectives
   of research
objectivity, 137, 158, 250–51
observation, 44, 120, 124, 139, 182–3, 250–
   65, 376
   direct, 252–3, 259–61

indirect, 252–3
methods, 257–62
naturalistic, 253–4
targets, 254–5
observer
effect, 257
training, 262
ontology, 114–16
open coding, 127
Open University, 23, 26
operational definitions, 18–19, 61, 80, 93,
  180, 237, 255–6, 263, 280
operational terms, *see* operational definitions
oral history, 119
ordinal data, 18, 304
ordinal scale, *see* ordinal data
organizational chart, 366
outcome measurement, 393

paradigm research, *see* qualitative research
parameters, 310
parametric statistics, 317–29
participant observation, 118–20, 137–8,
  337–38, *see also* observation, indirect
participant, research, *see* subject, research
PASCAL, 296
Pearson correlation coefficient, 216
peer review, 33
percentile, 313
PhD, *see* higher degree
phenomena, 127
phenomenology, 115
photograph, 368–9
physiological
data, 275–7
knowledge, 5
measurement, 275–87
pie chart, 305–7, 342, 364
pilot study, 17, 62, 94, 239, 285–6, 374, 376
placebo control group, 149
population, 15, 93, 140, 202, 303, 314
precision, *see* confidence
prediction, *see* hypothesis
predictive statements, 331
primary journals, 65–6
probability, 20, 309
density function, 309
distribution, 309, 324
procedure, 19–20

properties, 127, 130
proposal, preparing a research, *see* research,
  proposal
proposition, *see* hypothesis
prospective research, 14–15, 187–8
publication, writing for, 33, 377–83
punch card, 298–300
p-value, *see* significance level

qualitative research, 44–5, 113–22, 139,
  156–8, 376
quality assessment, 393
QUALPRO, 353, 355
quantitative
data, 46
measurement of, 17–18
research, 44–5, 135–44, 156–7
quartiles, 313, 315
quasi experiment, 140
questionnaire, 46, 138–40, 181–2, 236–49,
  292–3, 345, 376
closed end, *see* fixed alternative
design of, 238–9
fixed alternative, 138, 239, 240–41
length, 242
matrix, 241
open-ended, 139, 239–40
question sequence, 243
survey, 246–8
wording, 242–43
question, research
and aim of study, 61
asking the, 41–2, 53–63
changing the, 62–3
development of, 54, 57–8
finding a, 55–7
and hypothesis, 62
and literature review, 41–2, 62
need for, 54–5
primary, 55
secondary, 55, 62

random error, 211
randomization, 93, 141
random numbers, 206
range, 311, 313–15
ranking, 313
rating scale, 139, 239, 257–9
ratio data, 18

ratio scale. *see* ratio data

raw data, 376

recommendations, in research report, 81, 377

reductionism, 136–7

references, 86, 381–2

reflexivity, 114, 161

regression, *see* linear regression

relative frequency, 309

reliability, 18–19, 125, 181, 263, 283–4, 376
   inter-observer, 18, 263
   inter-rater, 18

repeated measures design, 145, 151
   with counterbalancing, 151

replication, 14, 55–6

reporting research, *see* disseminating research

reports, research,
   format, 373–77
   length, 374

research
   assistant, 10
   awareness, 9
   committee, *see* Ethics, committee
   contract, 373
   courses, 22
   defining, 3–4, 14
   design, 44–5, 92–3, 145
   and development, 12
   interest groups, 25
   interview, *see* interview
   involvement in, 9–11
   method, 375–6
   nature of, 3–5
   need for, 7–8
   proposal, 43–4, 89–101
      length, 100
      rejection of, 100
   purpose of, 5–7
   question, 6, 375–6
   setting, 142
   site, gaining access to, 44, 102–9
   studentships, 23
   subject, *see* subject, research
   training, 22–3
   units, 24

researcher
   identity of, 34–5
   responsibilities of, 383–4

resources, 96–8, 164, 175

respondent, *see* subject, research

response error, 211-12

response rates, 376

results, in research report, 20, 81
   falsifying, 33

retrospective research, 14–15, 186

Royal College of Midwives, ethical guidelines, 31

Royal College of Nursing
   ethical guidelines, 31
   Research Advisory Group, 25

sample, 15–16, 80, 93, 124–5, 140–41, 171, 181, 202–12, 303, 376
   behaviour, 260
   means, 146, 326
   random, 16, 141, 147, 204, 303
   representative, 303
   selection, 203–4, 206–7
   statistics, 202
   stratified, 16, 93
   variance, 314

sample size, 93, 125, 209–10, 303

sampling, *see* sample

sampling frame, 93, 204–6

saturation, 129

scale drawing, *see* blueprint

scaling method, 244

scatter diagram, *see* scatterplot

scatterplot, 305, 311–12, 236, 370

scientific
   enquiry, 4, 12, 119
   method, 4, 11, 40
   paper, 379–81
   principles, 3
   rules, 3, 6, 11

searching the literature, 43, 64–77

secondary journal, 65–6

semantic differential scale, *see* attitude, scales

semi-interquartile range, 311, 313–15

significance level, 320–25

simple case design, *see* single subject design

simple descriptive design, 184

single subject design, 145, 152–3

site, gaining access to, *see* research site, gaining access to

skewness, 311–12

Smith and Nephew scholarship, 27

Social Service Abstracts, 71
Society for Research in Rehabilitation, 25
Society for Social Medicine, 25
Society for Tissue Viability, 25
sociogram, 365–6
sorting, 131–2
spreadsheet, 341
SPSS, 305, 309, 313, 316, 342, 344, 346–7, 361
SPSS DOS, 343
SPSS VERSION 4 for MS DOS, 342
SPSS-X, 95
standard deviation, 305–6, 310–11, 313–14, 342
standard error, 313–14, 329
standard normal distribution, 310
statistical analysis, 136–7, 341–2
statistical methods, 20, 46
statistical power, 317
statistical significance, 319, 325
statistics, descriptive, *see* descriptive statistics
statistics, inferential, *see* inferential statistics
Steinberg Collection of Nursing Research, 66
subject index, library, 70
subjectivity, 114
subject, research, 16–17, 30, 33, 80, 103–4, 239
    availability of, 60
    human, 33
    selection of, 107–8
substantive codes, 126–7
summary, 90
summary statistics, 311–13, 326
summative evaluation, 192
supervision of research, 24
survey, 202–12
systematic enquiry, 3, 14
systematic error, 211–12

table, 305–6, 360–61, 376, 381
t-distribution, 322
t-table, 322, 324
terms, research, 14–21
TEXT BASE ALPHA, 352, 355
TEXT COLLECTOR, 352, 355
theoretical construct, 128

theoretical framework, 56–7, 114
theoretical sampling, 124–5
theory, 125, 332
    development, 123–4, 131
    general, 6
    generation, 129–30
    testing, 5–6
    writing, 132–33
thesis, 47, 373–4, 377–8, *see also* dissertation
Thurstone scale, see attitude, scales
thought listing, 222
time sample, 261
timetable, research, 59, 95
title, research, 60–61, 80, 90, 382
treatment group, *see* experimental group
triangulation, 136, 160, 336
truth, 136
t-test, 321–4
Type I error, 321
Type II error, 321

United Kingdom Central Council for Nursing, Midwifery and Health Visiting, (UKCC), 9, 11, 105–6
    Code of Professional Conduct, 31
utilization of research, 392–8

validity, 19, 125, 181, 237, 263, 284
    predictive, 19
Vancouver reference system, *see* numerical reference system
variability, measure of, 313–15
variable, 16, 93, 140, 180, 303, 305, 308
    binary, 304
    dependent, 17, 145
    extraneous, 140–41
    independent, 17, 145, 153
    ordinal, 304
    physiological, 279
    quantitative, 127, 305, 326
visual analogue scale, 182, 245, 304

word processor, 349
work plan, *see* timetable

χ^2-test, *see* chi-squared test

ZYINDEX, 352, 355